Colposcopy of Female Genital Tract

Sumita Mehta • Poonam Sachdeva
Editors

Colposcopy of Female Genital Tract

Springer

Editors
Sumita Mehta
Department of Obstetrics and Gynecology
Babu Jagjivan Ram Memorial Hospital
New Delhi
India

Poonam Sachdeva
Department of Obstetrics and Gynecology
Maulana Azad Medical College and Lok
Nayak Hospital
New Delhi
India

ISBN 978-981-10-1704-9 ISBN 978-981-10-1705-6 (eBook)
DOI 10.1007/978-981-10-1705-6

Library of Congress Control Number: 2016959470

Printed on acid-free paper

This Springer imprint is published by Springer Nature
The registered company is Springer Science+Business Media Singapore Pte Ltd.
The registered company address is 152 Beach Road, #22-06/08 Gateway East, Singapore 189721, Singapore

Foreword

It gives me immense pleasure to write the foreword for this book as it is edited by my two young and dynamic colleagues who have been associated with me for a long period and are trained by me.

Congratulations!

The need of the hour is that more and more gynaecologists take interest in the prevention of cervical cancer. It will not only help in decreasing the burden of this disease but also help in reducing the morbidity and mortality caused by cervical cancer. Over the years, the practice of medicine is becoming more and more evidence based, and the same applies to the treatment of preinvasive lesions of the cervix. If a gynaecologist with average skills can be trained properly to treat the cases in the preinvasive stage, the need for treatment at full-fledged oncology centres can be avoided.

This book deals with screening methods for cervical cancer, like cytology, visual methods and HPV testing. Colposcopy of the cervix, vagina and vulva has also been described. The pitfalls of colposcopy in infections and pregnancy have also been discussed in a precise way. Case discussions will help the learner to chalk out the treatment of a particular case in the proper manner. This publication will help the students, practising gynaecologists and oncologists in understanding the algorithm in the management of preinvasive lesions.

The chapters are comprehensive, up to date and educative. I wish all the best to the editors and authors who have contributed to this book.

New Delhi, India

Swaraj Batra

Preface

Cervical cancer is the fourth most common cancer in women, and a large majority of the global burden of this disease occurs in the less developed countries. Out of the total new cases detected worldwide in 2013, more than one-fifth occurred in India. This is a disease which affects women in their prime and adversely impacts their social and economic health along with their physical health. Cervical cancer is one of the diseases that can be detected in the preinvasive stage through routine screening methods. Timely diagnosis and treatment of preinvasive disease can prevent invasive cancer and also the morbidity and mortality associated with it.

Keeping this intention, we have arranged this book into three different parts with 16 chapters, covering all aspects of cervical pre-malignant disease. Part 1 covers the normal anatomy and physiology of the cervix, as it is very important to know the normal to differentiate it from what is abnormal. A chapter on pathology of preinvasive lesions is also included. Part 2 examines in detail how invasive cervical cancer is largely preventable if preinvasive lesions are detected early using effective screening methods. This section includes a chapter on screening via conventional cytology and treatment algorithms if abnormal cytology is detected. Furthermore, visual screening methods which have emerged as an important screening tool in low-resource settings have also been discussed in detail. Tests for detection of HPV infection and the clinical implications thereof are also elucidated. A chapter on primary prevention of HPV infection, the cause of the majority of cervical cancers, using HPV vaccination is also included.

Part 3 is exclusively on colposcopy. There are separate chapters on the tissue basis of colposcopy, the technique of colposcopy, the terminology and grading systems in practice, and colposcopic appearance of intraepithelial lesions. All the chapters that describe the colposcopic features in detail have abundant pictures and illustrations to facilitate easy comprehension. There is a chapter on colposcopy of the vulva and vagina too because intraepithelial lesions of the lower genital tract are multifocal and interrelated. The management of intraepithelial lesions using ablative and excisional methods is also explained in detail.

We hope this book will serve as a comprehensive and practical guide for timely diagnosis and optimal treatment of cervical preinvasive disease to all practising gynaecologists, gynae oncosurgeons and postgraduate students which will go a long way in bringing down the incidence of cervical cancer.

New Delhi, India

Sumita Mehta
Poonam Sachdeva
Editors

About the Editors

Dr. Sumita Mehta is Specialist and In-charge, Department of Obstetrics & Gynecology at Babu Jagjivan Ram Memorial Hospital, Delhi, India. She is the secretary of Indian Society of Colposcopy and Cervical Pathology. She has also been the editor of Association of Obstetricians & Gynecologists of Delhi and is a reviewer for many international journals like EJORB, IJOC, and JCDR.

Her area of special interest is in the field of gynecologic oncology, especially cervical cancer. She has conducted several colposcopy workshops all over India and has delivered numerous lectures in various academic forums. She is the author of 7 books and has over 75 publications in national and international journals of repute. Her peers hold her in high esteem for her academic and professional acumen.

Dr. Poonam Sachdeva is Specialist, Obstetrics & Gynecology at Lok Nayak Hospital attached to Maulana Azad Medical College, Delhi, India. Her area of interest is preventive oncology and high-risk obstetrics. She has conducted many live workshops on colposcopy all over India. She has contributed chapters in various books and is also the author of many publications in national and international journals. She is also the editor of *Labor Ward Protocols* and *Scientific Proceedings of AICOG*. She is an active member of national societies like FOGSI, AOGD, NARCHI, and ISCCP and has participated as organizing team and faculty in various conferences. It has been her dream to publish this book to highlight the original work of various authors from all over India. Endless efforts of Dr. Sumita Mehta have made this dream come true.

Contents

Contributors

Krishna Agarwal, MS Department of Obstetrics and Gynecology, Maulana Azad Medical College and Lok Nayak Hospital, Delhi, India

Pakhee Aggarwal, MS (O&G), MICOG, MRCOG (London) Commonwealth Fellow in Gyne Oncology, Delhi, India

Department of Obstetrics and Gynecology, Fortis Healthcare (Fortis Memorial Hosp, Gurgaon, Flt Lt Rajan Dhall Hospital and Aashlok Hospital Delhi), Delhi, India

Raksha Arora, MD Department of Obstetrics and Gynecology, Santosh Medical College, Ghaziabad, UP, India

Poorva Badkur, MS Department of Obstetrics and Gynecology, NSCB Govt. Medical College, Jabalpur, MP, India

Sweta Balani, MS Department of Obstetrics and Gynecology, Sant Parmanand Hospital, Delhi, India

Bharti Bharani, MS Dysplasia Clinic, Indore, India

Vani Bharani, MD Dysplasia Clinic, Indore, India

Sruthi Bhaskaran, MS Department of Obstetrics and Gynecology, University College of Medical Sciences and Guru Teg Bahadur Hospital, Delhi, India

Sumiti Mehta Dixit, DGO Department of Obstetrics and Gynecology, Babu Jagjivan Ram Memorial Hospital, Delhi, India

Anshul Grover, DGO, DNB Department of Obstetrics and Gynecology, Babu Jagjivan Ram Memorial Hospital, Delhi, India

Sheenam Jain, MBBS Department of Obstetrics and Gynecology, Santosh Medical College, Ghaziabad, UP, India

Satinder Kaur, MD, DNB Fellowship Gyne Oncology and Diploma Advanced Gyne Endoscopy, Consultant Gyne Oncologist, Dharamshila Hospital and Research Centre, Delhi, India

Sumita Mehta, DGO, DNB, MAMS, MICOG Department of Obstetrics and Gynecology, Babu Jagjivan Ram Memorial Hospital, Delhi, India

Aruna Nigam, MS Department of Obstetrics and Gynecology, Hamdard Institute of Medical Sciences and Research, Jamia Hamdard, Delhi, India

Divya Pandey, MS Department of Obstetrics and Gynecology, Vardhman Mahavir Medical College and Safdarjung Hospital, Delhi, India

Upasna Pandit, MS Department of Obstetrics and Gynecology, Subharti Medical College, Meerut, India

Deepika Pannu, MS Department of Obstetrics and Gynecology, Vardhman Mahavir Medical College and Safdarjung Hospital, Delhi, India

Swati Priya, MS Department of Obstetrics and Gynecology, Maulana Azad Medical College and Lok Nayak Hospital, Delhi, India

Veena Rahatgaonkar, MD, DGO Department of Obsterician and Gynecologist and Colposcopist, Deenanath Mangeshkar Hospital and Research Center, Pune, India

Pikee Saxena, MD Department of Obstetrics and Gynecology, Lady Hardinge Medical College and Associated SSK Hospital, Delhi, India

Saritha Shamsunder, MD, FRCOG Department of Obstetrics and Gynecology, Vardhman Mahavir Medical College and Safdarjung Hospital, Delhi, India

Sumedha Sharma, MS Department of Obstetrics and Gynecology, Hamdard Institute of Medical Sciences and Research, Jamia Hamdard, Delhi, India

Kavita N. Singh, MS, PhD (Gyn.Oncology), FICOG Department of Obstetrics and Gynecology, NSCB Govt. Medical College, Jabalpur, MP, India

Anshuja Singla, DNB Department of Obstetrics and Gynecology, University College of Medical Sciences and Guru Teg Bahadur Hospital, Delhi, India

Mala Srivastava, DGO, DNB, MICOG Institute of Obstetrics and Gynecology, Sir Ganga Ram Hospital, New Delhi, India

Ankita Srivastava, MBBS Department of Obstetrics and Gynecology, Sri Aurobindo Institute of Medical Sciences, Indore, India

Amita Suneja, MD, MAMS Department of Obstetrics and Gynecology, University College of Medical Sciences and Guru Teg Bahadur Hospital, Delhi, India

Part I

Cervix

Anatomy and Physiology of Cervix

1

Anshul Grover and Divya Pandey

Understanding the normal Anatomy and Physiology of the uterine cervix helps us to identify the abnormal. To be aware of the dynamic nature of the Squamocoloumnar junction and the Transformation Zone forms the basis of an effective screening program for cancer of the cervix. In this chapter, we attempt to recapitulate both gross and microscopic anatomy of the uterine cervix and the physiology of the transformation zone.

1.1 Gross Anatomy

Uterine cervix is the lowermost part of the uterus (Fig. 1.1), which is fibromuscular in origin. The uterine cervix is cylindrical or conical in shape, measuring about 3–4 cm in length and ranges from 1 to 3 cm in diameter. It has two parts, the portio vaginalis and a supravaginal portion of the cervix.

The *portio vaginalis* cervix is the part of cervix protruding into the vagina and surrounded by vaginal fornices. The *supravaginal portion* of the cervix is not seen on vaginal examination as it lies above the vaginal mucosa reflection. A central canal, known as the cervical canal, runs along its length and connects the cavity of the body of the uterus with the lumen of the vagina. The portio vaginalis opens in the vagina through an opening known as external os. The supravaginal portion of

A. Grover
Department of Obstetrics and Gynecology, Babu Jagjivan Ram Memorial Hospital, Delhi, India
e-mail: anshul_abc@yahoo.com

D. Pandey (✉)
Department of Obstetrics and Gynecology, Vardhman Mahavir Medical College and Safdarjung Hospital, Delhi, India
e-mail: dr_devya1@yahoo.co.in

S. Mehta, P. Sachdeva (eds.), *Colposcopy of Female Genital Tract*,
DOI 10.1007/978-981-10-1705-6_1

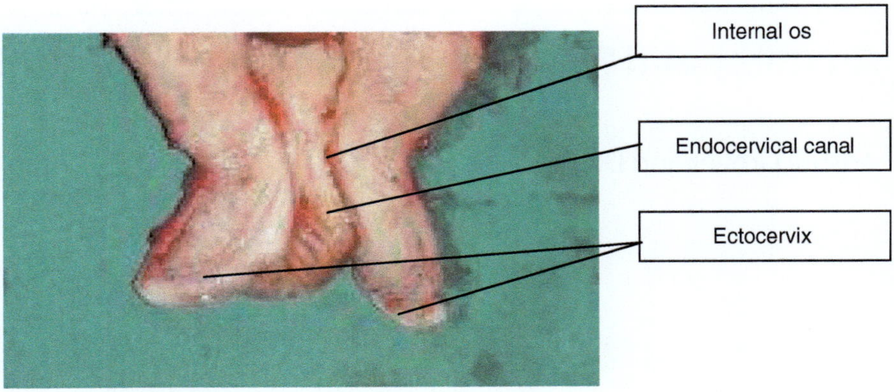

Fig. 1.1 Gross anatomy of cervix

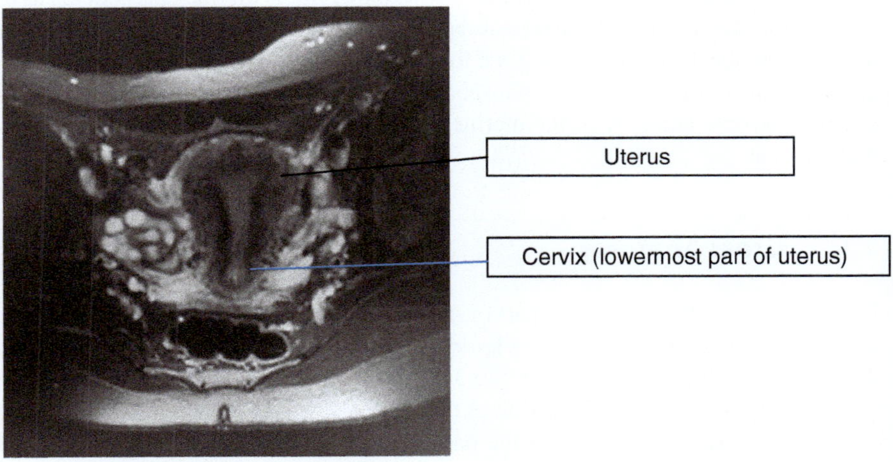

Fig. 1.2 Axial (T2 weighted) image of pelvis showing uterus and cervix

the cervix meets the uterine body at the level of internal os. It requires a certain amount of force to dilate the internal os in order to enter the uterine cavity as part of many surgical procedures. The mucosa lining the cervical canal is known as the endocervix. *External os* thus marks the junction between ectocervix and endocervix (Fig. 1.2).

The size and shape of cervix may vary according to the female's age, parity, and hormonal status. In parous woman, it may be bulky with wide gaping or transversely slit-like external os. In contrast, the os is pinpoint in nulliparous woman. The external os on an average is of 3–4 mm in diameter in a nulliparous woman. It is smooth textured, rich pink in color. The external os may contain clear or cloudy mucus depending on the menstrual phase. The canal joining the internal os and the external os is endocervical canal or endocervix. The endocervix is 3.5–4 cm long, red or orange-red in color. The mucosa of the endocervix is thrown into longitudinal folds. This increases the surface area of mucus secreting columnar cells, and the arrangement is known as *plica palmate*. From plica palmate, further branching folds emerge out peripherally, creating a palm tree-like pattern which is referred to as *arbor vitae*. Intervening in between these folds are clefts whose depth ranges from 1–2 mm to 1.2 cm.

The upper part of the cervix is separated from the bladder by cellular connective tissue known as parametrium, which also extends over the sides of the cervix. Posteriorly, the supravaginal cervix is covered by peritoneum, which runs onto the back of the vaginal wall and then turns upward and onto the rectum forming the recto-uterine pouch.

The cervical stroma is made of dense fibromuscular tissue through which lymphatic, vascular, and nerve supplies of the cervix pass to form a complex plexus.

1.1.1 Embryological Development

Cervix is derived from the two paramesonephric ducts also called the Müllerian ducts, in the sixth week of embryogenesis. During development, the outer parts of the two ducts fuse, forming a single urogenital canal, which further forms the uterus, cervix, and vagina.

The original squamous epithelium of the cervix is derived from the urogenital sinus, and the original columnar epithelium is derived from the paramesonephric duct. The point at which the two meet is called the squamocolumnar junction.

1.1.2 Vascular Supply

The arterial supply of the cervix is derived from internal iliac arteries via the cervical and vaginal branches of the uterine arteries. The cervical branch of the uterine arteries descend lateral to the cervix at 3 o'clock and 9 o' clock positions. The corresponding veins run parallel to the arteries and drain finally in the hypogastric venous plexus.

1.1.3 Lymphatics

Three channels facilitate lymphatic drainage from the cervix. The anterior and lateral part of the cervix drain into nodes along the uterine artery to the external iliac lymph nodes and finally into the para-aortic lymph nodes. The posterior and lateral cervix drains along the uterine arteries to the internal iliac lymph nodes and ultimately into the para-aortic lymph nodes. The posterior section of the cervix drains into the obturator and presacral lymph nodes.

1.1.4 Nerve Supply

The endocervix has rich neural innervation, while it is very poor in ectocervix. Therefore, procedures like cervical biopsy, electrocoagulation, and cryotherapy are easily and well tolerated by most women without the need of local anesthesia. The endocervix has abundant innervation by sympathetic or parasympathetic fibers emerging as S2–S3. These nerves travel along the uterosacral ligaments, which pass from the uterus to the anterior sacrum. Dilatation and curettage of the endocervix may sometimes lead to vasovagal reflex. To negate this reflex, atropine (anticholinergic) is often given by the anesthetist prior to the procedures involving dilatation of cervix.

1.2 Microanatomy

1.2.1 Ectocervix

Ectocervix or portio vaginalis cervix is covered with stratified squamous epithelium which is nonkeratinized. However, keratinization can occur after exposure to the environment as in cervical prolapse. This is opaque, pale pink and has 15–20 layers of cells. This epithelium can be native to the site (formed during embryonic period), known as original squamous epithelium, or it can be newly formed as a result of squamous metaplasia during adult period. In reproductive age group, the original squamous epithelium is pinkish, while newly formed metaplastic squamous epithelium is pinkish white on visual inspection.

It has four layers of cell types (from below upward) (Figs. 1.3 and 1.4):

1. *Basal cells:* This is a single layer of cells lying directly on the basement membrane, which separates the epithelium from underlying stroma. As these cells are immature and have active mitoses, the nucleocytoplasmic ratio is higher. The epithelial-stromal junction is usually straight. But sometimes it can be undulating with short projections of stroma at regular intervals, known as papillae. The portion of epithelium in between these papillae is called *rete pegs*.
2. *Parabasal* or *prickle cell layer:* This consists of several layers of cells, larger than basal cells, but with lesser nucleocytoplasmic ratio as cytoplasm is relatively more. It is named so because of the presence of intracellular bridges, and mitosis here is similar as in the basal layer.
3. *Intermediate layer:* It consists of glycogenated cells larger than the parabasal layer, and the cells appear clear due to the presence of cytoplasmic vacuolations. Still above this layer is a layer which consists of non-vacuolated, flattened cells with basophilic properties.
4. *Superficial layer:* It consists of progressively flatter and elongated cells without vacuoles but with small pyknotic nuclei and eosinophilic cytoplasm.

Overall, from basal to superficial layer, there is a gradual increase in the cell size with corresponding decrease in the nuclear size. The intermediate and superficial

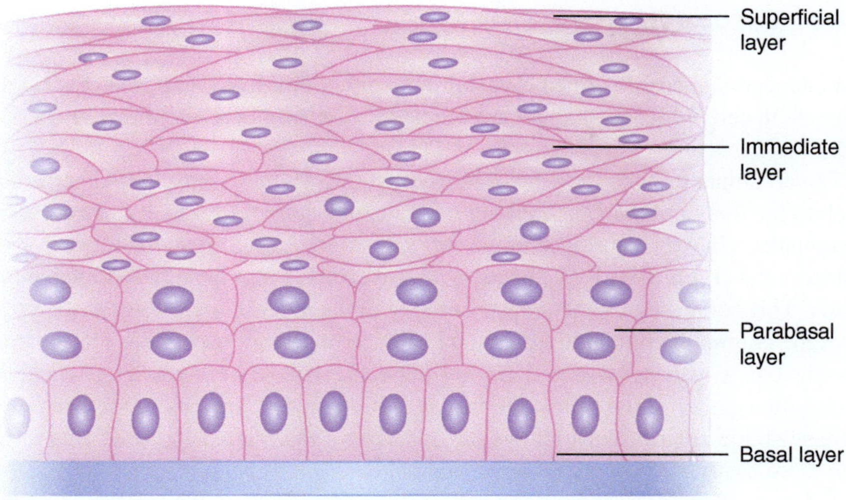

Fig. 1.3 Stratified squamous epithelium

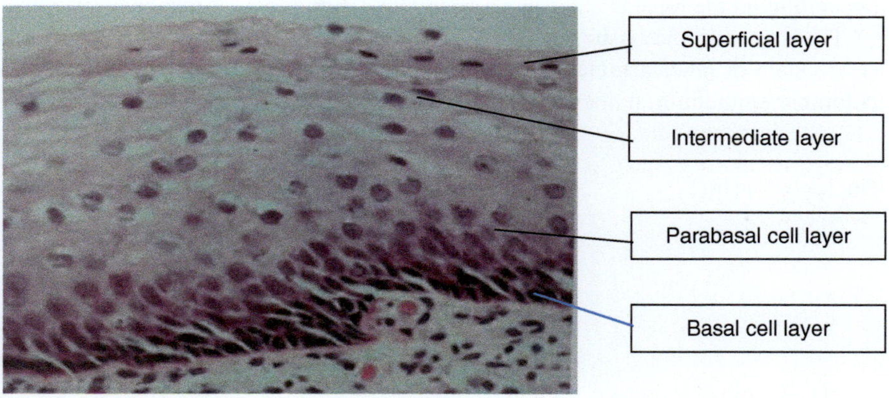

Fig. 1.4 Histological section from ectocervix showing nonkeratinizing stratified squamous epithelium (low power magnification)

layer cells have abundant cytoplasmic glycogen, which stains mahogany brown or black after Lugol's iodine and magenta after PAS stain application. This glycogenation of the intermediate and the superficial cell layer indicates normal maturation and development of the squamous epithelium.

Estrogen hormone is responsible for continuous remodeling of the squamous epithelium in the form of epithelial proliferation, maturation, and desquamation. In its absence, full maturation and glycogenation doesn't take place. Thus, in postmenopausal females, the cells don't mature beyond the parabasal stage and thus do not accumulate in multiple flat cell layers. As a result of which, the epithelium becomes thin and atrophic, which on visual inspection appears pale, often with subepithelial hemorrhagic spots since it is more prone for trauma.

1.2.2 Endocervix

The endocervical canal is lined by columnar epithelium. It is composed of a single layer of tall cells with dark staining nuclei close to the basement membrane (Figs. 1.5 and 1.6).

The columnar epithelium is not flattened but thrown into multiple folds protruding into the lumen of the canal, giving rise to papillary projections. It forms several invaginations into the substance of the cervical stroma, resulting in the formation of endocervical crypts (Fig. 1.7). These crypts traverse 5–8 mm from the surface of the cervix. This complex architecture, comprising of the mucosal infoldings and crypts, gives the columnar epithelium grainy appearance on visual inspection. The subepithelium has a well-developed capillary network. The vessels are intertwined in loops in the center of the villus. On visual examination, it appears reddish in color because single layer of cells allows the underlying vasculature in the stroma to be seen more easily.

The endocervix merges with the endometrial epithelium in the lower part of the body of the uterus. At its proximal or lower limit, it meets the squamous epithelium at the squamocolumnar junction. It covers a variable length of the portio vaginalis depending on the woman's age and reproductive, hormonal, or menopausal status.

The mucus in the tissue section is easily detectable using periodic acid-Schiff (PAS) stain or mucicarmine stain. As glycogenation and mitoses are absent in the columnar epithelium, it doesn't change color after application of Lugol's iodine.

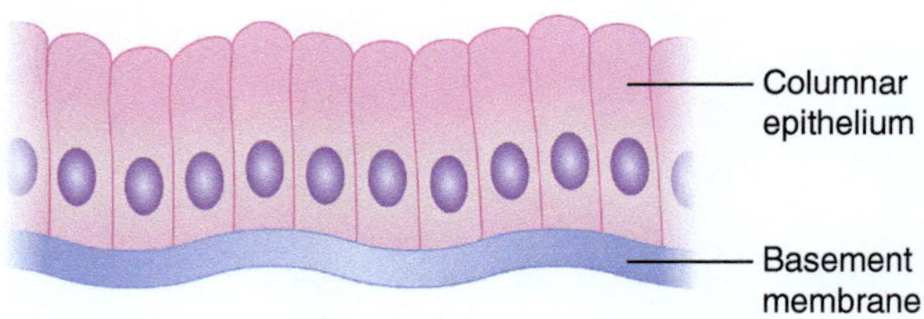

Fig. 1.5 Columnar epithelium

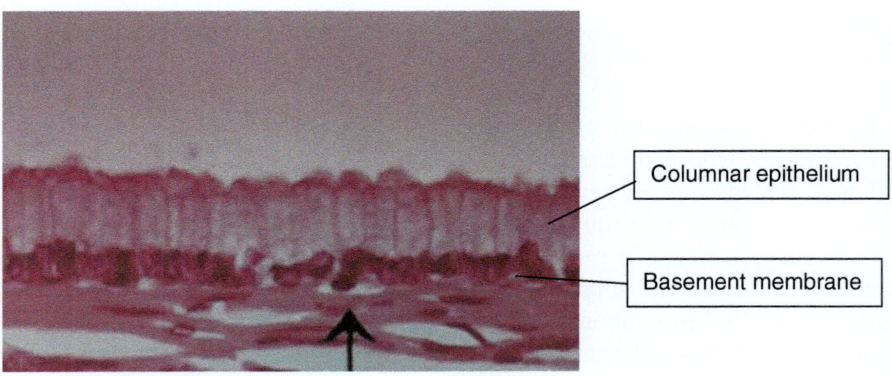

Fig. 1.6 Histological section from endocervix showing single-layered columnar epithelium (high power magnification)

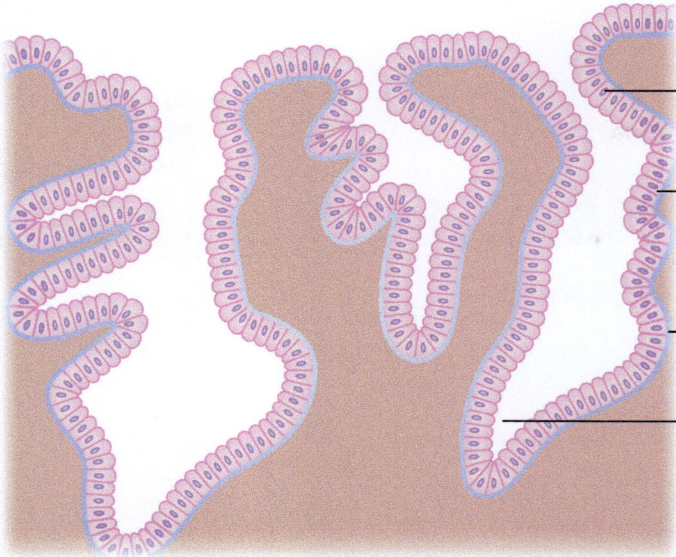

Fig. 1.7 Crypt of endocervix

1.2.3 Squamocolumnar Junction (SCJ)

The squamocolumnar junction (SCJ) is the interface between the original columnar epithelium and squamous cells (Figs. 1.8, 1.9, and 1.10).

Original SCJ is the interphase between the columnar epithelium and the original squamous epithelium laid down during embryogenesis and intrauterine life. It is the embryologically determined caudal extent of columnar epithelium. It is the junction from where transformation begins.

The location of the squamocolumnar junction in relation to the external os is variable depending on female's age, hormonal status, birth trauma, oral contraceptive use, and physiological conditions like pregnancy (Fig. 1.11).

During childhood and before menarche, the original SCJ is very close to the external os. However, after puberty and during reproductive period, under the effect of estrogen, the cervix enlarges and endocervical canal elongates, leading to the eversion of columnar epithelium of the endocervix onto the ectocervix. This condition is called ectopy which looks reddish on visual inspection. The terms "erosion and ulcer" should not be used in lieu of these and are misnomers. The eversion of columnar epithelium is more pronounced on anterior and posterior lips than on lateral lips, and this is a normal physiological occurrence in reproductive years. Occasionally it may even extend over to the vaginal fornix. The whole columnar epithelium and the underlying stroma are shifted in ectopy. This is the region in which physiological transformation to squamous metaplasia, as well as abnormal transformation during cervical carcinogenesis, takes place. Thus, the original SCJ is now located on ectocervix far from the external os.

The everted columnar epithelium when exposed to acidic vaginal pH undergoes squamous metaplasia. This metaplasia starts at the original SCJ and proceeds centripetally toward the external os throughout the reproductive period to menopause. Thus, a new SCJ is formed between the formed metaplastic squamous epithelium

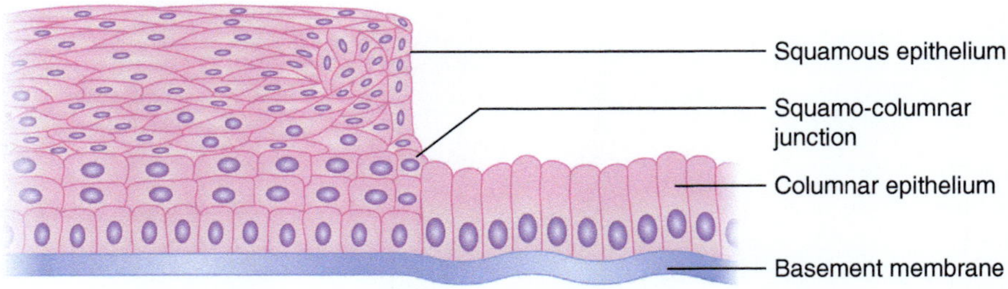

Fig. 1.8 Squamocolumnar junction

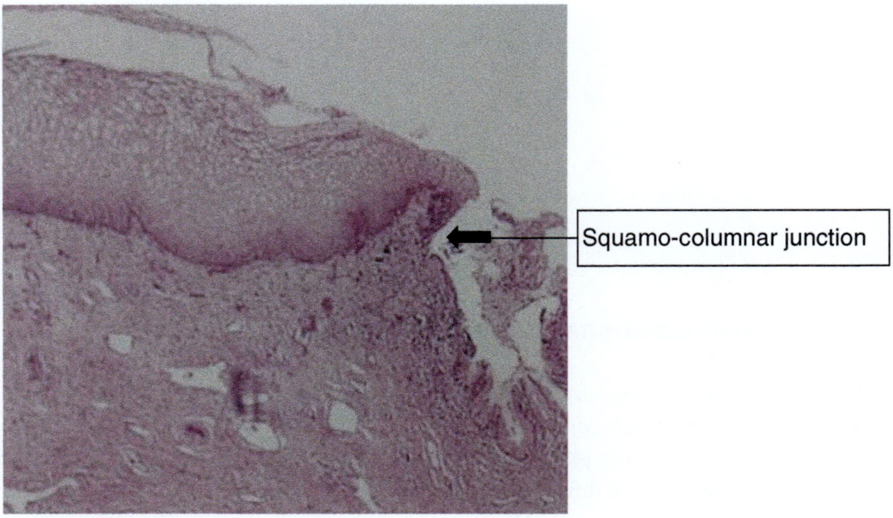

Fig. 1.9 Histology of squamocolumnar junction (low magnification)

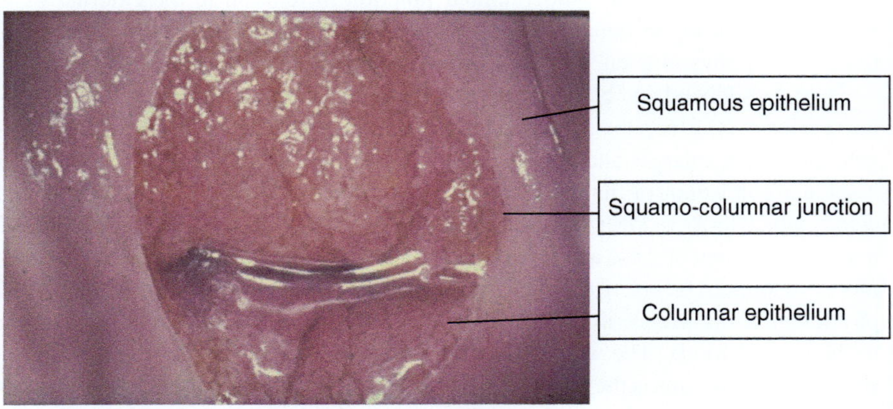

Fig. 1.10 Colposcopic view of squamocolumnar junction

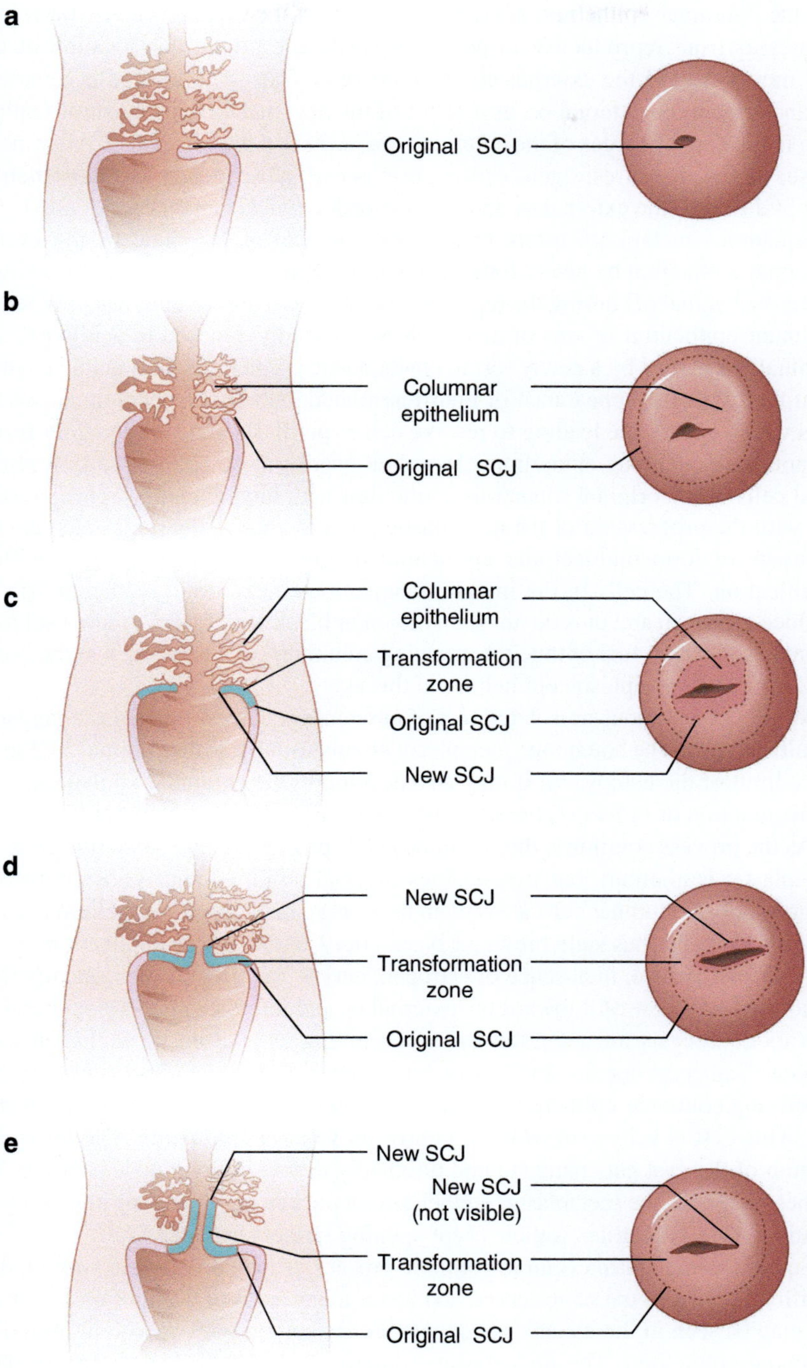

Fig. 1.11 Age-related changes of transformation zone location over cervix. (**a**) Before menarche. (**b**) After puberty and early reproductive age. (**c**) During reproductive age. (**d**) Perimenopausal age. (**e**) Postmenopausal age

and the columnar epithelium remaining everted on the ectocervix. As the woman progresses from reproductive to perimenopausal age group, this location of new SCJ moves toward the external os on ectocervix. Thus, it is located at a variable distances from the external os, as a result of the new metaplastic squamous epithelium in the exposed areas of the columnar epithelium in the ectocervix. After menopause, in absence of estrogen, cervix shrinks and subsequently the movement of new SCJ toward the external os and into the endocervical canal is accelerated.

Squamous metaplasia refers to the physiological replacement of the everted columnar epithelium by newly formed squamous epithelium which occurs owing to the acidic vaginal pH during the reproductive years and during pregnancy. When the columnar epithelium in area of ectropion is repeatedly exposed to acidic pH, it is eventually replaced by a newly formed metaplastic epithelium. This acidic environment results in the appearance of undifferentiated, cuboidal, subcolumnar reserve cells which proliferate leading to reserve cell hyperplasia and subsequently form a metaplastic squamous epithelium. Morphologically these reserve cells resemble basal cells of the original squamous epithelium with high nucleocytoplasmic ratio. But with the progression of the metaplastic process, these cells proliferate and differentiate to form multicellular epithelium of immature squamous cells without stratification. The cells in the immature squamous metaplastic epithelium do not produce glycogen and thus do not stain brown or black with Lugol's iodine solution. It may also contain foci of mucin containing columnar cells embedded in the immature squamous metaplastic epithelium in this stage.

Multiple continuous or isolated foci of immature squamous metaplasia may arise simultaneously. The squamous metaplasia begins usually at the original SCJ at the distal limit of the ectopy, but it may also develop in the columnar epithelium close to this junction or in foci scattered in the exposed columnar epithelium.

As the process continues, the squamous cells proliferate into immature stratified metaplastic epithelium, but it resembles original stratified squamous epithelium. Some residual columnar cells are seen in the mature metaplastic epithelium containing glycogen and thus stain brown or black after Lugol's iodine application.

After menopause, in absence of estrogen, cervix shrinks and subsequently there is movement of new SCJ toward the external os and into the endocervical canal.

Nabothian cysts are retention cysts developing as a result of occlusion of an endocervical crypt opening by the overlying metaplastic squamous epithelium. The underlying columnar epithelium continues to secrete mucus leading to cyst formation. This cyst is yellowish white or yellow on visual examination. The lining epithelium of the cyst gets flattened and ultimately destroyed by mucus pressure. The farthest extent of the metaplastic epithelium on the ectocervix is best known by the location of the Nabothian follicle crypt opening farthest from the SCJ.

Squamous metaplasia is an irreversible process. It may progress at varying rates in different areas of the same cervix, and hence many areas of widely differing maturity may be seen in the metaplastic squamous epithelium with or without islands of columnar epithelium. The metaplastic epithelium adjacent to the SCJ is made of immature metaplasia, while the mature metaplastic epithelium is found near the original squamocolumnar junction. In majority, the newly formed immature metaplastic epithelium develops into a mature squamous metaplastic epithelium, which is similar to the normal glycogen containing original squamous epithelium. However, in a minority of women, it may develop into an atypical, dysplastic epithelium. Certain oncogenic human papillomavirus (HPV) types may persistently infect the immature basal squamous metaplastic cells and transform them into atypical cells with nuclear and cytoplasmic abnormalities. The uncontrolled proliferation and multiplication of these atypical cells may lead to the formation of an abnormal dysplastic epithelium which may regress to normal, persist as dysplasia, or progress into invasive cancer after several years. It is also thought that some metaplasia may occur by in-growth of the squamous epithelium from the squamous epithelium of the ectocervix.

1.3 Transformation Zone

Transformation zone (TZ) refers to the dynamic area usually located on the ectocervix where the columnar epithelium has been replaced and/or is being replaced by the new metaplastic squamous epithelium. By definition it is the area between the original squamocolumnar junction and the current squamocolumnar junction. This process is most active during fetal development, around menarche, and during pregnancy. Local hormonal changes influence this process. In newborns and young females, the endocervical tissue tends to roll out from the cervical os. This is called cervical ectropion and corresponds to the original squamocolumnar junction. In a normal transformation zone, one finds remnants of gland openings and Nabothian cysts. With the decreasing levels of estrogen, in postmenopausal age, as the cervix shrinks, the TZ may move partially and later completely into the cervical canal (Fig. 1.12).

Understanding the TZ is of utmost importance because cervical cancer and its precursors typically begin within the TZ.

Transformation zone can be classified as normal TZ and atypical TZ:

Normal TZ is made of immature and/or mature squamous metaplasia with intervening areas or islands of columnar epithelium, with no signs of cervical carcinogenesis.

Atypical transformation zone (ATZ) is when dysplastic changes are seen in the transformation zone, which are indicative of cervical carcinogenesis.

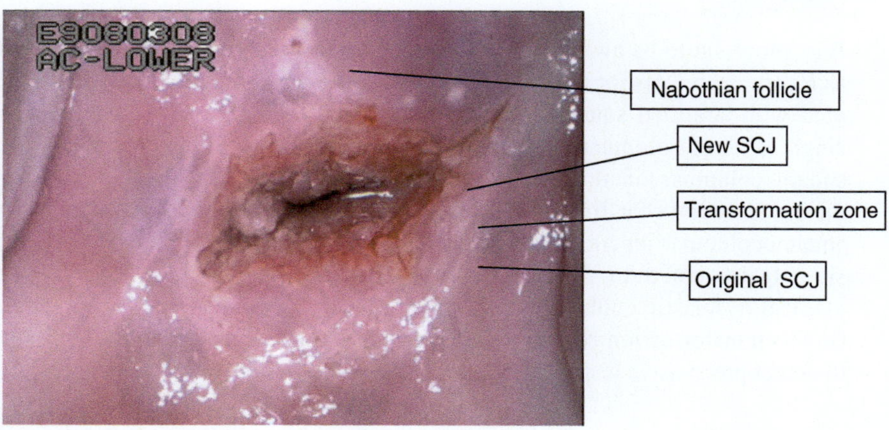

Fig. 1.12 Transformation zone

1.4 Congenital Transformation Zone (CTZ)

It is a common variant of squamous metaplasia, in which differentiation of the squamous epithelium is incomplete due to an interference with normal maturation. Excessive maturation is seen on the surface (as evidenced by keratinization), while delayed or incomplete maturation is seen in deeper layers. Clinically, it is seen as an extensive whitish-gray, hyperkeratotic area extending from the anterior and posterior lips of the cervix to the vaginal fornices. Gradual maturation of the epithelium may occur over several years. This type of transformation zone is seen in less than 5 % of women and is a variant of the normal transformation zone.

During early embryonic period, the cuboidal epithelium of the vaginal tube is replaced by the squamous epithelium, which begins at the caudal end of the dorsal urogenital sinus. This process finishes before birth and the entire length of vagina and the ectocervix is covered by squamous epithelium. This process proceeds very rapidly along the lateral walls and later in the anterior and posterior vaginal walls. If the epithelialization proceeds normally, the original squamocolumnar junction will be located at the external os at birth. However, if due to some reason this process is arrested or remains incomplete, the original squamocolumnar junction will be located distal to the external os or may rarely be located on the vaginal walls, particularly involving the anterior and posterior fornices. The cuboidal epithelium remaining here will undergo squamous metaplasia. This late conversion to squamous epithelium in the anterior and posterior vaginal walls, as well as the ectocervix, results in the formation of the congenital transformation zone.

Distinct features of congenital transformation zone are:

- Irregular dentate pattern akin to rete ridges of the skin at the lower margin or epithelial-stromal junction. Rarely the epithelial incursions are detached from the overlying epithelium, giving an impression of invasive buds.
- Absence of cytoplasmic glycogen (epithelium is iodine-negative on VILI).
- The histologic and colposcopic appearances of CTZ are identical to appearances seen post DES exposure.

Conclusion

It is important to be aware of the normal anatomy and physiology of the cervix as it forms the basis for an optimal cervical cancer screening. Ectocervix is covered with stratified squamous epithelium, while the endocervix is lined by a single layer of columnar epithelium, and where these two epithelia meet is the squamocolumnar junction. In the reproductive age group, this junction is located on the ectocervix far from the external os. The area between the old and new squamocolumnar junction is the transformation zone where squamous metaplasia is taking place. In a minority of women, this metaplasia may develop into atypical dysplastic epithelium under the influence of persistent HPV infection. So this transformation zone is the area which is examined under the colposcope to detect preinvasive lesions.

Key Points

- Cervix is the lowermost part of the uterus, which is fibromuscular in origin.
- The ectocervix or portio vaginalis is covered by multilayered stratified squamous epithelium which is nonkeratinized.
- The endocervix is lined by tall, columnar mucus secreting epithelium.
- Estrogen hormone is responsible for continuous remodeling of the squamous epithelium in the form of epithelial proliferation, maturation, and desquamation.
- Normal, matured squamous epithelium stains mahogany brown following application of Lugol's iodine due to glycogenation.
- Glycogenation and mitoses are absent in the columnar epithelium; therefore, it does not stain after application of Lugol's iodine.
- The squamocolumnar junction (SCJ) is the interface between the original columnar epithelium and squamous cells.
- The location of the squamocolumnar junction in relation to the external os is variable depending on female's age, hormonal status, birth trauma, oral contraceptive use, and physiological conditions like pregnancy.
- Ectopy is a condition of eversion of columnar epithelium of the endocervix onto the ectocervix under the effect of estrogen during reproductive period.
- Squamous metaplasia refers to the physiological replacement of the everted columnar epithelium by newly formed squamous epithelium.
- Transformation zone (TZ) is the dynamic area located on the ectocervix where the columnar epithelium has been replaced and/or is being replaced by the new metaplastic squamous epithelium.
- Cervical cancer and its precursors typically begin within the TZ.

Suggested Reading

1. Standring S. Gray's anatomy, the anatomical basis of clinical practice. 40th ed. Edinburgh: Churchill Livingstone/Elsevier; 2011, 2008.
2. Snell RS. Clinical anatomy by regions. 9th ed. Philadelphia: Wolters Kluwer/Lippincott Williams & Wilkins; 2012.
3. Bajka M, Manestar M, Hug J, et al. Detailed anatomy of the abdomen and pelvis of the human female. Clin Anat. 2004;17:252–60.
4. Abrahams PH, Boon JM, Spratt JD, Hutchings RT. Clinical atlas of human anatomy. 6th ed. London: Elsevier; 2008.
5. Baggish MS. Colposcopy of the cervix, vagina, and vulva: a comprehensive textbook. Philadelphia: Mosby; 2003.
6. Berek JS. Berek & Novak's gynecology. 16th ed. Philadelphia: Lippincott Williams & Wilkins; 2008.

7. Kumar V, Abbas AK, Fausto N, Aster JC. Robbins and Cotran pathologic basis of disease. 8th ed. Philadelphia: Saunders, Elsevier; 2010.
8. Coppleson M, Pixley EC. Colposcopy of vulva and vagina. In: Coppleson M, editor. Gynecologic oncology. Fundamental principles and clinical practice, vol. 1. 2nd ed. New York: Churchill Livingstone; 1992.
9. Apgar BS, Brotzman GL, Spitzer M. Colposcopy-principles and practice. An integrated textbook and atlas. Philadelphia: W.B. Saunders Company; 2002.

Pathology of Preinvasive Lesions of the Cervix

2

Satinder Kaur

Preinvasive intraepithelial lesions contain a group of proliferative lesions characterized by abnormal cytological and histological differentiation, maturation, and stratification of squamous or columnar epithelium. Microscopically they are characterized by nuclear atypia, increased mitotic activity, and the presence of atypical mitoses and cellular pleomorphism on all epithelium levels, regardless of the degree of cytoplasm maturation [1]. The intensity of these lesions varies in accordance with the extent of epithelial involvement. Since these lesions have a potential to develop into invasive carcinoma, pathological diagnosis plays a very important role in the management of these conditions. The fear of missing an invasive carcinoma leads to a tendency of overdiagnosis by the pathologist and overtreatment by the clinician. Hence, understanding the basic pathology and the use of correct terminology and standard management guidelines are the need of the hour. A good knowledge of the etiology, pathophysiology, and natural history of cervical intraepithelial neoplasia (CIN) provides a strong basis both for visual testing and for colposcopic diagnosis and understanding the principles of treatment of these lesions. This chapter describes the evolution of the classification systems of cervical squamous cell cancer precursors and the cytological and histological basis of their diagnosis.

2.1 Etiopathogenesis of Cervical Preinvasive Lesions

A number of risk factors that contribute to the development of cervical cancer precursors and cervical cancer have been identified. These include infection with certain oncogenic types of human papillomaviruses (HPVs), sexual intercourse at an early age, multiple sexual partners, multiparity, long-term oral contraceptive use,

S. Kaur, MD, DNB
Fellowship Gyne Oncology and , Diploma Advanced Gyne Endoscopy,
Consultant Gyne Oncologist, Dharamshila Hospital and Research Centre, Delhi, India
e-mail: satinder31@yahoo.com

S. Mehta, P. Sachdeva (eds.), *Colposcopy of Female Genital Tract*,
DOI 10.1007/978-981-10-1705-6_2

tobacco smoking, low socioeconomic status, infection with *Chlamydia trachomatis*, and micronutrient deficiency [2].

HPV DNA has been associated with cervical cancer in almost 99 % of cases in many studies. HPV types 16, 18, 31, 33, 35, 39, 45, 51, 52, 56, 58, 59, and 68 are strongly associated with CIN and invasive cancer, 16 and 18 being responsible for almost 70 % of cases. HPV infection is transmitted through sexual contact, and the risk factors therefore are closely related to sexual behavior (e.g., lifetime number of sexual partners, sexual intercourse at an early age) [3].

The HPV itself is made up of two distinct late regions, L1 and L2, as well as six distinct early regions, E1, E2, and E4 through E7 (Fig. 2.1). L1 and L2 are conserved regions within the HPV genome and are involved in capsid protein production. The E6 and E7 genes are regulators of cell growth and are able to directly transform cells into a malignant phenotype. The E6 protein binds the host p53 tumor suppressor protein and directs its degradation, resulting in effective silencing of *p53* function. This prevents apoptosis and predisposes the cell to further genetic damage [4]. Similarly, the E7 protein disrupts normal activity of the retinoblastoma gene, pRb, by making it unavailable for binding with E2F, a cellular transcription factor. Unbound E2F is able to directly stimulate cell cycling, which goes unchecked by pRb (and p53, if E6 is active) due to binding of E7. Again, this can lead to undetected genomic abnormalities and malignant transformation of the cell. E1 is typically involved in DNA replication, whereas E2 is involved in transcriptional regulation of HPV E6 and E7. E2 is a frequent site of DNA integration, allowing disruption of the E6–E7 genes. Disruption of these genes causes abnormal transcriptional control, allowing genetic alterations to go unchecked and aberrant growth to proceed unaltered [4].

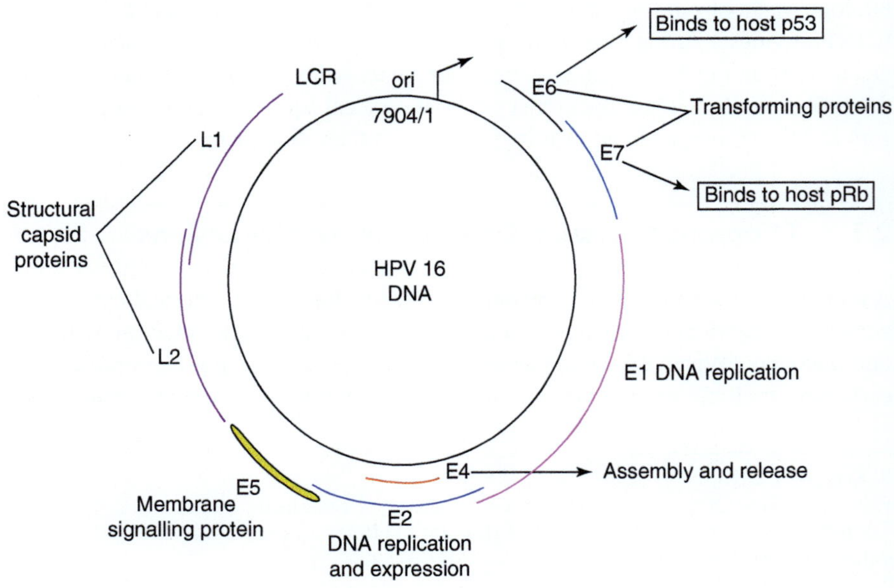

Fig. 2.1 HPV DNA: double-stranded DNA N 8000 base pairs. *LCR* long control region

HPV infection is believed to start in basal or parabasal cells of metaplastic epithelium. It is dependent on cellular interactions beyond simple cellular infection [5]. Typically, HPV enters the cytoplasm of the host and is sequestered in its circular form in particles called episomes. Here HPV replication can occur, filling the cellular cytoplasm with viral particles that appear as areas of perinuclear clearing by light microscopy, the process of koilocytosis. Once viral particles enter the nucleus, they can bind to cellular DNA and integrate into the host genome, causing genomic and proteomic alterations. HPV integration is a process that is biologically necessary but not always sufficient to cause neoplastic transformation.

2.2 Understanding the Pathology

Embryologically, the endocervix and upper vagina are derived from the mullerian ducts and covered by a single layer of mucus-secreting columnar epithelium. While in utero, this columnar lining in the vaginal tube is colonized by upward growth of stratified squamous epithelium derived from cloacal endoderm. This process of replacement of mature columnar epithelium by mature differentiated squamous epithelium is termed as squamous metaplasia. By birth, a distinct junction between the squamous cells and columnar cells is present on the outer portion of the cervix and is known as the squamocolumnar junction (SCJ) or more precisely the original squamocolumnar junction. In response to hormonal stimulation at menarche, further squamous metaplasia occurs, causing movement of the SCJ toward the endocervical canal. During the menopausal years, the SCJ is often in an endocervical location. The region of the cervix that has undergone metaplasia between the initial and current SCJ is known as the transformation zone (TZ). Cervical neoplasia invariably originates within this zone.

2.2.1 Dysplasia

The term dysplasia is a disorder of maturation and differentiation, in which there is an increase in population of immature cells which are restricted to the mucosal surface and have not invaded through the basement membrane to the deeper soft tissues. The term cervical dysplasia was originally coined in the late 1950s to designate the cervical epithelial atypia that is intermediate between the normal epithelium and CIS [6]. Thus, squamous metaplasia is the replacement of one type of normal epithelium by another type of normal epithelium, while dysplasia is the replacement of normal epithelium by abnormal epithelial cells. Dysplasia was further categorized into three groups – mild, moderate, and severe – depending on the degree of involvement of the epithelial thickness by the atypical cells. Subsequently, for many years, cervical precancerous lesions were reported using the categories of dysplasia and CIS and are still widely used in many countries.

A system of classification with separate classes for dysplasia and CIS was increasingly perceived as an arbitrary configuration, based upon the findings from a number of follow-up studies involving women with such lesions. It was observed that some cases of dysplasia regressed, some persisted, and others progressed to CIS. A direct correlation with progression and histological grade was observed. These observations led to the concept of a single, continuous disease process by which normal epithelium evolves into epithelial precursor lesions and onto invasive cancer. On the basis of the above observations, the term cervical intraepithelial neoplasia (CIN) was introduced in 1968 to denote the whole range of cellular atypia confined to the epithelium. CIN was divided into grades 1, 2, and 3 [7]. CIN 1 corresponded to mild dysplasia, CIN 2 corresponded to moderate dysplasia, and CIN 3 corresponded to both severe dysplasia and CIS.

In the 1980s, the pathological changes such as koilocytic or condylomatous atypia associated with human papillomavirus (HPV) infection were increasingly recognized. Koilocytes are atypical cells with a perinuclear cavitation or halo in the cytoplasm indicating the cytopathic changes due to HPV infection. This led to the development of a simplified two-grade histological system. Thus, in 1990, a histopathological terminology based on two grades of disease was proposed:

- Low-grade CIN comprising the abnormalities consistent with koilocytic atypia and CIN 1 lesions
- High-grade CIN comprising CIN 2 and 3

In CIN 1 there is good maturation with minimal nuclear abnormalities and few mitotic figures (Fig. 2.2). Undifferentiated cells are confined to the deeper layers (lower third) of the epithelium. Mitotic figures are present but not very numerous. Cytopathic changes due to HPV infection may be observed in the full thickness of the epithelium. CIN 2 is characterized by dysplastic cellular changes mostly restricted to the lower half or the lower two-thirds of the epithelium, with more marked nuclear abnormalities than in CIN 1 (Fig. 2.3). Mitotic figures may be seen throughout the lower half of the epithelium. In CIN 3, differentiation and stratification may be totally absent or present only in the superficial quarter of the epithelium with numerous mitotic figures (Fig. 2.4). Nuclear abnormalities extend

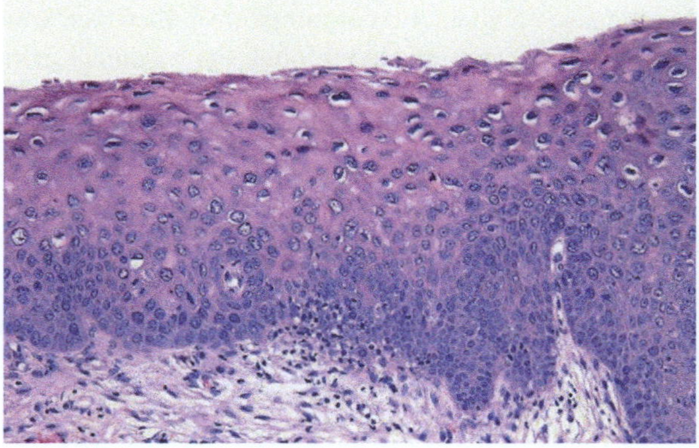

Fig. 2.2 CIN 1

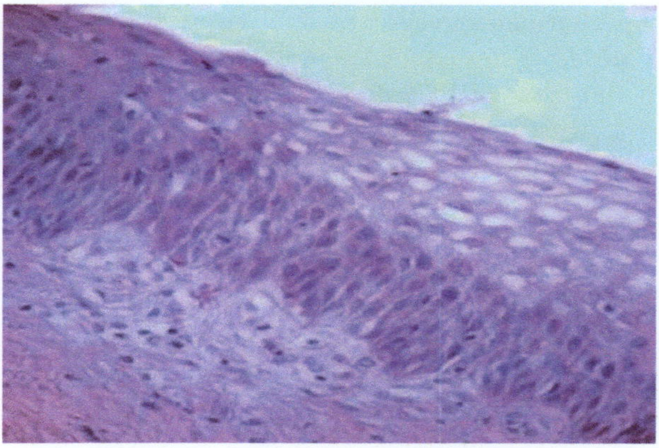

Fig. 2.3 CIN 2

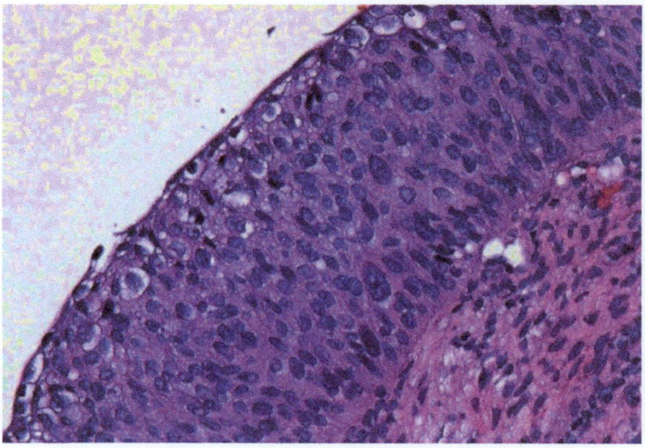

Fig. 2.4 CIN 3

throughout the thickness of the epithelium. Many mitotic figures have abnormal forms. The high-grade lesions were considered to be true precursors of invasive cancer [7].

In 1988, the US National Cancer Institute convened a workshop to propose a new scheme for reporting cervical cytology results [8, 10, 11]. The recommendations from this workshop and the subsequent revision in a second workshop held in 1991 became known as the Bethesda system (TBS) [9]. The main feature of TBS was the creation of the term squamous intraepithelial lesion (SIL) and a two-grade scheme consisting of low-grade squamous intraepithelial lesion (LSIL) and high-grade squamous intraepithelial lesion (HSIL). TBS classification combines flat condylomatous (HPV) changes and low-grade CIN (CIN 1) into LSIL, while the HSIL encompasses more advanced CIN such as CIN 2 and 3. TBS has become over a short period of time the internationally standardized method of cervical cytology reporting. The most recent review and revision of this terminology took place at the Bethesda Workshop in 2001.

Specimen adequacy

Satisfactory for evaluation (note the presence/absence of endocervical/transformation zone component)

Unsatisfactory for evaluation … (*specify reason*)

Specimen rejected/not processed (*specify reason*)

Specimen processed and examined but unsatisfactory for the evaluation of the epithelium

Abnormality because of (*specify reason*)

General Categorization (*Optional*)

Negative for intraepithelial lesion or malignancy

Epithelial cell abnormality

Others

Interpretation/Result

Negative for intraepithelial lesion or malignancy

Organisms

Trichomonas vaginalis

Fungal organisms morphologically consistent with *Candida* species

Shift in flora suggestive of bacterial vaginosis

Bacteria morphologically consistent with *Actinomyces* species

Cellular changes consistent with herpes simplex virus

Other nonneoplastic findings (*optional to report, list not comprehensive*)

Reactive cellular changes associated with:

Inflammation (includes typical repair)

Radiation

Intrauterine contraceptive device

Glandular cell status post-hysterectomy

Atrophy

Epithelial cell abnormalities

Squamous cells

Atypical squamous cells (ASC) of undetermined significance (ASCUS)

Cannot exclude HSIL (ASC-H)

Low-grade squamous intraepithelial lesion (LSIL) encompassing human papillomavirus/mild dysplasia/cervical intraepithelial neoplasia (CIN 1)

High-grade squamous intraepithelial lesion (HSIL) encompassing moderate and severe dysplasia and carcinoma in situ

CIN 2 and CIN 3

Squamous cell carcinoma

Glandular cell

Atypical glandular cells (AGC) (*specify endocervical and endometrial or not otherwise specified*)

Atypical glandular cells, favor neoplastic (*specify endocervical or not otherwise specified*)

Endocervical adenocarcinoma in situ (AIS)

Adenocarcinoma

Others (*list not comprehensive*)

Endometrial cells in a woman, ≥40 years of age
Automated review and ancillary testing (*include as appropriate*)
Educational notes and suggestions (*optional*)

In March 2012, the College of American Pathologists and American Society for Colposcopy and Cervical Pathology, in collaboration with 35 stakeholder organizations, convened a consensus conference called the Lower Anogenital Squamous Terminology (LAST) Project [12]. The recommendations of this project include using a uniform, two-tiered terminology to describe the histology of human papillomavirus-associated squamous disease across all anogenital tract tissues: vulva, vagina, cervix, penis, peri-anus, and anus. These important observations resulted in a number of changes in recommendations for reporting HPV-associated squamous histopathology of lower anogenital tract sites, including the cervix. The group recommended using terms familiar to clinicians and decided on a two-tiered system similar to that used for reporting cervical cytology. Lesions are now categorized as high grade or low grade followed by the phrase "squamous intraepithelial lesion." Acronyms like the Bethesda system (LSIL and HSIL) are used. During transition to the new terminology and at the clinician's request, the diagnosis may be further supplemented with existing "(-IN)" terminology for each lower anogenital site. If the -IN qualifier is used, it has to be reported in parentheses after the main diagnosis. For example, a cervical biopsy previously reported as "CIN 2" will now be reported as "HSIL" or "HSIL (CIN 2)." A prior "CIN 3" now would be reported as "HSIL" or as "HSIL (CIN 3)." Because the LAST Project terminology parallels cytology reporting, healthcare providers must ensure that the report received refers to either a cytologic or histopathologic specimen. The use of similar terminology was not intended to alter the role of cytology as a screening test or to imply that cytology can substitute for histologic diagnosis.

The advantages of the binary terminology consist in the fact that this type of terminology reflects our current understanding of the biology of precancerous lesions; it can be used both in cytopathologic diagnosis and in the histopathological one, while at the same time reflecting the current clinical attitude according to which patients with LSIL and satisfactory colposcopy may be simply monitored, while patients with HSIL must be treated [3]:

Dysplasia terminology	Original CIN terminology 1968	Modified CIN terminology 1990	LAST Project terminology 2012
Normal	Normal	Normal	Within normal limits Benign cellular changes (infection or repair) ASCUS/AGUS
Atypia	Koilocytic atypia, flat condyloma, without epithelial change	Low-grade CIN	LSIL
Mild dysplasia/dyskaryosis	CIN 1	Low-grade CIN	LSIL

Dysplasia terminology	Original CIN terminology 1968	Modified CIN terminology 1990	LAST Project terminology 2012
Moderate dysplasia	CIN 2	High-grade CIN	HSIL
Severe dysplasia	CIN 3	High-grade CIN	HSIL
Carcinoma in situ	CIN 3	High-grade CIN	HSIL
Invasive carcinoma	Invasive cancer	Invasive cancer	Invasive cancer

CIN cervical intraepithelial neoplasia, *LSIL* low-grade squamous intraepithelial lesion, *HSIL* high-grade squamous intraepithelial lesion, *ASCUS* atypical squamous cells of undetermined significance, *AGUS* atypical glandular cells of undetermined significance

2.3 Cervical Glandular Intraepithelial Neoplasia (CGIN)

The presence of cervical glandular intraepithelial neoplasia is increasing in real forms. CGIN is divided into low-grade and high-grade categories. In WHO terminology, low-grade CGIN corresponds to glandular dysplasia and high-grade CGIN to adenocarcinoma in situ (AIS) [13, 14].

Low-grade CGIN is a poorly reproducible diagnosis, as the morphological features are not well described. There is usually little nuclear atypia or mucin depletion, but the nuclei are hyper-chromatic with occasional mitotic figures and apoptotic bodies (Fig. 2.5). The apoptotic bodies are a useful aid to diagnosis because they are seldom identified in non-neoplastic endocervical glandular lesions. However, the natural history is not known with little evidence that this is a precursor of high-grade CGIN and there are no clear management guidelines. Hence, it is managed as per high-grade CGIN. This has led to controversy whether the term low-grade CGIN should ever be used.

CGIN has two main variants: intestinal type and tubal/ciliated type.

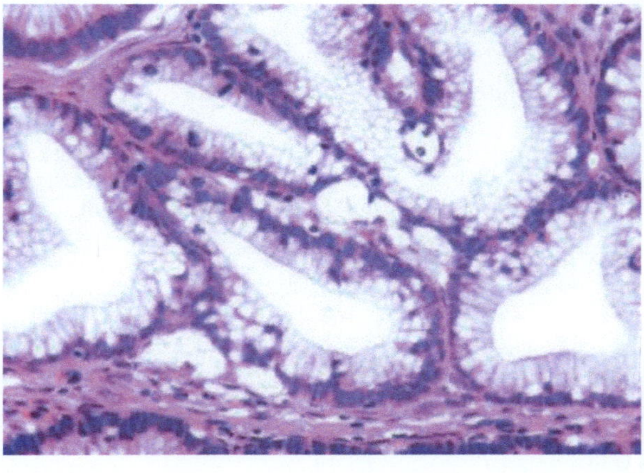

Fig. 2.5 Low-grade CGIN

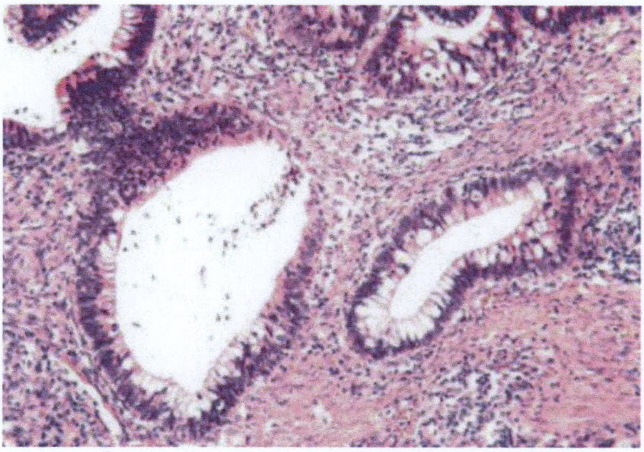

Fig. 2.6 Intestinal-type CGIN

Intestinal CGIN The most common variant of CGIN is the intestinal type with goblet cells. Paneth cells and/or neuroendocrine cells occur more uncommonly [15, 16]. Intestinal differentiation in CGIN is usually a focal finding in association with usual-type CGIN; in one study, intestinal differentiation was present in 29 % of cases of CGIN, always in association with usual type [15]. When intestinal-type epithelium with goblet cells is present in the cervix, this almost always indicates a premalignant or malignant endocervical glandular lesion, although the nuclear features of malignancy may be subtle because of compression by intracytoplasmic mucin globules; truly "benign" intestinal metaplasia occurs rarely in the cervix [17]. One study showed that intestinal-type CGIN is more likely than the usual type to be associated with early invasion [16] (Fig. 2.6).

Tubal/Ciliated CGIN Occasional examples of CGIN contain cilia and are referred to as being of tubal or ciliated type [18]. This rare variant of CGIN usually occurs in association with usual type. The main differential diagnosis is tubo-endometrial metaplasia with a degree of nuclear atypia. Apoptotic bodies are a useful diagnostic clue to CGIN.

2.3.1 Stratified Mucin-producing Intraepithelial Lesion (SMILE)

This is described as a lesion, which exhibits morphological overlap between CGIN and cervical intraepithelial neoplasia (CIN) and has been suggested to be a form of adenosquamous carcinoma in situ [19]. SMILE occasionally occurs in pure form (unassociated with a premalignant or malignant squamous or glandular lesion) and is best regarded and reported by the pathologist as a form of high-grade reserve cell dysplasia. Histologically SMILE may involve both the surface and underlying crypt epithelium. There is a morphological overlap with both CIN and CGIN. The epithelium is stratified similarly to CIN, but mucin, in the form of discrete vacuoles or cytoplasmic clearing, is present throughout the full epithelial thickness (Fig. 2.7).

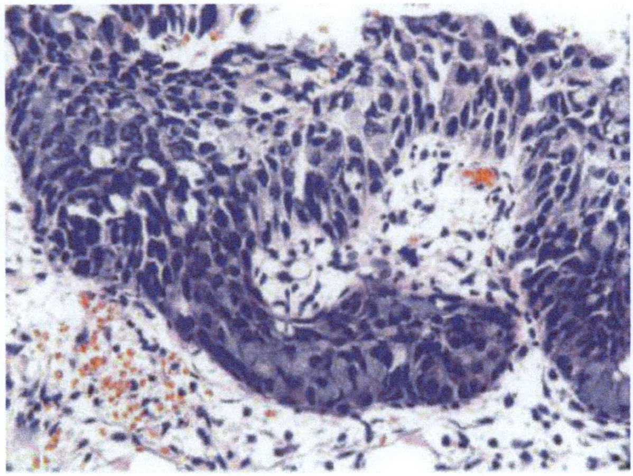

Fig. 2.7 SMILE

2.4 Immunohistochemistry Markers in the Diagnosis of Preinvasive Lesions

Relationship of HPV with the host cell cycle has identified several biomarkers including p16, Ki-67, and ProExTMC (TriPath Imaging, Inc., Burlington, NC) that are overexpressed in HPV-infected cells. These markers can be used as adjuncts to histopathology to improve the detection and grading of HPV-associated CIN [20–22]. They are especially useful in cases of histopathological dilemmas like CIN 2.

p16, a tumor suppressor, is a kinase inhibitor that regulates transition from the G_1 to the S phase of the cell cycle [23]. The cellular kinase inhibitor p16INK4a is strongly overexpressed in transforming HR-HPV infections due to the disruption of a pRb-controlled negative feedback loop by the viral oncogene E7. p16INK4a overexpression is thus considered as a surrogate marker for deregulated E7 expression and hence for transforming HPV infections [24, 25]. The conjunctive use of p16INK4a immuno-histochemistry together with H&E stained sections has improved the interobserver agreement in the evaluation of cervical specimens and is thus widely used as an adjunctive test in routine histology [26] (Fig. 2.8).

Ki-67 is a cell proliferation indicator that is expressed during all phases of the cell cycle except G_0 [27]. MIB-1 is a monoclonal antibody that targets the Ki-67 antigen. In normal and metaplastic squamous epithelium, MIB-1 positivity is confined to the parabasal cell layer [28]. Since HPV-associated lesions have an increased rate of cellular proliferation as compared with normal squamous or glandular epithelium, MIB-1 can be used to detect the increased activity and distinguish benign atypia from dysplasia [28].

Topoisomerase IIa (TOP2A) is a nuclear enzyme involved in DNA replication. Its expression is related to the cell cycle, with the lowest levels of expression occurring in G_0 and G_1 phases of the cell cycle. Gene expression profiling studies have

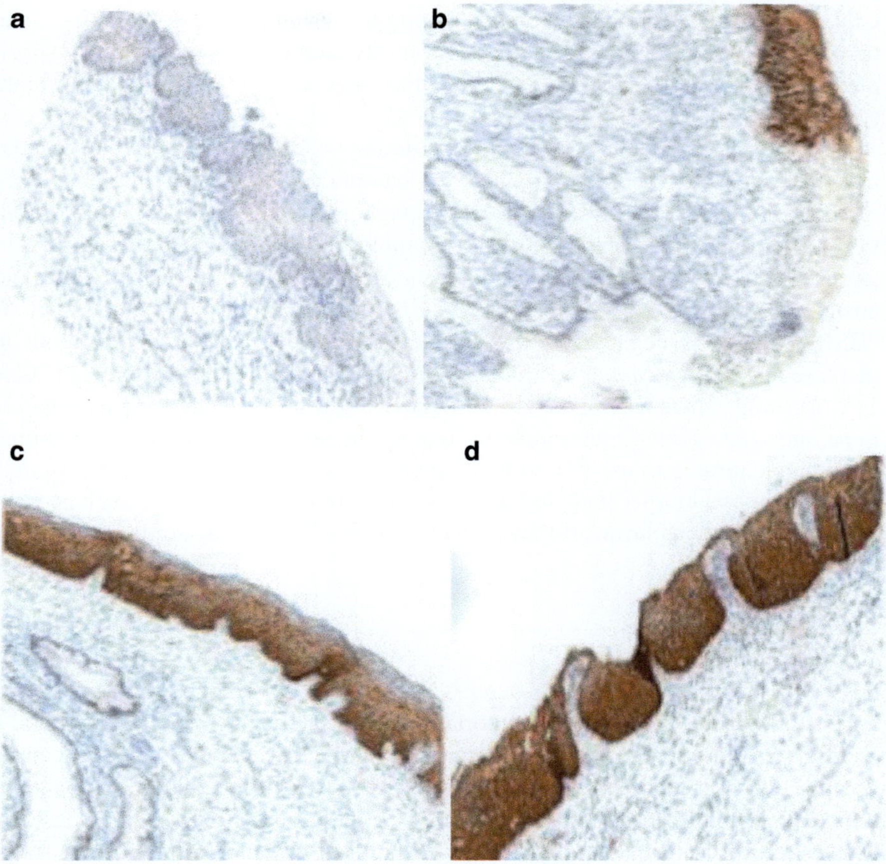

Fig. 2.8 p16 staining: (**a**) normal, (**b**) CIN1, (**c**) CIN2, and (**d**) CIN3

shown increased expression of TOP2A in cervical cancer cell lines and invasive cervical cancer [29, 30]. Immunohistochemical analysis has also shown increased TOP2A protein expression levels in CIN and cervical cancer compared with normal cervical epithelium [31, 32].

Minichromosome maintenance (MCM2) is a member of the DNA licensing protein family, which is involved with licensing DNA for replication, and thus is a marker of proliferation [33]. ProExC is an immunocytochemical assay composed of two monoclonal antibodies directed against TOP2A and MCM2 protein. Studies using ProExC have described the characteristic staining patterns seen in CIN [34], which seem to increase with increasing grades of disease [35].The staining pattern in high-grade CIN shows strong nuclear staining in more than 50% of dysplastic cells, whereas in low-grade CIN, varying degrees of scattered positive cells are observed [34].In a combined approach with p16 immunostaining, ProExC demonstrates higher specificity but lower sensitivity than p16 staining for detection of

CIN3þ [35], suggesting that a combined approach using these two biomarkers can be used together to distinguish CIN 2/3 from its mimics in cervical biopsy specimens [35].The utility of ProExC for diagnosis of low-grade CIN is more contentious.

The Lower Anogenital Squamous Terminology (LAST) Project recommendations include very specific guidelines for laboratory use of IHC markers. They recommend against the use of a panel of diagnostic immunostains in most situations. The only recommendation is p16 staining to confirm a diagnosis of a high-grade lesion when entertaining a diagnosis of CIN 2 based on hematoxylin and eosin morphology. If a "CIN 2" specimen is p16 positive, it will be classified as "HSIL"; if p16 is negative, it will be classified as "LSIL." This will result in increased specificity of diagnosing HSIL. Many clinicians currently manage "CIN 1–2" as a high-grade lesion; the use of p16 will allow lesion testing as p16 negative to be managed as low-grade squamous intraepithelial lesion (LSIL). An additional recommendation is to use p16 to facilitate diagnosis when a potential high-grade lesion cannot be morphologically differentiated from a benign mimic such as reactive squamous metaplasia, atrophy, reparative epithelial changes, or tangential sectioning [12].

2.5 Summary

An accurate diagnosis of CIN is important for clinical management because CIN 1 and CIN 2/3 lesions are treated differently. Histological diagnosis of CIN can be complicated by the variety of cellular changes that can be associated with inflammation, pregnancy, and hormonal therapies, which can mimic precancerous lesions. This makes histological diagnosis prone to subjectivity and variability, which is clearly reflected in the poor intra- and interobserver agreement between pathologists. Incorporation of biomarkers into diagnostic strategies has the potential to improve current cervical screening performance and management of disease. We believe a combined approach of histological diagnosis and biomarkers has the potential to stratify women into different diagnostic categories associated with different levels of risk and manage them accordingly.

Key Points

- Invasive squamous cell cervical cancers are preceded by a long phase of preinvasive disease, collectively referred to as cervical intraepithelial neoplasia (CIN).
- CIN may be categorized into grades 1, 2, and 3 depending upon the proportion of the thickness of the epithelium showing mature and differentiated cells.

- More severe grades of CIN (2 and 3) reveal a greater proportion of the thickness of the epithelium composed of undifferentiated cells.
- Persistent infection with one or more of the oncogenic subtypes of human papillomaviruses (HPVs) is a necessary cause for cervical neoplasia.
- A uniform, two-tiered terminology to describe the histology of human papillomavirus-associated squamous disease across all anogenital tract tissues, vulva, vagina, cervix, penis, peri-anus, and anus, has been suggested. This parallels the Bethesda system.
- The combined interpretation of hematoxylin and eosin and p16INK4a staining can significantly improve the accuracy of interpreting and grading cervical lesions on biopsy samples.
- The precursor lesion arising from the columnar epithelium is referred to as adenocarcinoma in situ (AIS). AIS may be associated with CIN in one-to two-thirds of cases.

Bibliography

1. Muntean M, Simionescu C, Taslica R, et al. Cytological and histopathological aspects concerning pre-invasive squamous cervical lesions. Curr Health Sci J. 2010;36(1):26–32.
2. Castellsagué X, Muñoz N. Cofactors in human papillomavirus carcinogenesis–role of parity, oral contraceptives, and tobacco smoking. J Natl Cancer Inst Monogr. 2003;31:20–8.
3. Ferenczy A, Franco E. Persistent human papillomavirus infection in cervical neoplasia. Lancet Oncol. 2002;3:11–6.
4. Sonnex C. Human papillomavirus infection with particular reference to genital disease. J Clin Pathol. 1998;51:643–8.
5. Doorbar J. Molecular biology of human papillomavirus infection and cervical cancer. Clin Sci (Lond). 2006;110:525–41.
6. Reagan JW. Dysplasia of the uterine cervix. In: Gray LA, editor. Dysplasia, Carcinoma in Situ and Microinvasive Carcinoma. Springfield: Thomas;1965.
7. Richart RM. Natural history of cervical intraepithelial neoplasia. Clin. Obstet. Gynecol. 1967;10:748.
8. National Cancer Institute workshop. The 1988 Bethesda System for reporting cervical/vaginal cytologic diagnosis. JAMA 1989;262:931–4.
9. National cancer Institute Workshop. The 1991 Bethesda System for reporting cervical/vaginal cytologic diagnosis. Acta Cytologica 1993;37:115–24.
10. Soloman D. The 1988 Bethesda System for reporting cervical/ vaginal cytologic diagnosis. Acta Cytologica 1989;33:567–74.
11. Kurman RJ, Malkisian GD Jr, Sedlis A, et al. From Papanicolaou to Bethesda:the rationale for a new cervical cytologic classification. Obstet Gynecol 1991;77:779–82.
12. Waxman GA, Chelmow D, Darragh TM, et al. Revised terminology for cervical histopathology and its implications for management of high-grade squamous intraepithelial lesions of the cervix. Obstet Gynecol. 2012;120(6):1465–71.
13. Tavassoli FA, Devilee P, editors. World Health Organization classification of tumors: pathology and genetics. Tumors of the breast and female genital organs. Lyon: IARC Press; 2003.
14. Fox H, Buckley CH, Al-Nafussi AI, et al. Histopathology reporting in cervical screening. NHS Cervical Screening Programme (NHSCSP), Sheffield, England. Publication no. 10; Apr 1999.

15. Jaworski RC, Pacey NF, Greenberg ML, et al. The histologic diagnosis of adenocarcinoma in situ and related lesions of the cervix uteri. Cancer. 1988;61:1171–81.
16. Mc Cluggage WG, Shah R, Connolly LE, McBride HA. Intestinal- type cervical adenocarcinoma in situ and adenocarcinoma exhibit a partial immunophenotype with consistent expression of CDX2. Int J Gynecol Pathol. 2008;27:92–100.
17. Nicolae A, Goyenaga P, McCluggage WG, Preda O, Nogales FF. Endometrial intestinal metaplasia: a report of two cases, including one associated with cervical intestinal and pyloric metaplasia. Int J Gynecol Pathol. 2011;30:492–6.
18. Schlesinger C, Silverberg SG. Endocervical adenocarcinoma in situ of tubal type and its relation to atypical tubal metaplasia. Int J Gynecol Pathol. 1999;73:305–11.
19. Park JJ, Sun D, Quade BJ, et al. Stratified mucin producing intraepithelial lesions of the cervix: adenosquamous or columnar cell neoplasia? Am J Surg Pathol. 2000;24:1414–9.
20. Hu L, Guo M, He Z, Thornton J, McDaniel LS, Hughson MD. Human papillomavirus genotyping and p16INK4a expression in cervical intraepithelial neoplasia of adolescents. Mod Pathol. 2005;18:267–73.
21. Kelly D, Kincaid E, Fansler Z, Rosenthal DL, Clark DP. Detection of cervical high-grade squamous intraepithelial lesions from cytologic samples using a novel immunocytochemical assay (ProEx C). Cancer. 2006;108:494–500.
22. Klaes R, Benner A, Friedrich T, et al. p16INK4a immunohistochemistry improves interobserver agreement in the diagnosis of cervical intraepithelial neoplasia. Am J Surg Pathol. 2002;26:1389–99.
23. Ortega S, Malumbres M, Barbacid M. Cyclin D–dependent kinases INK4 inhibitors and cancer. Biochim Biophys Acta. 2002;1602:73–87.
24. Sano T, Oyama T, Kashiwabara K, Fukuda T, Nakajima T. Expression status of p16 protein is associated with human papillomavirus oncogenic potential in cervical and genital lesions. Am J Pathol. 1998;153:1741–8.
25. von Knebel Doeberitz M. New molecular tools for efficient screening of cervical cancer. Dis Markers. 2001;17:123–99.
26. Horn LC, Reichert A, Oster A, Arndal SF, Trunk MJ, Ridder R, et al. Immunostaining for p16INK4a used as a conjunctive tool improves inter-observer agreement of the histologic diagnosis of cervical intraepithelial neoplasia. Am J Surg Pathol. 2008;32:502–12.
27. Indinnemo M, Cicchini C, Stazi A, et al. Immunohistochemical assessment of Ki-67 as prognostic cellular proliferation marker in anal canal carcinoma. J Exp Clin Cancer Res. 2000;19:471–5.
28. al-Saleh W, Delvenne P, Greimers R, et al. Assessment of Ki-67 antigen immunostaining in squamous intraepithelial lesions of the uterine cervix. Correlation with the histologic grade and human papillomavirus type. Am J Clin Pathol. 1995;104(2):154–60.
29. Santin AD, Zhan F, Bignotti E, et al. Gene expression profiles of primary HPV16- and HPV18-infected early stage cervical cancers and normal cervical epithelium: identification of novel candidate molecular markers for cervical cancer diagnosis and therapy. Virology. 2005;20(331):269–91.
30. Chen Y, Miller C, Mosher R, et al. Identification of cervical cancer markers by cDNA and tissue micro arrays. Cancer Res. 2003;15:1927–35.
31. Davidson B, Goldberg I, Lerner-Geva L, et al. Expression of topoisomerase II and Ki-67 in cervical carcinoma–clinicopathological study using immunohistochemistry. APMIS. 2000;108:209–15.
32. Shi J, Liu H, Wilkerson M, et al. Evaluation of p16, MCM2, DNA Topoisomerase IIA and ProExC in cervical squamous intraepithelial lesions. Lab Investig. 2007;87 Suppl 1:214A.
33. Bell SP, Dutta A. DNA replication in eukaryotic cells. Annu Rev Biochem. 2002;71:333–74.
34. Walts AE, Bose S. p16, Ki67, and BD ProEx C immunostaining: a practical approach for diagnosis of cervical intraepithelial neoplasia. Hum Pathol. 2009;40:957–64.
35. Guo M, Baruch AC, Silva EG. Efficacy of p16 and ProExC immunostaining in the detection of high-grade cervical intra- epithelial neoplasia and cervical carcinoma. Am J Clin Pathol. 2011;135:212–20.

Part II

Screening for Cervical Cancer

Visual Inspection Methods for Cervical Cancer Prevention

3

Swati Priya and Krishna Agarwal

3.1 Introduction

Cervical cancer is the most common cancer in Indian women, accounting for about 1,320,000 new cases each year and 73,000 deaths per year. One-fourth of global cervical cancer-related mortality occurs in India [1].

Cervical cancer is easily preventable by screening due to long preinvasive stage and reliable, easy, and effective treatment. Pap smear has been the traditional method of screening for cervical precancer and cancer all over the world with national screening programs in place in the Western countries. Newer methods of screening like high-risk human papillomavirus (HPV) DNA testing and aided visual methods are being increasingly used nowadays [2].

However, lack of resources and poorly organized health system account for no screening program and high incidence of cervical cancer in our country. Therefore, we need screening methods which are cheaper, require less expertise, and are reasonably reliable. Visual inspection methods, visual inspection with acetic acid (VIA) and visual inspection with Lugol's iodine (VILI), have been proven to be promising alternatives.

Several methods of visual screening are being used for screening in India and various parts of the world, and their effectiveness for the detection of premalignant and malignant lesions of the cervix is being evaluated. These methods are simple and can be performed by any trained health worker, are comparatively inexpensive, do not require too well-equipped laboratory infrastructure, and provide immediate results, thus enabling the use of "screen-and-treat" policy. The various visual examination methods are unaided visual inspection, visual inspection after the application of acetic acid (VIA), VIA with magnification (VIAM), and visual inspection after the application of Lugol's iodine (VILI). Out of these visual methods, simple

S. Priya • K. Agarwal (✉)
Department of Obstetrics and Gynecology, Maulana Azad Medical College and Lok Nayak Hospital, Delhi, India
e-mail: drkrishna.agarwal@gmail.com

S. Mehta, P. Sachdeva (eds.), *Colposcopy of Female Genital Tract*,
DOI 10.1007/978-981-10-1705-6_3

visual inspection methods with acetic acid (VIA) and with Lugol's iodine (VILI) are the most commonly used.

It is seen that VIA and VILI highlight precancerous lesions so they can be viewed with the "naked eye" and thus shift the identification of premalignant lesions from the *laboratory to the clinic*. Visual methods eliminate the need for laboratories and transport of specimens, require very little equipment, and provide women with immediate test results and also treatment at the same visit. A range of medical professionals can effectively perform the procedure, provided they receive adequate training and supervision.

The accuracy of VIA in identifying precancerous lesions is similar to cervical cytology, but cytology provides higher specificity (fewer false positives) than VIA. Visual inspection with acetic acid (VIA) is easy to perform and less expensive than Pap smear, but since they are observer dependent, they have a wide range of sensitivity and specificity. Several studies have found that VIA has a sensitivity of 76–97 % and specificity of 37–64 % [3, 4]. VILI has a sensitivity of around 89 % and a specificity of around 77 % [4]. Thus, it is seen that aided visual tests have a high sensitivity but low specificity. One of the limitations of VIA is that results are highly dependent on the accuracy of an individual's interpretation. So, initial training and quality control are important. Increased false positives are particularly important in a screen-and-treat setting, since overtreatment and resulting impairment of fertility are more likely.

It is seen that visual methods are reliable screening methods for the identification of premalignant and malignant lesions in low-resource countries. Recently, trials and various pilot projects involving medical personnel and paramedics are ongoing using VIA/VILI as screening method for premalignant and malignant lesions.

3.2 Visual Inspection with Acetic Acid (VIA)

Visual inspection with acetic acid (VIA) involves naked-eye examination of the cervix using bright light source, 1 min after dabbing the cervix with 3–5 % acetic acid, using cotton swab or spray. This enables easy differentiation of premalignant or malignant lesions, as they turn acetowhite on acetic acid application.

3.2.1 Principle

Acetowhiteness due to acetic acid application is caused by reversible coagulation of intracellular nuclear proteins and cytokeratins. Rapid coagulation of proteins due to penetration of acetic acid and thus enhanced opacity and reflection of light from superficial layers of the epithelium occurs in abnormal cells (cervical intraepithelial neoplasia and cancer) as compared to the normal epithelium in which superficial layers are sparsely nucleated. The areas of abnormal cells undergo maximum coagulation due to higher content of nuclear proteins. As a result, normal subepithelial vessel pattern (pinkish hue) is obliterated, and the epithelium turns white (Figs. 3.1, 3.2, and 3.3).

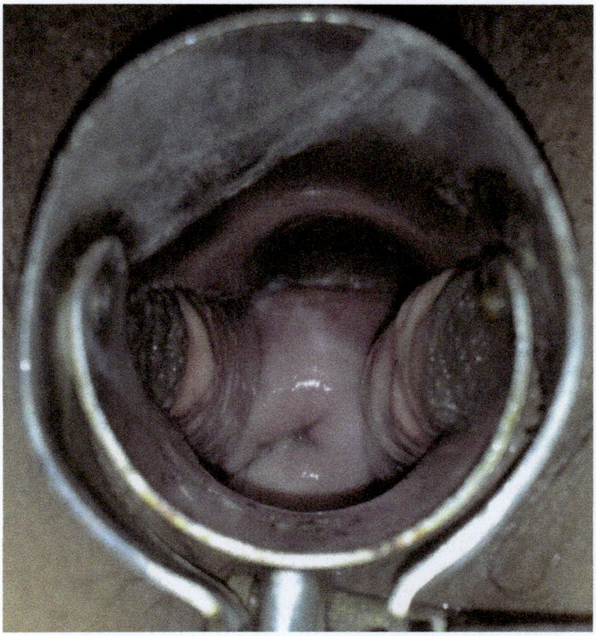

Fig. 3.1 VIA: Normal cervix and no acetowhite area

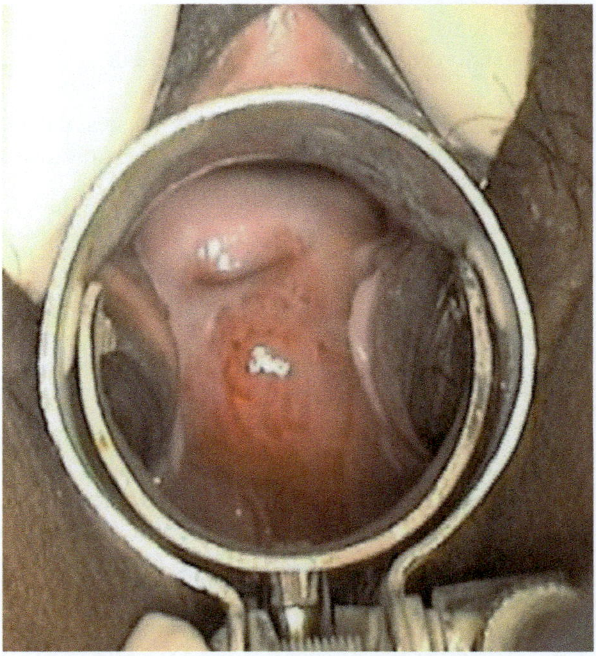

Fig. 3.2 VIA: Low-grade lesion; faint shady acetowhite areas are seen at 11 and 7 o'clock (biopsy done from these areas showed mild dysplasia)

The rapid acetowhiteness of high-grade lesions can be explained by large number of dysplastic cells having more nucleoproteins in superficial layers of the epithelium.

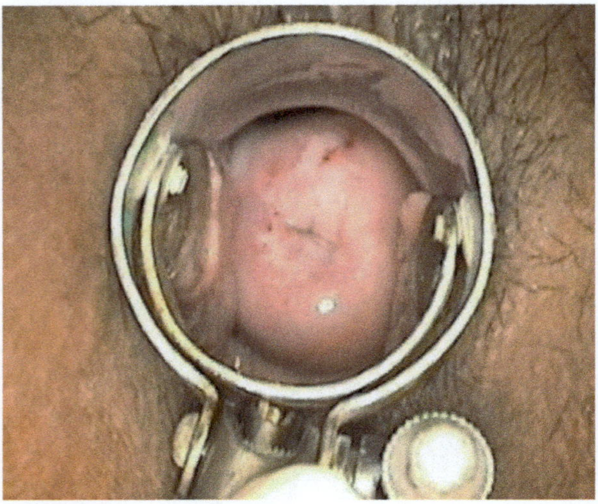

Fig. 3.3 VIA: High-grade lesion-circumferential opaque acetowhite areas with well-defined margins

Acetowhiteness may also occur in various conditions such as:

- Immature squamous metaplasia
- Congenital transformation zone
- Leukoplakia
- Condyloma
- Inflamed, regenerating cervical epithelium

Acetowhiteness of these conditions is thin, less pale, translucent, and without well-defined margins and takes longer to appear and disappears more rapidly than CIN.

3.2.2 Procedure

For making freshly prepared 3–5 % acetic acid solution, 3–5 ml of glacial acetic acid is mixed with 95–97 ml of distilled water. After explaining the procedure to the woman, written content is taken. The perineum and external genitalia are inspected for lesions. The cervix is exposed by sterile speculum in good light, torch, or halogen lamp. The external os, columnar epithelium, squamous epithelium, squamocolumnar junction, and transformation zone are identified. Acetic acid is dabbed by sterile cotton swab and the cervix is inspected for acetowhite areas after 1 min. Acetic acid can be reapplied if in doubt, taking care not to induce bleeding. Several studies have found that VIA has a sensitivity of 76–97 % and specificity of 37–64 % [3, 4].

3.3 Visual Inspection with Lugol's Iodine (VILI)

3.3.1 Principle

VILI involves the use of Lugol's iodine to aid inspection of the cervix with the naked eye. Mature squamous cells store glycogen resulting in black or dark mahogany-brown

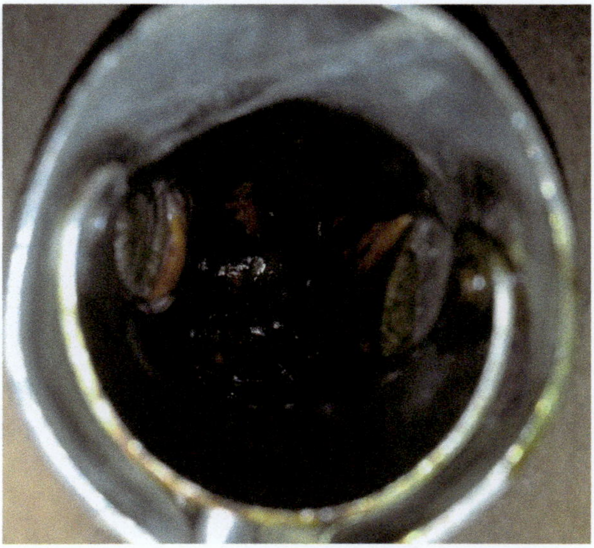

Fig. 3.4 VILI: Normal cervix

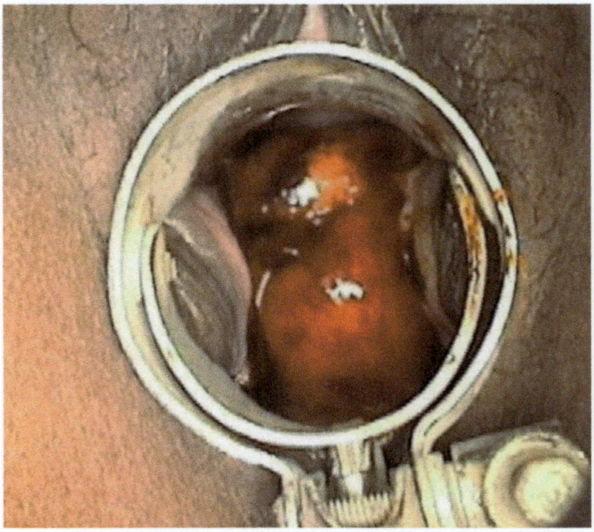

Fig. 3.5 VILI: Low-grade lesion and iodine-negative area seen at 12–1 o'clock position (biopsy from this lesion showed mild dysplasia)

staining. Immature squamous cells and metaplastic epithelium have small amounts of glycogen depending on the grade of maturity resulting in patchy staining. Neoplastic squamous epithelium contains little or no glycogen and does not stain with iodine.

3.3.2 Procedure

After explaining the procedure to the woman and taking written informed consent, the cervix is dabbed with Lugol's iodine and inspected under bright light. Due to low glycogen content, premalignant and malignant lesions of the cervix are mustard yellow, while normal areas take up dark mahogany-brown stain (Figs. 3.4, 3.5, and 3.6).

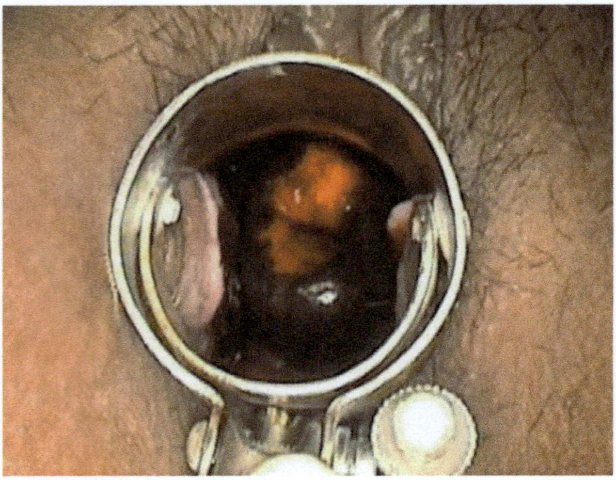

Fig. 3.6 VILI: High-grade lesion. Distinct iodine-negative areas are seen at 12 and at 6 o'clock positions (biopsy from these areas showed severe dysplasia)

The sensitivity of VILI, reported in various studies, ranges from 56.7 to 91.7 % and is higher than that of cytology. The specificity of VILI is reported to be less than cytology, ranging from 76.2 to 89.3 % [5–9].

3.4 Visual Inspection After Acetic Acid Application and Under Magnification (VIAM)

This is VIA done under low magnification using magnification devices. It is also called gynoscopy, aided visual inspection, or VIAM. VIAM has similar sensitivity and specificity as compared with VIA and does not have any added benefit over VIA as noted in the Mumbai cervix cancer trial [5].

3.5 VIA and VILI as a Screening Method

VIA has been analyzed as a promising alternative to more laboratory-dependent and expensive cytology. VIA has shown to have a low specificity compared to cytology and a high rate of false positives in several studies [10–12].

VIA clearly scores over cytology in low-resource settings, in terms of increased screening coverage, easy and improved follow-up care, and overall program quality [13]. As fewer specialized medical personnel and lesser infrastructure, training, and equipment are required in screening with VIA, cervical cancer screening can be easily performed successfully in more remote and less equipped health-care settings leading to higher coverage. Moreover, the results of VIA are available immediately, making it possible to screen-and-treat women during the same visit. This ensures the administration of treatment at the same visit and thus reduces the number of women who may miss out on treatment because they are not able to return to the clinic at another time. Certain benign conditions like inflammation, cervical condyloma, and leukoplakia can give false-positive results of VIA test [12, 14]. VIA has a low positive predictive value resulting in overdiagnosis and overtreatment [15].

The lesions above the endocervical canal which cannot be visualized represent a major problem especially for postmenopausal women where the transformation zone recedes inside the endocervical canal [16].

Various studies have demonstrated the low cost and ease of screening with acetic acid as an alternative to exfoliative cytology and human papillomavirus (HPV) DNA testing in areas where adequate infrastructure is not available.

VIA has also successfully been used in conjugation with cryotherapy, a relatively simple and inexpensive method of treating cervical lesions, thus enabling administration of treatment at a single visit.

Shastri et al. screened women in age group 35–64 years and with no prior history of cancer. VIA was performed by primary health workers and community-based, nonmedical trained personnel who provided basic health-care services in rural India. The primary health workers who screened the women included in the study were local women with at least a tenth grade education and good communication skills. The workers received 4 weeks of intensive training at the beginning of the study, and 1-week refresher courses every year, and screened about 76,000 women in two groups (one group who followed screening protocol and the other group random screening) each in rural India over a period of about 15 years. The test was performed by applying vinegar to the cervix using a cotton swab. After 60 seconds, the cervix was examined using a lamp. Premalignant lesions turn white when vinegar is applied.

It was observed that cervical cancer mortality was reduced by 31 % over a period of 15 years among women screened with biennial visual inspection with vinegar, by primary health workers in this study [17]. The researchers estimated that this strategy could prevent 22,000 cervical cancer deaths every year in India and close to 73,000 in resource-poor countries worldwide where there is little or no access to Pap screening. Cervical cancer is responsible for more than 250,000 deaths worldwide annually.

Goldie et al. have shown that screening women once in a lifetime at the age of 35 years with one or two visit screening strategies involving VIA would reduce the lifetime risk of cervical cancer by approximately 25–36 % [18].

In an observation made in Maharashtra state, encouraging community participation was observed among women educated about the screening using visual methods. About 89 % participation for screening and 79 % for postscreening diagnostic confirmation have been reported. So, visual methods are considered reasonable alternatives to cytology.

Although studies have shown chances of overdiagnosis if visual screening is used as a screening method, several studies have shown that screening by visual methods doesn't lead to overdiagnosis [13]. It has been shown in studies comparing women undergoing screening by visual methods and unscreened women that cancer was often diagnosed at an earlier stage in the screening group, and there was a 7 % reduction in the overall death rate, although the difference was not statistically significant. In Indian women where incidence of premalignant and malignant lesions of the cervix is high, there are fewer chances of visual-aided screening to lead to overdiagnosis and thus overtreatment [19].

In high-income countries, screening for precancerous and cancerous cells using Pap smear has reduced cervical cancer incidence and deaths by 80 %. In India, however, large-scale Pap smear screening and HPV DNA testing have limited coverage due to paucity of resource infrastructure and medical personnels [19].

In 1996, the Indian Council of Medical Research estimated that even if number of existing Pap smear facilities in India were multiplied 12 times, they would only be able to provide a single round of screening to 25 % of eligible women in 10 years. In 2006, the government of India constituted a committee with assistance from the World Health Organization to develop guidelines for population-wide cervical cancer screening in India. This committee again observed that Pap smear-based cervical screening was not feasible in India except at a few centers. Thus, aided visual methods are of great importance in resource-poor countries like India.

Key Points

1. Aided visual methods (VIA and VILI) are important screening methods for premalignant and malignant lesions in low-resource countries.
2. In visual inspection with acetic acid, the cervix is examined under bright light source 1 min after the application of 3–5 % acetic acid.
3. Aided visual methods have advantage over cytology in being simple, low-cost procedure, requiring no laboratory equipments or technician, and immediate result acquisition for treatment at the same setting.
4. In a few studies, false-positive rates of VIA are found to be high, leading to overdiagnosis and overtreatment. In India, however, due to high prevalence of precancerous and cancerous cervical lesions in the population, VIA is proved to be an accurate screening procedure, with little overdiagnosis and overtreatment.
5. VILI involves diagnosis of abnormal iodine-negative areas after the application of Lugol's iodine on the cervix as compared to normal glycogen-containing epithelium which takes up mahogany-brown stain.
6. Once in a lifetime screening by visual methods at 35 years has demonstrated to reduce mortality due to cervical cancer by 31 %.
7. These methods can facilitate reliable "see-and-treat protocols" in low-resource and less well-equipped areas.

References

1. Ferlay J, Soerjomataram I, Ervik M, Dikshit R, Eser S, Mathers C, Rebelo M, Parkin DM, Forman D, Bray, F. GLOBOCAN 2012 v1.0, cancer incidence and mortality worldwide: IARC cancer base no. 11. Lyon: International Agency for Research on Cancer; 2013. Available from: http://globocan.iarc.fr.
2. Chase DM, Kalouyan Marlene BS, Di Saia P. Colposcopy to evaluate abnormal cervical cytology in 2008. Am J Obstet Gynaecol. 2009;200(5):472–80.

3. Karrberg C, Ryd W, Strander B, Branstorm M, Radberg T. Histological diagnosis and evaluation of the Swede score colposcopic system in a large cohort of pregnant women with atypical cervical cytology or cervical malignancy signs. Acta Obstet Gynecol Scand. 2012;91:952–8.
4. Hopman EH, Helmerhorst TJM. Colposcopic findings and nomenclature. CME J Gynecol Oncol. 2005;10:11–3.
5. Shastri SS, Dinshaw K, Amin G, Goswami S, Patil S, Chinoy R, et al. Concurrent evaluation of visual, cytological, HPV testing as screening methods for the early detection of cervical neoplasia in Mumbai, India. Bull World Health Organ. 2005;83(3):186–94.
6. Goel A, Gandhi G, Batra S, Bhambhani S, Zutshi V, Sachdeva P. Visual inspection of the cervix with acetic acid for cervical intraepithelial lesions. Int J Gynecol Obstet. 2005;88(1):25–30.
7. Sarian LO, Derchain SF, Naud P, Roteli-Martins C, Longatto-Filho A, Tatti S, et al. Evaluation of visual inspection with acetic acid (VIA), Lugol's iodine (VILI), cervical cytology and HPV testing as cervical screening tools in Latin America. J Med Screen. 2005;12(3):142–9.
8. Sankarnarayanan R, Chatterjee R, Shastri S, Wesley R, Basu P, Mahe C, et al. Accuracy of human papillomavirus testing in the primary screening of cervical neoplasia: results from a multicentric study in India. Int J Cancer. 2004;112:341–7.
9. Lugoma GS, Mahmud S, Samih H, Liaras J. Visual inspection as a cervical cancer screening method in a primary health care setting in Africa. Int J Cancer. 2006;119:1389–95.
10. IARC. Handbooks of cancer prevention. Cervical cancer screening. Lyon: IARC Press; 2005.
11. Jeronimo J, et al. A multicountry evaluation of care HPV testing, visual inspection with acetic acid, and papanicolaou testing for the detection of cervical cancer. Int J Gynecol Cancer. 2014;24(3):576–85.
12. Longatto-Filho A, et al. Performance characteristics of Pap test, VIA, VILI, HR-HPV testing, cervicography, and colposcopy in diagnosis of significant cervical pathology. Virchows Arch. 2012;460(6):577–85.
13. Luciani S, Winkler J. Cervical cancer prevention in Peru: lessons learned from the TATI demonstration project. Washington, DC: Pan American Health Organization; 2006.
14. Labani S, et al. CareHPV cervical cancer screening demonstration in a rural population of North India. Eur J Obstet Gynecol Reprod Biol. 2014;176:75–9.
15. Ajenifuja KO, et al. A population-based study of visual inspection with acetic acid (VIA) for cervical screening in rural Nigeria. Int J Gynecol Cancer. 2013;23(3):507–12.
16. International Agency for Research on Cancer. A practical manual on visual screening for cervical neoplasia. Lyon: IARC; 2003.
17. Shastri SS, Mittra I, Mishra GA, Gupta S, Dikshit R, Singh S, Badwe RA. Effect of VIA screening by primary health workers: randomized controlled study in Mumbai, India. J Natl Cancer Inst. 2014; 106(3):dju009. doi: 10.1093/jnci/dju009.
18. Goldie SJ, Gaffikin L, Goldhaber-Fiebert JD, Gordillo-Tobar A, Levin C, Mahé C, et al. Cost-effectiveness of cervical-cancer screening in five developing countries. Alliance for Cervical Cancer Prevention Cost Working Group. N Engl J Med. 2005;353:2158–68.
19. Sankaranarayanan R, Basu P, Wesley R, Mahe C, Keita N, Gombe Mbalwa CC, et al. Accuracy of visual screening for cervical neoplasia: Results from an IARC multicentre study in India and Africa. Int J Cancer. 2004;112:341–7.

4 Cytology as a Screening Tool

Vani Bharani and Bharti Bharani

4.1 Introduction

In 1928, Georgios Nikolaou Papanikolaou (Fig. 4.1), a Greek physician, made a monumental breakthrough when he discovered abnormal cells under the microscope in a uterine cancer patient's vaginal fluid. Dr. Papanikolaou had previously demonstrated the existence of a menstrual cycle by examining vaginal smears of guinea pigs. Eventually, he became interested in the menstrual cycle of women; it was doing this work that he observed these abnormal cells.

Medical history has consistently shown that change is hard and breakthroughs often unwelcome. Papanikolaou's work was met with skepticism and resistance from the scientific community. It took over a decade to validate the diagnostic potential of the vaginal smear. In 1943 Papanikolaou and gynecologist Dr. Herbert Traut published their findings and conclusions in the famous monograph *Diagnosis of Uterine Cancer by the Vaginal Smear*. This diagnostic procedure was named the Pap test [2].

With 528,000 new cases per year, cervical cancer is now the fourth most common cancer affecting women worldwide after breast, colorectal, and lung cancer. Eighty percent of the global burden falls in areas with low-income countries especially of sub-Saharan Africa. Over a fifth of newly diagnosed cases are from India [3].

In sub-Saharan Africa, 34.8 new cases of cervical cancers are diagnosed per 100,000 women annually, and 22.5 per 100,000 women die from the disease, while in North America these figures are as low as 6.6 and 2.5 per 100,000 women,

V. Bharani, MD (✉) • B. Bharani, MS (✉)
Dysplasia Clinic, 119, Ravindra Nagar, Indore, India
e-mail: vanibharani@gmail.com; bhartibharani@gmail.com

S. Mehta, P. Sachdeva (eds.), *Colposcopy of Female Genital Tract*,
DOI 10.1007/978-981-10-1705-6_4

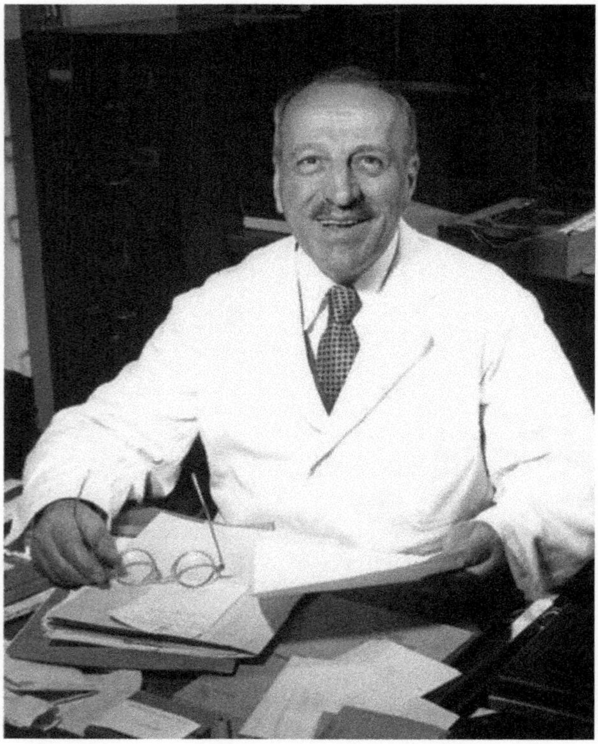

Fig. 4.1 Georgios Nikolaou Papanikolaou, Born 13 May 1883 in Kymi, Euboea, Kingdom of Greece. Died 19 February 1962 [1, 2]

respectively. The drastic reduction in the incidence of cervical cancer in North America and Oceania over the past 50 years is attributed to widespread use of the Pap test for screening [3].

4.2 Screening for Cervical Cancer

Most of the premalignant and malignant lesions of the cervix are of the squamous type. Human papillomavirus (HPV) types 16 and 18 are the dominant oncotypes in squamous lesions, but type 18 is relatively more important in glandular lesions. HPV infections occur in the transformation zone, an area which undergoes physiological metaplasia from glandular to squamous epithelium at the onset of adolescence. Persistent infection produces perturbation of the cell-cycle controls, resulting in cervical intraepithelial neoplasia (CIN). At their mildest (CIN 1), these lesions are generally no more than manifestations of HPV infection, but at their most severe (CIN 3), the risk of progression to cancer is high. The risk in CIN 1 lesions is about 1 %, while it is 5 % and 12 % among those with CIN 2 and CIN 3, respectively [4]. The progression to invasive carcinoma is a slow process, giving a wide opportunity for detection by exfoliative cytology [5–8].

4.3 Cervical Cytology

Papanikolaou devised a class system for reporting cervical smears, intended to convey degree of suspicion that the patient had cancer: class I, the absence of atypical or abnormal cells; class II, atypical cytology but no evidence of malignancy; class III, cytology suggestive of but not conclusive for malignancy; class IV, cytology strongly suggestive of malignancy; and class V, cytology conclusive for malignancy. Later descriptive terms borrowed from histologic classifications of preinvasive squamous lesions were used (Fig. 4.2).

The dysplasia nomenclature divided lesions into carcinoma in situ; high-risk lesion of immature, undifferentiated atypical cells; and dysplasia, considered to be a low-risk lesion. In the 1960s, Dr. Ralph Richart challenged the duality of dysplasia/carcinoma in situ and proposed a new term, cervical intraepithelial neoplasia (CIN), which was graded from 1 to 3. Due to lack of universal application,

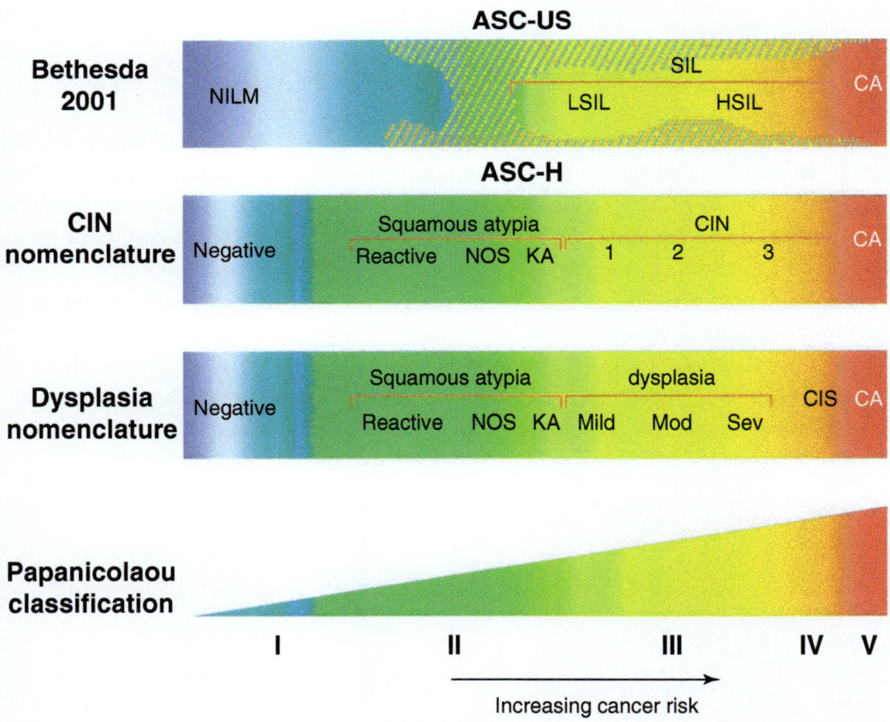

Fig. 4.2 Classifications for cervical cytology: The graded shades of colors emphasize a morphologic continuum of cytologic findings with indiscrete transitions, *blue* negative, *green* equivocal, *yellow* low-grade intraepithelial abnormalities, *orange* high-grade intraepithelial abnormalities, and *red* carcinoma. The categories of atypical squamous cells of undetermined significance (ASC-US) and atypical squamous cells that cannot exclude high-grade squamous intraepithelial lesion (ASC-H) are represented by *dots*. *NILM* negative for intraepithelial lesion, *HSIL* high-grade intraepithelial lesion, *CA* cancer, *NOS* not otherwise specified, *KA* koilocytic atypia, *CIN* cervical intraepithelial neoplasia, *CIS* carcinoma in situ [9]

a uniform system was needed for grouping in studies and evolving treatment protocols. Developed in 1988 and revised in 2001, the Bethesda system for reporting cervical cytology accomplished these goals. The name for preinvasive squamous lesions was changed to squamous intraepithelial lesion, subdivided into only two grades, low and high. This paradigm shift from the CIN concept was based on HPV biology. Low-grade lesions are transient infections that carry little risk for oncogenesis, whereas most high-grade lesions are associated with viral persistence and a significant potential for progression to invasive cancer [10].

4.4 The Bethesda System (TBS) [11, 12]

The Bethesda system is a standardized framework for reporting cervical cytology that includes a descriptive diagnosis and an evaluation of specimen adequacy. It provides a clear guidance for clinical management.

4.4.1 Satisfactory or Unsatisfactory Smear

Smears are reported as "satisfactory for evaluation" or "unsatisfactory for evaluation." Minimal squamous cellularity requirements for a specimen to qualify as "satisfactory" are 8,000 to 12,000 well-visualized squamous cells for conventional smears and 5,000 squamous cells for liquid-based preparations. A comment on the presence or absence of endocervical/transformation zone component is also included. There should be at least ten well-preserved endocervical or squamous metaplastic cells (Fig. 4.3).

Samples that cannot be accessioned, for example, broken or unlabelled slide, are labeled as unsatisfactory. Certain smears are designated as unsatisfactory following microscopic evaluation. Specimens with more than 75 % of epithelial cells obscured

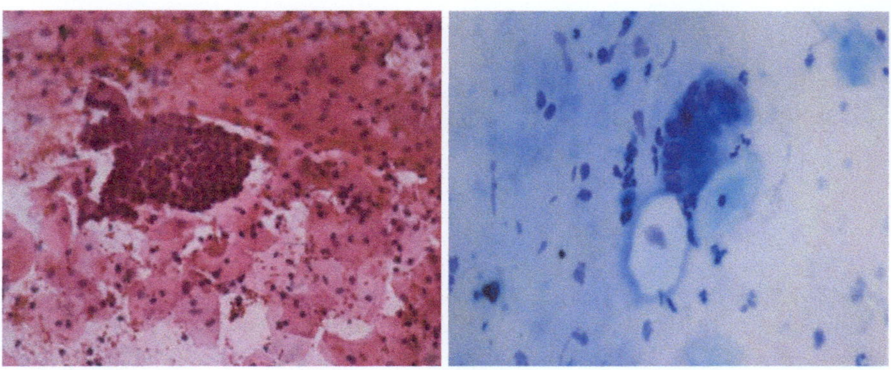

Fig. 4.3 Clusters of endocervical cells. A minimum of ten well-preserved endocervical or squamous metaplastic cells are an indicator of transformation zone or endocervical sampling (Courtesy Dr. Satish Phatak)

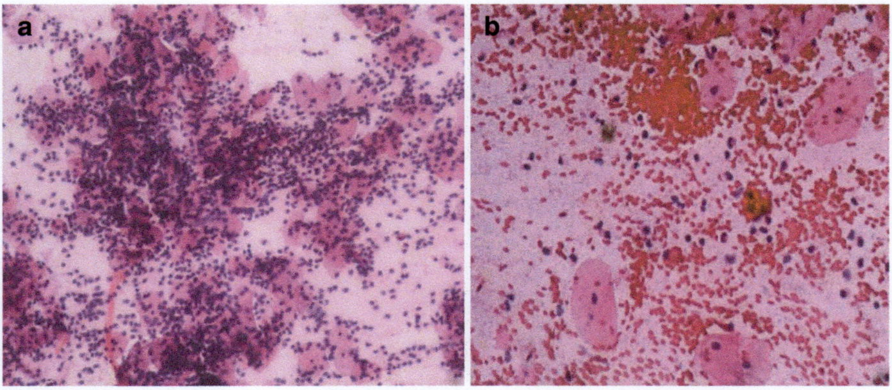

Fig. 4.4 Squamous cells obscured by polymorphs (**a**) and blood (**b**) (Courtesy Dr. Satish Phatak)

by blood or inflammation are "unsatisfactory." A specimen is considered "partially obscured" when 50–75 % of the epithelial cells cannot be visualized. Evaluation of specimen adequacy is considered to be the single most important quality assurance component of the Bethesda system (Fig. 4.4).

4.4.2 General Categorization

This is an optional component of the Bethesda system, to allow clinicians to triage reports readily. Smears with no abnormality or reactive changes are categorized as "negative for intraepithelial lesion or malignancy." Categories for epithelial abnormalities and other morphologic findings that may indicate some increased risk like benign-appearing endometrial cells in a woman >40 years of age are included.

4.4.3 Interpretation/Result

4.4.3.1 Negative for Intraepithelial Lesion or Malignancy

Specimens for which no epithelial abnormality is identified are reported as "negative for intraepithelial lesion or malignancy." Organisms like *Trichomonas vaginalis*, *Candida* species, shift in flora suggestive of bacterial vaginosis, *Actinomyces* species, and herpes simplex virus are also reported. Reporting nonneoplastic findings like reactive cellular changes associated with inflammation, radiation, intrauterine contraceptive device, or atrophy are optional.

4.4.3.2 Epithelial Cell Abnormalities: Squamous Cells

The first category is *atypical squamous cells* to designate "cellular abnormalities that are more marked than those attributable to reactive changes but that quantitatively or qualitatively fall short of a definitive diagnosis of 'squamous intraepithelial lesion' (SIL)." This class is further subdivided into two atypical squamous cells of

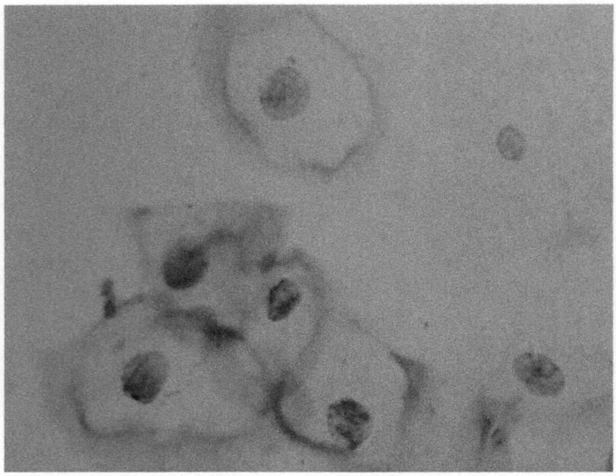

Fig. 4.5 Atypical squamous cells of undetermined significance: designate cellular abnormalities that are more marked than reactive changes but fall short of a definitive diagnosis of squamous intraepithelial lesion (Courtesy Dr. Satish Phatak)

undetermined significance (*ASC-US*) and atypical squamous cells that cannot exclude high-grade squamous intraepithelial lesion (*ASC-H*) (Fig. 4.5). The qualifier "undetermined significance" indicates that some cases of ASC-US are associated with underlying CIN 2 or 3. ASC-H includes approximately 5–10% of ASC cases and reflects a mixture of true HSIL and its mimics. Estimates suggest that 10–20% of women with ASC have underlying CIN 2 or 3 and that 1 in 1000 may have invasive cancer [13].

Low-grade squamous intraepithelial lesions (LSILs) affect intermediate or superficial cells, which show nuclear enlargement, moderate variation in nuclear size, and slight irregularities in nuclear shape and contour. LSIL encompasses lesions previously described as koilocytosis and mild dysplasia (CIN 1). Classic koilocytes have large, sharply defined perinuclear cytoplasmic cavities surrounded by dense rims of cytoplasm (Fig. 4.6). LSILs are low-risk intraepithelial lesions majority of which regress spontaneously.

High-grade squamous intraepithelial lesions (HSILs) carry a significant risk for progression to cervical cancer. HSIL is usually a lesion of smaller, less mature squamous cells. Nuclear-to-cytoplasmic ratio, hyperchromasia, irregular chromatin distribution, and membrane contour irregularity are all more severe than in LSIL. HSIL encompasses lesions previously described as moderate dysplasia (CIN 2) and as severe dysplasia/carcinoma in situ (CIN 3) (Fig. 4.7).

Classic *squamous cell carcinoma* shows abundant necrotic debris: a granular, amorphous precipitate with nuclear debris and red blood cells called "tumor diathesis." This is associated with hyperchromatic crowded groups of atypical cells or abundant atypical keratinized cells with unusual shapes ("tadpoles," "fiber cells") (Fig. 4.8).

4.4.3.3 Epithelial Cell Abnormalities: Glandular Cells

Similar to the ASC, *atypical glandular cells* include glandular cells that demonstrate changes beyond benign reactive processes but are insufficient to be labeled as

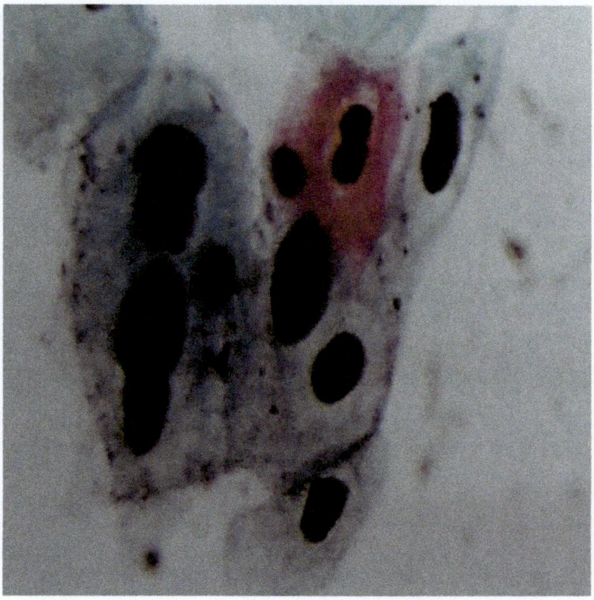

Fig. 4.6 Koilocyte: HPV-infected, intermediate, or superficial cells with perinuclear cytoplasmic cavities (Courtesy Dr. Satish Phatak)

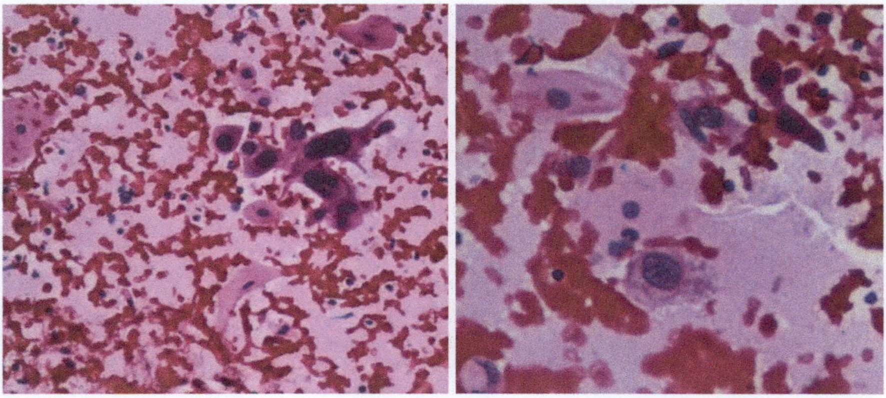

Fig. 4.7 High-grade squamous intraepithelial lesions (HSIL): high nuclear-to-cytoplasmic ratio, hyperchromasia, irregular chromatin distribution, and membrane contour irregularity (Courtesy Dr. Satish Phatak)

in situ or invasive adenocarcinoma. These are further classified to indicate their origin as endocervical or endometrial origin whenever possible.

Endocervical adenocarcinomas, in situ and invasive, are high-grade lesions that demonstrate nuclear enlargement, hyperchromasia, stratification, and mitotic activity. Invasive carcinoma shows additional features of invasion, including prominent nucleoli and tumor diathesis.

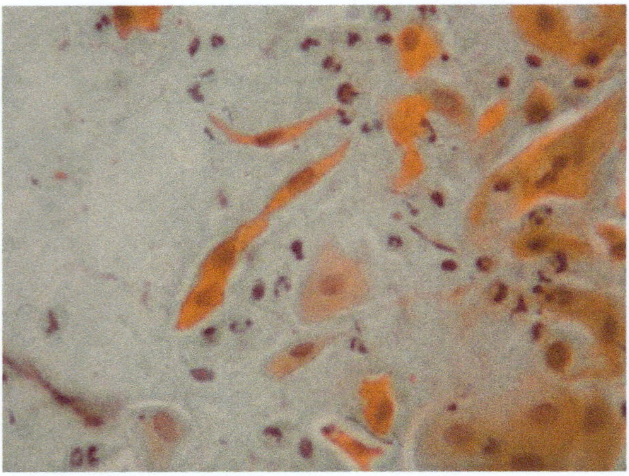

Fig. 4.8 Squamous cell carcinoma: atypical keratinized cells with abnormal shapes (Courtesy Dr. Satish Phatak)

Endometrial adenocarcinoma yields fewer cells than endocervical lesions, which are directly sampled. The cytologic features vary according to the grade of tumor. Tumor diathesis is often difficult to appreciate.

An intermediate category of *atypical endocervical cells that favor neoplastic* includes smears with atypical features not amounting to an interpretation of AIS but conveys a significant level of concern.

4.4.4 Others

Additional findings like endometrial cells if seen in a woman 40 years of age or older are noted, regardless of the date of the last menstrual period. Although usually benign in nature, the presence of endometrial cells, if not associated with menses or after menopause, may indicate risk for an endometrial abnormality.

4.4.5 Automated Review and Ancillary Testing

Instrumentation and automated review result are included in cytology report if the slide is scanned by automated computer systems. The assay and result of an ancillary molecular test performed are also added when appropriate.

4.4.6 Educational Notes and Suggestions

These are optional in a report; format and style vary according to preferences of the laboratory and clinicians.

4.5 Sample Collection [14]

Adequate sample collection and proper submission to the laboratory with appropriate clinical information play a pivotal role in cervical cytology reporting. Majority of false negatives are attributed to improper sample collection or lack of skill and knowledge of the individual who obtains the specimen [15–17].

4.5.1 Patient Preparation

Collection of sample is planned approximately 2 weeks (10–18 days) after the first day of menstrual period. The woman is instructed against the use of douche, tampons, birth control foams, jellies, or other vaginal creams or vaginal medications for 48 h prior to the test. Also, she is advised to refrain from intercourse 48 h prior to the test.

4.5.2 Test Requisition

The requisition form must include patient details including name, age, menstrual status (LMP, hysterectomy, pregnant, postpartum, hormone therapy), and previous abnormal cervical cytology result and previous treatment, biopsy, or surgical procedure. The source of specimen, e.g., cervical and vaginal, should be mentioned along with the history of the use of hormone/contraceptive use and relevant clinical findings (abnormal bleeding, grossly visible lesion, etc.).

4.5.3 Labeling the Sample

The glass slide or specimen vial must be labeled with patient's first and last names at the time of the collection of sample. For glass slides a solvent-resistant pen or pencil can be used on the frosted end of the slide. For liquid-based samples, the information is affixed to the vial.

4.5.4 Visualization of the Cervix for the Collection of an Adequate Sample

The smear is collected before bimanual examination and application of acetic acid or Lugol's iodine. A sterile bivalve speculum of appropriate size is inserted into the vagina without lubrication in the dorsolithotomy position. Warm water or water-soluble jelly may be used to facilitate insertion. The jelly should not be applied on the tip of the speculum. Excess mucus or other discharge should be removed gently with ring forceps holding a folded gauze pad. A well-placed speculum would allow visualization of the os and ectocervix. The transformation zone may be easily visualized in some patients, while it may be high in the endocervical canal in others. The position of transformation zone varies in an individual over time as well. Various factors influence the position of transformation zone including changes in vaginal pH; hormonal changes including pregnancy, childbirth, and menopausal status; and hormonal therapy. Cervical stenosis in postmenopausal patients or postradiation therapy may prevent visualization of the transformation zone. It is important to sample the endocervix in these patients. A sample from the vaginal cuff is sufficient in a post-hysterectomy setting.

4.5.5 Collection Devices

Several devices including endocervical brushes, wooden and plastic spatulas, and plastic "broom-type" samplers are available for sampling. Plastic spatulas are preferred over wooden as they retain cellular material [18]. Also the use of moistened cotton-tipped swab results in incomplete sampling as cells adhere to the cotton and do not transfer well to the glass slide. Overall, the cytobrush and spatula together provide the best specimen quality for cervical cytology [19].

4.5.6 Collection of Samples for Conventional Smear Preparation Using the Spatula and Endocervical Brush

The ectocervix is sampled first using a plastic spatula. The notched end of the spatula that corresponds to the contour of the cervix is rotated 360° around the circumference, retaining the sample on the upper surface. The endocervical brush is inserted in the endocervical canal so that some bristles are still visible, rotated 45°–90°, and removed. Now the sample on the spatula is spread evenly and thinly lengthwise by single uniform motion on one half of glass slide. The endocervical brush is rolled along the remaining half. Forceful smearing in multiple directions is avoided. The entire slide is then rapidly fixed in alcohol and the collection devices are discarded. The vaginal fornix and ectocervix should always be sampled before the endocervix/transformation zone. If the order is reversed, bleeding secondary to abrasion from the brush may obscure the cellular material (Fig. 4.9).

4.5.7 Collection of Samples for Liquid-Based Preparations Using the Spatula and Endocervical Brush

The ectocervix and endocervix are sampled using the same procedure as for conventional smears. However, the spatula and the endocervical brush with the cellular material are rinsed in the specimen vial and then discarded.

4.5.8 Collection of Sample Using the "Broom-Like" Device

The broom-like brush ("broom") has a flat plastic strips contoured to conform to the cervix, with longer strips in the middle. The endocervix and ectocervix can be sampled simultaneously. The long middle strips are inserted into the os until the shorter

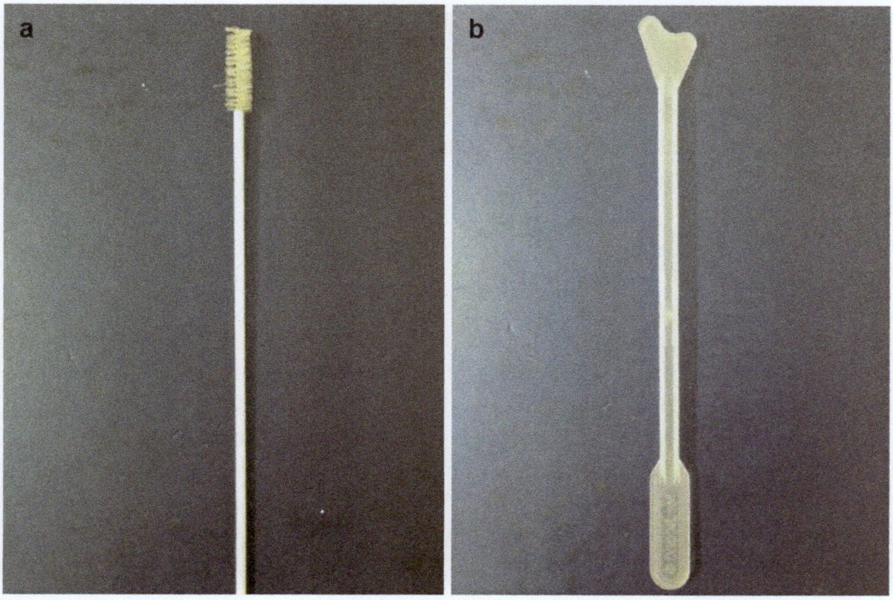

Fig. 4.9 (**a**) Endocervical brush and (**b**) Ayres spatula

outer strips bend against the ectocervix. It is rotated 360° in the same direction five times while maintaining gentle pressure. To transfer the material, each side of the broom is stroked once across the slide in a painting motion on the glass slide. The slide is rapidly fixed and the broom is then discarded. In the case of liquid-based preparations, the broom is rinsed in the specimen vial after the collection of sample.

4.5.9 Cell Fixation for Conventional Smears

Immediate fixation of smears by immersing the slide in alcohol or spraying with fixative is essential to prevent air-drying. Air-drying obscures cellular detail and compromises specimen evaluation. If the specimen is immersed in alcohol, it can be transported to the laboratory in the same container. Alternatively, smear can be immersed in alcohol for 2–3 min, removed, and allowed to air-dry and then placed in a container for transport to the laboratory. This technique requires the use of a separate container for each specimen and changing or filtering the alcohol between specimens.

Quality-controlled cytology fixatives can also be used. Generally, spray fixatives should be 6–10 inches (15–25 cm) from the glass slide when applied.

4.5.10 Variability in Specimen Collection

No consensus has been reached regarding the use of one or two slides for cervical cytology. The use of one slide decreases the number of slides to be screened, reduces costs, and requires less space for storage [20, 21].

4.5.11 Laboratory Sample Processing

The modified Papanicolaou method is recommended for the staining of gynecologic cytology slides. The method uses hematoxylin as a nuclear stain and two cytoplasmic counterstains, OG-6 and EA. This staining provides transparency of the cytoplasm and a clear visualization of cellular morphology.

4.6 Liquid-Based Cytology

In 1996, the Food and Drug Administration (FDA) approved the ThinPrep™ (Cytyc Corporation, Boxborough, MA) as an alternative to the conventional cervicovaginal smear. This was followed in 1999 by the approval of AutoCyte PREP™ (now known as SurePrep™) (TriPath Imaging, Burlington, NC). In these methods, cervical cells are immersed in a conserving liquid before being fixed on the slide. This avoids desiccation and reduces the quantity of obscuring material like blood and mucus. These preparations were originally developed to minimize cell overlap to improve identification of abnormal cells by automated screeners [9, 22, 23].

4.6.1 ThinPrep [9, 22, 23]

This is a filter-based cell concentration technique. Sample is collected in CytoLyt solution, a methanol-based fixative, which is both hemolytic and mucolytic. A 20 mm diameter cylinder with a polycarbonate thin filter attached to one end is introduced into the specimen vial and rotated. This disaggregates mucus, blood, and other debris and breaks up large cell clusters and homogenizes the cell suspension. A gentle vacuum is applied to the cylinder so that erythrocytes and debris to pass through the filter pores and the cells adhere to the filter. The cylinder is pressed against a positively charged slide, and air pressure is applied to transfer the cells to the slide. The slide is immediately dropped into 95 % ethanol. The entire procedure takes about 70 s per slide (Fig. 4.10).

4.6.2 SurePath [9, 22, 23]

This is a density gradient-based cell enrichment process. Sample is collected in an ethanol-based preservative fluid, which also lyses blood. In contrast to the ThinPrep method, the tip of the collection device is snipped and submitted with the sample vial. The larger fragments are disaggregated, and the sample is mixed with a density gradient reagent with polysaccharide solution that acts to trap small particulates and debris. A cell pellet is obtained after centrifugation which is resuspended, and the sedimentation is repeated. A robotic arm transfers the sample to a glass slide.

Various studies and meta-analysis have demonstrated that LBC shows similar sensitivity and specificity as conventional smears in detection of high-grade cervical

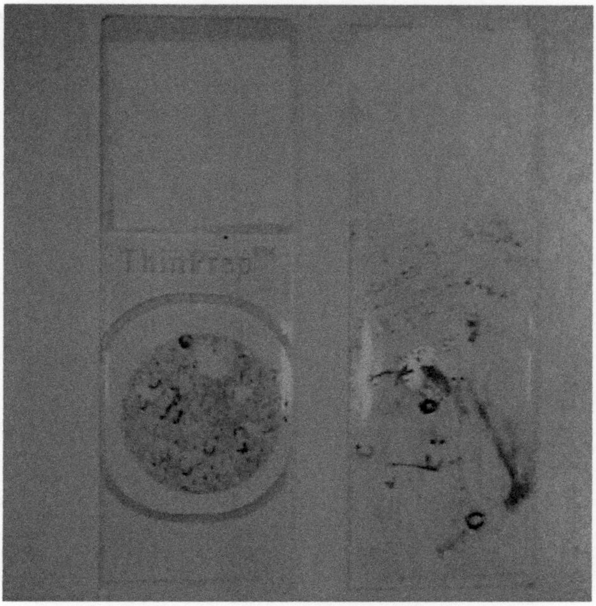

Fig. 4.10 Conventional cytology slide and ThinPrep slide: uniform spread of sample in a diameter of 20 mm in ThinPrep smear

intraepithelial neoplasia, although a fall in specificity is seen when ASC-US is the threshold for colposcopy [24, 25]. In the largest randomized control trial, the sensitivity and positive predictive value of LBC and conventional smears were comparable [26, 27]. However, there were significantly less unsatisfactory smears with LBC preparations [28]. Though specimen adequacy is improved with LBC, the identification of endocervical cells as a marker of transformation zone sampling becomes difficult [29, 30]. Several studies report higher detection and more accurate categorization of glandular lesions by LBC as compared to conventional smears [31, 32].

A clear advantage of LBC is improved visualization of cells so the slides are less fatiguing to read and require less to screen. A study reported that the time needed for reading a LBC slide was half as compared to a conventional cytology slide [33].

Yet another advantage of LBC is the use of residual material in the vial for the preparation of additional slides, molecular testing of infectious agents, DNA cytometry, and DNA ploidy analysis. The additional sample can be used in cases showing undetermined nuclear atypia, questionable grade of the lesion, and excess or scarcity of cells, blood, or exudates [34, 35].

4.7 Automation in Cervical Cytology

Automated cytology screening devices have been under development since the 1950s. The chief purpose of automation is to reduce the labor required for manual screening. These devices classify a set percentage of cervical smears as negative which do not require human review. Automation provides a more rapid, accurate, and standardized screening while reducing the labor. It also reduces errors caused by human fatigue and detects lesions when the sample contains a lesser number of abnormal cells [36]. High cost of equipment and the implementation of the technology make its use difficult principally in developing nations.

BD FocalPoint guided screening (GS) imaging system is one such FDA-approved instrument. The device uses algorithms to measure cellular features such as nuclear size, integrated optical density, nuclear-to-cytoplasmic ratio, and nuclear contour. The smear is assigned a score that is used to rank slides for likelihood of an abnormality. It identifies up to 25 % of slides as requiring no further human review [22, 23].

4.8 Target Population and Interval of Screening

The screening recommendations vary among various international bodies. The American College of Obstetricians and Gynecologists (ACOG) currently recommends screening starting at age 21, every 2 years for most women under age 30 and every 3 years for women 30 and older who have three negative prior screenings. They recommend cessation of screening at age 65 or 70, depending on a woman's screening history [37]. The American Cancer Society (ACS), American Society for Colposcopy and Cervical Pathology (ASCCP), and American Society for Clinical Pathology (ASCP) also recommend initiation of screening at 21 years but recommend screening every 3 years for all women between 21 and 65 years. Both guidelines recommend against the use of HPV co-testing in women <30 years of age. For women between 30 and 65 years who wish to lengthen the screening interval, cytology with HPV contesting once every 5 years is an acceptable option [38].

4.9 Role of Cytology in Screening

Reviews on the accuracy of cervical cytology show sensitivity of 47–62 % and the specificity of 60–95 % in detecting CIN 2–3 [39–41], while in studies from various developing countries, a sensitivity of 44–78 % and a specificity of 91–96 % have been reported [42–47]. With low to moderate sensitivity, the value of cervical cytology in decreasing incidence of and mortality from cervical cancer can be attributed to organized screening programs with repeated testing at regular intervals, high population coverage, and quality control procedures. Additionally cytology screening requires well-trained personnel for collection, preparation, and staining and final reporting of smear. Laboratory infrastructure, with quality control for processing slides and microscopy, and a system for communicating the results to the women are also needed. Reliable and efficient testing requires high-quality training, continuing education, and proficiency testing of personnel. With the need for trained personnel, laboratory infrastructure, facility for delivery results, and financial resources, cytology is not a viable option in many developing countries [48, 49].

Tests like visual inspection with 3–5 % acetic acid (VIA), magnified visual inspection with acetic acid (VIAM), and visual inspection with Lugol's iodine (VILI) have been evaluated to a lesser extent. VIA and VILI are promising approaches, particularly in low-resource settings. A major advantage is immediate availability of results after visual testing. Uniform criteria for reporting still remain to be established. Quality control, close monitoring of test positivity, and periodic retraining are essential to maintain good standards of visual testing. The addition of visual tests to cytology improves sensitivity but decreases specificity. A study from Mumbai showed an increase in sensitivity of cytology from 57.4 to 83.3 % by the addition of VIA to cytology as an adjunctive test, but the specificity decreased from 98.6 to 87.4 %. The combination of cytology and VILI also improved test sensitivity significantly but reduced the specificity [50].

HPV testing alone or in addition with cytology is a promising approach. Cross-sectional studies indicate a sensitivity of 94 % or greater by HPV co-testing with cytology, which is a significant improvement over cytology alone [51]. Currently it is far more expensive than other screening tests and requires sophisticated laboratory infrastructure, including testing equipment, storage facilities for samples, and trained technicians.

4.10 Indian Scenario

Lack of awareness about the disease, low socioeconomic status, illiteracy, inadequate and inaccessible medical facilities, and paucity of an organized screening program have together contributed to unabated progress of cervical cancer to mammoth proportions in developing countries like India. Efforts to improve awareness of the population have resulted in early detection of and improved survival from cervical cancer in a backward rural region in Western India [52, 53].

A large population and limited and variable resources and infrastructure in different parts of the country preclude a national cytology-based screening program. As an alternative, the National Cancer Control Program has suggested the use of VIA as the immediate option for cervical cancer control initiatives. They recommend screening of women in the age group of 30–59 years at the primary health centers, with a repeat after 5 years for VIA-negative cases. The management of VIA-positive cases is to be done at the district hospital with Pap smear and colposcopy [54].

Key Points

1. The premalignant lesions of the cervix are amenable to early detection and treatment.
2. Organized cytology-based screening programs have markedly reduced the mortality and morbidity associated with cervical cancer in developed world.
3. The Bethesda system for reporting has aided in uniform grouping of the patients and evolution of standard treatment protocols.
4. The introduction of liquid-based cytology has significantly reduced the frequency of unsatisfactory smears while maintaining a comparable sensitivity and specificity to conventional cytology.
5. Twenty percent of 528,000 new cases of cervical cancer detected annually worldwide are from India.
6. Lack of skilled manpower, standardized laboratories, and an organized screening program preclude the use of cytology in Indian scenario.
7. Visual inspection with acetic acid (VIA) is an affordable alternative suitable for immediate application in population-based screening program in India.

References

1. Anniversaries: George Papanicolaou – Weill Medical College. Available at http://weill.cornell.edu/archives/blog/2012/03/anniversaries-george-papanicolaou.html. Accessed 5 Sept 2014.
2. Georgios Papanikolaou – Wikipedia, the free encyclopedia. Available at http://en.wikipedia.org/wiki/Georgios_Papanikolaou. Accessed 5 Sept 2014.
3. World Health Organization, International Agency for Research on Cancer Latest world cancer statistics: global cancer burden rises to 14.1 million new cases in 2012: marked increase in breast cancers must be addressed. From: www.iarc.fr/en/media-centre/pr/2013/pdfs/pr223_E.pdf. Accessed 5 Sept 2014.
4. Pinto AP, Crum CP. Natural history of cervical neoplasia: defining progression and its consequence. Clin Obstet Gynecol. 2000;43(2):352–62. Review.
5. Jastreboff AM, Cymet T. Role of the human papilloma virus in the development of cervical intraepithelial neoplasia and malignancy. Postgrad Med J. 2002;78(918):225–8. Review.
6. Kitchener HC, Castle PE, Cox JT. Chapter 7: achievements and limitations of cervical cytology screening. Vaccine. 2006;24 Suppl 3:S3/63–70. Review.
7. Arends MJ, Buckley CH, Wells M. Aetiology, pathogenesis, and pathology of cervical neoplasia. J Clin Pathol. 1998;51(2):96–103. Review.
8. Cox JT. Epidemiology of cervical intraepithelial neoplasia: the role of human papillomavirus. Baillieres Clin Obstet Gynaecol. 1995;9(1):1–37. Review.
9. Comparison of four cytologic classifications for squamous cells. Available at http://jncimono.oxfordjournals.org/content/2003/31/72/F2.expansion.html. Accessed 6 Sept 2014.
10. Cibas ES. Cervical and vaginal cytology. In: Cibas ES, Ducatman BS, editors. Cytology diagnostic and clinical correlates. 3rd ed. Atlanta: Elsevier Health Sciences; 2009. p. 1–36.
11. Solomon D, Davey D, Kurman R, Moriarty A, O'Connor D, Prey M, Raab S, Sherman M, Wilbur D, Wright Jr T, Young N, Forum Group Members, Bethesda 2001 Workshop. The 2001 Bethesda System: terminology for reporting results of cervical cytology. JAMA. 2002; 287(16):2114–9. Review.

12. Solomon D, Nayar R, editors. The Bethesda system for reporting cervical cytology definitions, criteria, and explanatory notes. 2nd ed. New York: Springer; 2004.
13. Solomon D, Schiffman M, Tarone R, for the ALTS Group. Comparison of three management strategies for patients with atypical squamous cells of undetermined significance: baseline results from a randomized trial. J Natl Cancer Inst. 2001;93:293–9.
14. Cervical Cytology Practice Guidelines TOC. Available at http://www.cytopathology.org/cervical-cytology-practice-guidelines-toc/. Accessed 10 Sept 2014.
15. McGoogan E, Colgan TJ, Ramzy I, et al. Cell preparation methods and criteria for sample adequacy: IAC Task Force Summary. Acta Cytol. 1998;42:25–32.
16. Vooijs GP, Elias A, Van der Graaf Y, Poelen-van de Berg M. The influence of sample takers on the cellular composition of cervical smears. Acta Cytol. 1986;35:251–7.
17. Thompson D. Adequate "pap" smears: a guide for sampling techniques in screening for abnormalities of the uterine cervix. Toronto: Laboratory Proficiency Testing Program of Canada; 1989.
18. Rubio CA. The false negative smear. Obstet Gynecol. 1997;49:576–80.
19. Boon ME, Guilloud JC, Rietverd WJ. Analysis of five sampling methods for the preparation of cervical smears. Acta Cytol. 1989;33:843–8.
20. Saitas VL, Hawthorne C, Cater J, Bibbo M. Single slide versus double slide: a comparative study. Diagn Cytopathol. 1995;12:317–20.
21. Quakenbush SR. Single slide Pap smear: an acceptable alternative to the double-slide Pap smear. Diagn Cytopathol. 1999;20:317–20.
22. Thomas Cox J. Primary and secondary prevention: HPV vaccination and cervical cancer screening. In: Mayeaux EJ, Thomas Cox J, editors. Modern colposcopy textbook and atlas. 3rd ed. Philadelphia: Wolters Kluwer; 2012. p. 539–69.
23. Collaço LM, Zardo L. Cytologic screening programs. In: Bibbo M, Wilbur D, editors. Comprehensive cytopathology. 3rd ed. Philadelphia: Saunders; 2008. p. 47–57.
24. Ronco G, Cuzick J, Pierotti P, Cariaggi MP, Dalla Palma P, Naldoni C, Ghiringhello B, Giorgi-Rossi P, Minucci D, Parisio F, Pojer A, Schiboni ML, Sintoni C, Zorzi M, Segnan N, Confortini M. Accuracy of liquid based versus conventional cytology: overall results of new technologies for cervical cancer screening: randomised controlled trial. BMJ. 2007;335(7609):28.
25. Arbyn M, Bergeron C, Klinkhamer P, Martin-Hirsch P, Siebers AG, Bulten J. Liquid compared with conventional cervical cytology: a systematic review and meta-analysis. Obstet Gynecol. 2008;111(1):167–77. Review.
26. Siebers AG, Klinkhamer PJ, Grefte JM, Massuger LF, Vedder JE, Beijers-Broos A, Bulten J, Arbyn M. Comparison of liquid-based cytology with conventional cytology for detection of cervical cancer precursors: a randomized controlled trial. JAMA. 2009;302(16):1757–64.
27. Siebers AG, Klinkhamer PJ, Arbyn M, Raifu AO, Massuger LF, Bulten J. Cytologic detection of cervical abnormalities using liquid-based compared with conventional cytology: a randomized controlled trial. Obstet Gynecol. 2008;112(6):1327–34.
28. Marino JF, Fremont-Smith M. Direct-to-vial experience with AutoCyte PREP in a small New England regional cytology practice. J Reprod Med. 2001;46(4):353–8.
29. Lee KR, Ashfaq R, Birdsong GG, Corkill ME, McIntosh KM, Inhorn SL. Comparison of conventional Papanicolaou smears and a fluid-based, thin-layer system for cervical cancer screening. Obstet Gynecol. 1997;90(2):278–84.
30. Obwegeser JH, Brack S. Does liquid-based technology really improve detection of cervical neoplasia? A prospective, randomized trial comparing the ThinPrep Pap Test with the conventional Pap Test, including follow-up of HSIL cases. Acta Cytol. 2001;45(5):709–14.
31. Bai H, Sung CJ, Steinhoff MM. ThinPrep Pap Test promotes detection of glandular lesions of the endocervix. Diagn Cytopathol. 2000;23(1):19–22.
32. Hecht JL, Sheets EE, Lee KR. Atypical glandular cells of undetermined significance in conventional cervical/vaginal smears and thin-layer preparations. Cancer. 2002;96(1):1–4.
33. Cheung AN, Szeto EF, Leung BS, Khoo US, Ng AW. Liquid-based cytology and conventional cervical smears: a comparison study in an Asian screening population. Cancer. 2003;99(6):331–5.
34. Longatto Filho A, Pereira SM, Di Loreto C, et al. DCS liquid-based system is more effective than conventional smears to diagnosis of cervical lesions: study in high-risk population with biopsy based confirmation. Gynecol Oncol. 2005;97(2):497–500.

35. Dahl MB, Ejersbo D, Holund B. Cause and follow-up of inadequate cervical smears in the county of Funen. Ugeskr Laeger. 2002;164(37):4280–3.
36. Sherman ME. Chapter 11: future directions in cervical pathology. J Natl Cancer Inst Monogr. 2003;31:72–9. Review.
37. Committee on Practice Bulletins—Gynecology. ACOG practice bulletin number 131: screening for cervical cancer. Obstet Gynecol. 2012;120(5):1222–38.
38. Massad LS, Einstein MH, Huh WK, Katki HA, Kinney WK, Schiffman M, Solomon D, Wentzensen N, Lawson HW, 2012 ASCCP Consensus Guidelines Conference. 2012 updated consensus guidelines for the management of abnormal cervical cancer screening tests and cancer precursors. Obstet Gynecol. 2013;121(4):829–46.
39. Fahey MT, Irwig L, Macaskill P. Meta-analysis of Pap test accuracy. Am J Epidemiol. 1995;141:680–9.
40. Mitchell MF, Schottenfeld D, Tortolera-Luna G, Cantor SB, Richards-Kortum R. Colposcopy for the diagnosis of squamous intraepithelial lesions: a meta-analysis. Obstet Gynecol. 1998;91:626–31.
41. Nanda K, McCrory DC, Myers ER, Bastian LA, Hasselblad V, Hickey JD, et al. Accuracy of the Papanicolaou test in screening for and follow-up of cervical cytologic abnormalities: a systematic review. Ann Intern Med. 2000;132:810–9.
42. University of Zimbabwe/JHPIEGO Cervical Cancer Project. Visual inspection with acetic acid for cervical cancer screening: test qualities in a primary-care setting. Lancet. 1999;353: 869–73.
43. Denny L, Kuhn L, Pollack A, Wainwright H, Wright T. Evaluation of alternative methods of cervical cancer screening in resource poor settings. Cancer. 2000;89:826–33.
44. Wright Jr TC, Denny L, Kuhn L, Pollack A, Lorinez A. HPV DNA testing of self-collected vaginal samples compared with cytologic screening to detect cervical cancer. JAMA. 2000;283:81–6.
45. Denny L, Kuhn L, Pollack A, Wright Jr TC. Direct visual inspection for cervical cancer screening: an analysis of factors influencing test performance. Cancer. 2002;94:1699–707.
46. Cronjé HS, Parham GP, Cooreman BF, de Beer A, Divall P, Bam RH. A comparison of four screening methods for cervical neoplasia in a developing country. Am J Obstet Gynecol. 2003;188:395–400.
47. Sankaranarayanan R, Thara S, Anjali S, Roy C, Shastri SS, Mahe C, et al. Accuracy of conventional cytology: results from a multicentre screening study in India. J Med Screen. 2004;11: 77–84.
48. Sankaranarayanan R, Gaffikin L, Jacob M, Sellors J, Robles S. A critical assessment of screening methods for cervical neoplasia. Int J Gynaecol Obstet. 2005;89 Suppl 2:S4–12. Review.
49. Sankaranarayanan R, Budukh AM, Rajkumar R. Effective screening programmes for cervical cancer in low- and middle-income developing countries. Bull World Health Organ. 2001;79(10):954–62.
50. Shastri SS, Dinshaw K, Amin G, Goswami S, Patil S, Chinoy R, Kane S, Kelkar R, Muwonge R, Mahé C, Ajit D, Sankaranarayanan R. Concurrent evaluation of visual, cytological and HPV testing as screening methods for the early detection of cervical neoplasia in Mumbai, India. Bull World Health Organ. 2005;83(3):186–94.
51. Wright TC, Schiffman M, Solomon D, Cox JT, Garcia F, Goldie S, et al. Interim guidance for the use of human papillomavirus DNA testing as an adjunct to cervical cytology for screening. Obstet Gynecol. 2004;103:304–9.
52. Jayant K, et al. Improved stage at diagnosis of cervical cancer with increased cancer awareness in a rural Indian population. Int J Cancer. 1995;63:161–3.
53. Jayant K, et al. Survival from cancer in Barshi registry, rural India. In: Sankaranarayanan R, Black RJ, Parkin DM, editors. Cancer survival in developing countries, IARC scientific publications no. 145. Lyon: International Agency for Research on Cancer; 1988. p. 69–77.
54. Guidelines for cervical cancer screening programme. Available at http://screening.iarc.fr/doc/WHO_India_CCSP_guidelines_2005.pdf. Accessed 12 Sept 2014.

5 Management Recommendations in Abnormal Cytology

Amita Suneja and Upasna Pandit

Organized screening with Papanicolaou smear has reduced the prevalence of invasive cervix cancer in developed world, and in the recent screening guidelines, HPV as a co-test after 30 years of age has been added to Pap smear. The goal of screening is to find persistent HPV infection, detect and treat high-grade CIN, i.e. CIN 2 and 3 (with no margin of error), and not to miss invasive cancer.

In this chapter, cytology requiring further evaluation will be discussed in three categories:

1. Epithelial cell abnormalities as per revised Bethesda system
2. Unsatisfactory Pap smear as defined by Bethesda system
3. Negative cytology with positive HPV

5.1 Epithelial Cell Abnormalities as per Revised Bethesda System

Epithelial cell abnormalities are listed in Table 5.1 [1]. American Society for Colposcopy and Cervical Pathology (ASCCP) has laid down comprehensive, evidence-based consensus guidelines to aid clinicians in managing women with abnormal cervical cytology, cervical intraepithelial neoplasia (CIN) and adenocarcinoma in situ (AIS) and can be downloaded from www.asccp.org [2]. These are based on risk analysis. The risk of having CIN 3 based on cytology alone and cytology plus HPV test is given in Tables 5.2 and 5.3 [3–5].

A. Suneja (✉)
Department of Obstetrics and Gynecology, University College of Medical Sciences and Guru Teg Bahadur Hospital , Delhi, India
e-mail: amita_suneja@yahoo.co.in

U. Pandit
Subharti Medical College, Meerut, India

S. Mehta, P. Sachdeva (eds.), *Colposcopy of Female Genital Tract*,
DOI 10.1007/978-981-10-1705-6_5

Table 5.1 Epithelial cell abnormality as per Bethesda system

Epithelial cell abnormalities
Squamous cell
Atypical squamous cells (ASC)
Of undetermined significance (ASC-US)
Cannot exclude HSIL (ASC-H)
Low-grade squamous intraepithelial lesion (LSIL)
Encompassing: human papillomavirus/mild dysplasia/cervical
Intraepithelial neoplasia (CIN) 1
High-grade squamous intraepithelial lesion (HSIL)
Encompassing: moderate and severe dysplasia, carcinoma in situ
CIN 2 and CIN 3
Squamous cell carcinoma
Glandular cell
Atypical glandular cells (AGC) (specify endocervical, endometrial or not otherwise specified)
Atypical glandular cells, favour neoplastic (specify endocervical or not otherwise specified)
Endocervical adenocarcinoma in situ (AIS)

Table 5.2 Risk of CIN 3 based on cytology alone

Pap –ve (%)	ASC-US (%)	LSIL (%)	ASC-H (%)	AGC (%)	HSIL (%)
0.2	2.6	5.3	18	8.7	48

Table 5.3 Risk of CIN 3 based on cytology and HPV co-test

	Pap –ve	ASC-US	LSIL	ASC-H	AGC	HSIL
HPV –ve	0.08	0.45	2.1	3.8	1.1	29
HPV +ve	3.5	6.8	6.2	25	34	50

5.1.1 Atypical Squamous Cells of Undetermined Significance (ASC-US) [2, 6–8]

Management of Women Aged 25 Years or Older

Guidelines for workup of ASC-US are based on the following observations:

ASC-US is the most common cytologic abnormality. It carries the lowest risk of CIN 3+, partly because one third to two thirds are not HPV associated. In fact, the risk of CIN 3+ was 2 %, low enough to justify annual rather than semi-annual cytology to identify women with CIN 3+. Triage using HPV genotyping was considered. Women with ASC-US who also had HPV-16 or HPV-18 detected had approximately twice the risk of CIN 3+ as women with ASC-US and high-risk HPV types other than 16 or 18.

Management

Option 1

For women with ASC-US cytology, HPV testing is preferred. For women with HPV-negative ASC-US whether from reflex HPV testing or co-testing, repeat co-testing at 3 years is recommended. For women with HPV-positive ASC-US, colposcopy is recommended. Triaging ASC-US cytology with HPV reduces the referrals for colposcopy by 50 %.

When colposcopy does not identify CIN in women with HPV-positive ASC-US, co-testing at 12 months is recommended. It is recommended that HPV testing in follow-up after colposcopy not be performed at intervals of less than 12 months. If the co-test is HPV negative and cytology negative, return for age-appropriate testing in 3 years is recommended. If all tests are negative at that time, routine screening is recommended.

Option 2

For women with ASC-US cytology and no HPV result, repeat cytology at 1 year is acceptable. If the result is ASC-US or worse, colposcopy is recommended; if the result is negative, return to cytology testing at 3-year intervals is recommended.

In our centre, we opt for HPV test if the patient can afford, because this is not available in our hospital setting. Repeat Pap smear at 1 year is offered if patient is reliable for follow-up. Though guidelines don't suggest colposcopy as the first option for the work up of ASC-US cytology, we offer colposcopy as first choice to patients who cannot afford HPV testing and are noncompliant. Depending on the availability of facility at one's centre, one can individualize the management.

5.1.1.1 ASC-US in Special Populations

Women Aged 21–24 Years

For women aged 21–24 years with ASC-US, cytology alone at 12-month intervals is preferred, but reflex HPV testing is acceptable. If reflex HPV testing is performed with ASC-US and the HPV result is positive, repeat cytology in 12 months is recommended.

Immediate colposcopy or repeat HPV testing is not recommended. If reflex HPV testing is performed and is negative, return for routine screening with cytology alone in 3 years is recommended.

Follow-Up

For women with ASC-H or HSIL+ (HSIL, atypical glandular cells [AGC] or cancer) at the 12-month follow-up, colposcopy is recommended. For women with ASC-US or worse at the 24-month follow-up, colposcopy is recommended. For women with two consecutive negative results, return to routine screening is recommended.

Women Aged 65 Years and Older
Postmenopausal women with ASC-US should be managed in the same manner as women in the general population, except when considering exit from screening for women aged 65 years and older. HPV-negative ASC-US is considered abnormal for these women as they have a higher risk for cervical cancer during follow-up than women with negative co-testing, suggesting that they need continued screening. Additional surveillance is recommended with repeat screening in 1 year; co-testing is preferred, but cytology is acceptable.

Pregnant Women
Management options for pregnant women with ASC-US are identical to those described for nonpregnant women, with the exception that deferring colposcopy until 6 weeks postpartum is acceptable. Endocervical curettage in pregnant women is unacceptable. For pregnant women who have no cytologic, histologic or colposcopically suspected CIN 2+ at the initial colposcopy, postpartum follow-up is recommended.

5.1.2 Low-Grade Squamous Intraepithelial Lesion [2, 9, 10]

Low-grade squamous intraepithelial lesions are highly associated with HPV infection, with HPV positivity of 77 %. High rate of HPV positivity in LSIL does not favour reflex HPV testing to select women for colposcopy. The ASC-US-LSIL Triage Study showed that the natural history of LSIL approximates that of HPV-positive ASC-US. Women with LSIL at ages 21–24 years carry a lower risk of CIN 3+ than older women.

Management of Women with LSIL
For women with LSIL cytology and either no HPV test or a positive HPV test, colposcopy is recommended. If co-testing shows HPV-negative LSIL, repeat co-testing at 1 year is preferred, but colposcopy is acceptable. If repeat co-testing at 1 year is elected and if the cytology is ASC-US or worse or the HPV test is positive (i.e. if the co-testing result is other than HPV negative, cytology negative), colposcopy is recommended. If the co-testing result at 1 year is HPV negative and cytology negative, repeat co-testing after 3 years is recommended. If all tests are negative at that time, routine screening is recommended.

5.1.2.1 LSIL in Special Populations

Women Aged 21–24 Years
For women with LSIL who are aged 21–24 years, follow-up with cytology at 12-month intervals is recommended. Colposcopy is not recommended. For women with ASC-H or HSIL+ at the 12-month follow-up, colposcopy is recommended. For women with ASC-US or worse at the 24-month follow-up, colposcopy is

recommended. For women with two consecutive negative results, return to routine screening is recommended.

Pregnant Women
For pregnant women with LSIL, colposcopy is preferred. Endocervical curettage in pregnant women is unacceptable. For pregnant women aged 21–24 years, follow-up according to the guidelines for management of LSIL in women aged 21–24 years is recommended. Deferring colposcopy until 6 weeks postpartum is acceptable. For pregnant women who have no cytologic, histologic or colposcopically suspected CIN 2+ at the initial colposcopy, postpartum follow-up is recommended. Additional colposcopic and cytologic examinations during pregnancy are unacceptable for these women.

Postmenopausal Women
Acceptable options for the management of postmenopausal women with LSIL and no HPV test include obtaining HPV testing, repeat cytologic testing at 6 and 12 months and colposcopy. If the HPV test is negative or if CIN is not identified at colposcopy, repeat cytology in 12 months is recommended. If either the HPV test is positive or repeat cytology is ASC-US or greater, colposcopy is recommended. If two consecutive repeat cytology tests are negative, return to routine screening is recommended.

Many times cytologic abnormality of LSIL in menopausal women is due to vaginal mucosal atrophy; in that case, it is prudent to treat with local oestrogen cream for 3 weeks or oral conjugated oestrogens and then repeat the cytology.

5.1.3 Atypical Squamous Cells, Cannot Exclude High-Grade Squamous Intraepithelial Lesion (ASC-H) [2, 11]

ASC-H have a higher risk for CIN 3+ than ASC-US or LSIL although risk is lower than HSIL (Table 5.2). The risk of is also true for women aged 21–24 years, although their risk of CIN 3+ is lower than that for older women with ASC-H. There is high rate of HPV detection in women with ASC-H making reflex HPV testing unsuitable. Also, the 5-year cancer risk among women with HPV-negative ASC-H is 2 %, which is too high to justify observation.

For women with ASC-H cytology, colposcopy is recommended regardless of HPV result. Reflex HPV testing is not recommended.

5.1.3.1 ASC-H in Special Populations

Women Aged 21–24 Years
Colposcopy is recommended. Further management should follow guidelines for women aged 21–24 years with HSIL.

5.1.4 High-Grade Squamous Intraepithelial Lesion

For women with HSIL cytology, immediate colposcopy with endocervical assessment is recommended. Triage using either a programme of repeat cytology alone or HPV testing is unacceptable. If colposcopy is adequate, transformation zone is 1 or 2, or the lesion is seen in its entirety, one can treat the lesion with large loop electrosurgical excision (LEEP). This will provide the diagnosis and treatment as well. This is the only condition where "see and treat" policy can be given. If immediate treatment is not acceptable, colposcopically directed biopsy should be taken from most abnormal area and women with CIN 2, and CIN 3 should be managed according to the appropriate guidelines. If no lesion is identified on colposcopy or it is type 3 transformation zone, a diagnostic excisional procedure is recommended.

Ablation is unacceptable when colposcopy has not been performed, when CIN 2,3 is not identified histologically and when the endocervical assessment identifies CIN 2 or CIN 3.

5.1.4.1 HSIL in Special Populations

Women Aged 21–24 Years

Colposcopy is recommended. If CIN 2,3 is identified histologically, management is done accordingly. When CIN 2 or more is not identified histologically, observation for up to 24 months using both colposcopy and cytology at 6-month intervals is recommended, provided the colposcopic examination is adequate and endocervical assessment is negative or CIN 1.

If during follow-up a high-grade colposcopic lesion is identified or HSIL cytology persists for 1 year, biopsy is recommended. If HSIL persists for 24 months without identification of CIN 2+, a diagnostic excisional procedure is recommended. A diagnostic excisional procedure is recommended for this age group with HSIL when colposcopy is unsatisfactory or CIN 2, CIN 3, CIN 2,3 or ungraded CIN is identified on endocervical sampling. After two consecutive negative cytology results and no evidence of high-grade colposcopic abnormality, return to routine screening is recommended.

Pregnant Women with HSIL

Immediate colposcopy is recommended with biopsy of lesions suspicious for CIN 2,3 or cancer. Colposcopy should be repeated no earlier than 6 weeks postpartum if no CIN 2,3 is found. For pregnant women with CIN 2,3, repeat cytology and colposcopy may be performed every 12 weeks with repeat biopsy if the lesion worsens or cytology suggests invasion.

5.1.5 Atypical Glandular Cells, Cytologic Adenocarcinoma In Situ and Benign Glandular Changes [2, 12, 13]

AGC are uncommon. AGC are found with polyps, metaplasia and also neoplasias, including adenocarcinomas of the endometrium, cervix, ovary and fallopian tube. The risk of neoplasia is higher when AGC favour neoplasia or frank AIS are reported. In women younger than 35 years of age with AGC, the risk of CIN 2+ is higher than carcinoma, so a thorough assessment of AGC is warranted at all ages. AGC are most commonly associated with squamous lesions, as glandular and squamous lesions often coexist.

Benign-appearing endometrial cells and stromal cells or histiocytes are rarely associated with premalignant lesions or cancer in young women. However, in postmenopausal women, these changes can be associated with an approximately 5 % risk of clinically important pathology including endometrial adenocarcinoma.

Management of Women with AGC or Cytologic AIS

For initial workup of women with all subcategories of AGC and AIS except atypical endometrial cells, colposcopy with endocervical sampling is recommended regardless of HPV result. Accordingly, triage by reflex HPV testing is not recommended, and triage using repeat cervical cytology is unacceptable. Endometrial sampling is recommended in conjunction with colposcopy and endocervical sampling in women 35 years of age and older with all subcategories of AGC and AIS. Endometrial sampling is also recommended for women younger than 35 years with clinical indications suggesting they may be at risk for endometrial neoplasia. These include unexplained vaginal bleeding or conditions suggesting chronic anovulation. For women with atypical endometrial cells, initial evaluation limited to endometrial and endocervical sampling is preferred, with colposcopy acceptable either at the initial evaluation or deferred until the results of endometrial and endocervical sampling are known; if colposcopy is deferred and no endometrial pathology is identified, colposcopy is then recommended.

Subsequent Management

For women with AGC not otherwise specified cytology in whom CIN 2+ is not identified, co-testing at 12 and 24 months is recommended. If both co-tests are negative, return for repeat co-testing in 3 years is recommended. If any test is abnormal, colposcopy is recommended.

If CIN 2+ but no glandular neoplasia is identified histologically during the initial workup of a woman with atypical endocervical, endometrial or glandular cells not otherwise specified, management should be according to the 2012 consensus guidelines for the lesion found.

For women with AGC "favour neoplasia" or endocervical AIS cytology, if invasive disease is not identified during the initial colposcopic workup, a diagnostic excisional procedure is recommended. It is recommended that the type of diagnostic excisional procedure used in this setting provides an intact specimen with interpretable margins. Endocervical sampling after excision is preferred.

5.1.5.1 AGC or Cytologic AIS in Special Populations

Pregnant Women

The initial evaluation of AGC in pregnant women should be identical to that of nonpregnant women except that endocervical curettage and endometrial biopsy are unacceptable.

Women Aged 21–24 Years

It is recommended that ASCCP guidelines for management of AGC be followed for all women, including those aged 21–24 years.

Management of Benign Glandular Changes

For asymptomatic premenopausal women with benign endometrial cells, endometrial stromal cells or histiocytes, no further evaluation is recommended. For postmenopausal women with benign endometrial cells, endometrial assessment is recommended. For posthysterectomy patients with a cytologic report of benign glandular cells, no further evaluation is recommended.

5.2 Unsatisfactory Cytology [14–22]

5.2.1 Unsatisfactory Cytology

Unsatisfactory cytology is unreliable for detecting epithelial abnormalities. Studies have found a higher risk of disease in women with unsatisfactory cytology. Cytology is usually rendered unsatisfactory by obscuring blood, inflammation or other processes. Instead of conventional Pap smear, liquid-based media control obscuring factors in processing. Using liquid-based media, unsatisfactory results are because of insufficient squamous cells.

Specimen collection techniques effective to minimize unsatisfactory cytology are extended-tip spatulas, spatulas plus brushes and brooms.

With HPV co-testing although the risk of high-grade disease is low in women with negative HPV test result, some currently available HPV tests lack a control for epithelial cellularity, so a negative HPV test cannot be relied upon as the HPV test may be falsely negative because of an insufficient sample.

Management

For women with an unsatisfactory cytology result and no, unknown or a negative HPV test result, repeat cytology in 2–4 months is recommended. Triage using reflex HPV testing is not recommended. It is prudent to treat atrophy or obscuring inflammation when a specific infection is present.

For women aged 30 years and older who are co-tested and have unsatisfactory cytology and a positive HPV test, repeat cytology in 2–4 months or colposcopy is acceptable.

Colposcopy is recommended for women with two consecutive unsatisfactory cytology tests.

5.2.2 Cytology Reported as Negative But with Absent or Insufficient EC/TZ Component

In cytology reported as negative but with absent or insufficient EC/TZ (endocervical/transformation zone) component, the cellularity is adequate for interpretation, but there is lack of endocervical or metaplastic cells, suggesting that the squamocolumnar junction may not have been adequately sampled. Missing the disease was a concern in the past in such cytology which is not logical. Prior guidelines had recommended early repeat cytology. However, women with absent or insufficient EC/TZ component not only have fewer cytologic abnormalities, they also do not have a higher risk for CIN 3+ over time than women with a satisfactory EC/TZ component. Instead, there are lower rate of cytologic abnormality as these women are usually older and have lower risk of CIN 3+. HPV testing offers an added margin of safety for women aged 30–64 years as it is independent of transformation zone sampling.

Repeat cytology in 3 years is acceptable if HPV testing is not performed.

If the HPV test is done and is negative, return to routine screening is recommended.

If the HPV test is positive, repeating both tests in 1 year is acceptable. Genotyping is also acceptable; if HPV type 16 or type 18 is present, colposcopy is recommended. If HPV type 16 and type 18 are absent, repeat co-testing in 12 months is recommended.

For women aged 21–29 years with negative cytology and absent or insufficient EC/TZ component, routine screening is recommended. HPV testing is unacceptable.

5.3 Negative Cytology with a Positive HPV Test [2–5]

HPV testing is not indicated for younger women but is the preferred screening modality for women aged 30–64 years. Even women with negative cytology and with oncogenic HPV are at higher risk for later CIN 3+ than women with negative HPV tests. This sufficiently justifies early return for retesting. Persistent HPV positivity increases the risk of CIN 3+ further. However, since most HPV infections are cleared, it is also logical to observe to allow clearance. Nevertheless, CIN 3+ does occur during observation, requiring balancing risks arising from intervention for HPV that may yet be cleared against the risks of disease. HPV-16 particularly increases the risk for CIN 3+. HPV-18 is associated with cervical adenocarcinomas, which are less efficiently detected by cytology.

Management of Women Testing HPV Positive But Cytology Negative

For women 30 years of age and older with HPV-positive but cytology-negative co-testing, repeat co-testing at 1 year is acceptable. At 1-year repeat co-test, if the HPV test is positive or cytology is ASC-US or worse, colposcopy is recommended. If the 1-year repeat co-test result is HPV negative and cytology negative, repeat co-testing in 3 years is recommended.

HPV genotyping is also acceptable. If HPV-16 or HPV-18 tests are positive, colposcopy is recommended. If HPV-16 and HPV-18 tests are negative, repeat co-testing in 1 year is recommended.

5.4 Summary of Essential Changes from Prior Management Guidelines

- More strategies incorporate co-testing to reduce follow-up visits. Pap-only strategies are now limited to women younger than 30 years, but co-testing is expanded even to women younger than 30 years in some circumstances. Women aged 21–24 years are managed conservatively.
- For ASC-US cytology, immediate colposcopy is not an option. The serial cytology option for ASC-US incorporates cytology at 12 months, not 6 and 12 months, and then if negative, cytology every 3 years.
- HPV-negative and ASC-US results should be followed with co-testing at 3 years rather than 5 years.
- HPV-negative and ASC-US results are insufficient to allow exit from screening at age 65 years.
- Cytology reported as unsatisfactory requires repeat even if HPV negative.
- Cytology reported as negative but lacking endocervical cells can be managed without early repeat.
- Genotyping triages HPV-positive women with HPV type 16 or type 18 to earlier colposcopy only after negative cytology; colposcopy is indicated for all women with HPV and ASC-US, regardless of genotyping result.

References

1. Solomon D, Davey D, Kurman R, et al. The 2001 Bethesda system: terminology for reporting results of cervical cytology. JAMA. 2002;287(16):2114–9. doi:10.1001/jama.287.16.2114.
2. Guidelines – American Society for colposcopy and cervical pathology. www.asccp.org/guidelines.
3. Katki HA, Kinney WK, Fetterman B, Lorey T, Poitras NE, Cheung L, et al. Cervical cancer risk for women undergoing concurrent testing for human papillomavirus and cervical cytology: a population-based study in routine clinical practice. Lancet Oncol. 2011;12:663Y72.
4. Katki HA, Schiffman M, Castle PE, Fetterman B, Poitras NE, Lorey T, et al. Five-year risks of CIN 3+ and cervical cancer among women who test Pap-negative but are HPV-positive. J Low Genit Tract Dis. 2013;17:S56–63.
5. Katki HA, Schiffman M, Castle PE, Fetterman B, Poitras NE, Lorey T, et al. Five-year risk of cervical cancer and CIN3 for HPV-positive and HPV-negative high-grade Pap results. J Low Genit Tract Dis. 2013;17:S50–5.
6. Stoler MH, Wright TC, Sharma A, Apple R, Gutekunst K, Wright TL. High-risk human papillomavirus testing in women with ASC-US cytology: results from the ATHENA HPV study. Am J Clin Pathol. 2011;135:466–75.
7. Einstein MH, Martens MG, Garcia FA, Ferris DG, Mitchell AL, Day SP, et al. Clinical validation of the Cervista HPV HR and 16/18 genotyping tests for use in women with ASC-US cytology. Gynecol Oncol. 2010;118:116–22.
8. Guido R, Schiffman M, Solomon D, Burke L, for the ASCUS/LSIL Triage Study (ALTS) Group. Post-colposcopy management strategies for women referred with low-grade squamous intraepithelial lesions of human papillomavirus DNA-positive atypical squamous cells of undetermined significance: a two-year prospective trial. Am J Obstet Gynecol. 2003;188:1401–5.

9. Moore G, Fetterman B, Cox JT, Poitras N, Lorey T, Kinney W, et al. Lessons from practice: risk of CIN3 or cancer associated with an LSIL or HPV-positive ASC-US screening result in women aged 21–24. J Low Genit Tract Dis. 2010;14:97–102.
10. Arbyn M, Sasieni P, Meijer CJ, Clavel C, Koliopoulos G, Dillner J. Clinical applications of HPV testing: a summary of meta-analyses. Vaccine. 2006;24 Suppl 3:S78–89.
11. Katki HA, Gage JC, Schiffman M, Castle PE, Fetterman B, Poitras NE, et al. Follow-up testing after colposcopy: five-year risk of CIN 2+ after a colposcopic diagnosis of CIN 1 or less. J Low Genit Tract Dis. 2013;5:S69–77.
12. Zhao C, Florea A, Onisko A, Austin RM. Histologic follow-up results in 662 patients with Pap test findings of atypical glandular cells: results from a large academic women's hospital laboratory employing sensitive screening methods. Gynecol Oncol. 2009;114:383–9.
13. Simsir A, Carter W, Elgert P, Cangiarella J. Reporting endometrial cells in women 70 years and older: assessing the clinical usefulness of Bethesda 2001. Am J Clin Pathol. 2005;123:571–5.
14. Hoda RS, Loukeris K, Abdul-Karim FW. Gynecologic cytology on conventional and liquid-based preparations: a comprehensive review of similarities and differences. Diagn Cytopathol. 2012;41(3):257–78. doi:10.1002/dc.22842.
15. Hock YL, Ramaiah S, Wall ES, Harris AM, Marston L, Marshall J, et al. Outcome of women with inadequate cervical smears followed up for five years. J Clin Pathol. 2003;56:592–5.
16. Ransdell JS, Davey DD, Zaleski S. Clinicopathologic correlation of the unsatisfactory Papanicolaou smear. Cancer. 1997;81:139–43.
17. Siebers AG, Klinkhamer PJJM, Vedder JEM, Arbyn M, Bulten J. Causes and relevance of satisfactory and satisfactory but limited smears of liquid-based compared with conventional cervical cytology. Arch Pathol Lab Med. 2012;136:76–83.
18. Buntinx F, Brouwers M. Relation between sampling device and detection of abnormality in cervical smears: a meta-analysis of randomized and quasi-randomised studies. BMJ. 1996;313:1285–90.
19. Martin-Hirsch P, Jarvis G, Kitchener H, Lilford R. Collection devices for obtaining cervical cytology samples. Cochrane Database Syst Rev 2000;CD001036.
20. Huang A, Quinn M, Tan J. Outcome in women with no endocervical component on cervical cytology after treatment for high-grade cervical dysplasia. Aust N Z J Obstet Gynaecol. 2009;49:426–8.
21. Mitchell HS. Longitudinal analysis of histologic high-grade disease after negative cervical cytology according to endocervical status. Cancer. 2001;93:237–40.
22. Zhao C, Austin RM. Human papillomavirus DNA detection in ThinPrep Pap test vials is independent of cytologic sampling of the transformation zone. Gynecol Oncol. 2007;107:231–5.

HPV Detection and Clinical Implications

6

Sumita Mehta and Sumiti Mehta Dixit

6.1 Background

Human papillomaviruses (HPV) are known as the primary cause of cervical cancer. Most HPV infections resolve spontaneously, but those that persist may lead to the development of precancerous abnormalities and, if left untreated, may progress to cancer. Papillomaviruses are members of large family of viruses known as *Papovaviridae*. HPV is a relatively small virus containing non-enveloped double-stranded (ds) DNA. HPV genome is functionally divided into three regions: early region (E), late region (L), and long control region (LCR) [1] (Fig 6.1).

Early Region (E): It constitutes about 50 % of the viral genome and is one of the protein coding regions for early viral life cycle. E1 and E2 encode proteins for viral DNA replication and regulate the transcription of E6 and E7. E4 helps in the release of virions from infected cell. E5 interacts with various transmission proteins which promote cell growth. *E6 and E7 are viral oncogenes, which induce cell immortalization and transformation of the host cell.*

Late Region: It forms about 40 % of the viral genome and is expressed late in the viral life cycle. This region encodes two structural proteins of the viral icosahedral capsid. L1 is responsible for the formation of major capsid proteins and L2 for minor capsid proteins.

S. Mehta (✉) • S.M. Dixit
Department of Obstetrics and Gynecology,
Babu Jagjivan Ram Memorial Hospital,
Delhi, India
e-mail: sumitadr@gmail.com

S. Mehta, P. Sachdeva (eds.), *Colposcopy of Female Genital Tract*,
DOI 10.1007/978-981-10-1705-6_6

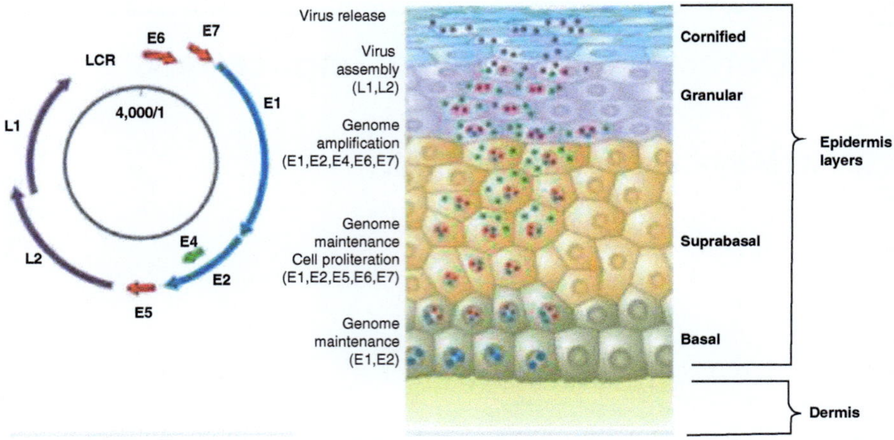

Fig 6.1 HPV genome and life cycle of the virus [2]

Long Control Region (LCR): It's a noncoding regulatory region which constitutes approximately 10% of the HPV genome. It controls DNA replication and transcription by protein coding regions, i.e., early and late regions.

The life cycle of HPV begins with the entry of virus into the basal epithelium of the host. The entry of virus requires mild abrasion or microtrauma. The virus replicates in the basal cell and gradually migrates upward to the surface epithelium. Late viral genes appear at this stage, and virions are released to restart the cycle. The viral genome remains extrachromosomal during replication in normal life cycle, in benign lesions, and in early dysplasia, but for development of precancer and invasive malignancies, viral DNA integrates into the host genome.

Approximately 190 different types of HPV viruses have been known. There are 30 types of HPV which target the genital mucosa; out of which 15 are high-risk or oncogenic types (16, 18, 31, 33, 35, 39, 45, 51, 52, 56, 58, 59, 68, 73, and 82) [3]. HPV types 16 and 18, together, account for more than 70% of cervical precancers and cancer cases, followed by HPV 45, 31, and 33. Non-oncogenic low-risk types especially HPV 6 and HPV 11 account for 90% of benign genital warts. Many HPV strains are structurally and functionally similar. HPV 16 is closely related to HPV 31, 33, 35, 52, and 58, and HPV 18 is related to HPV 45.

Most infections resolve spontaneously but may persist in some women leading to persistence and progression to precancerous lesions and invasive cancer in untreated women over a period of 5–15 years. The prevalence of HPV infection peaks at the age of 18–28 years, after which it declines. Approximately 90% of lesions regress spontaneously within 12–36 months. The prevalence of hrHPV infections in women above 30 years of age is around 10%. Older women with persistence are more likely to be at risk of invasive cancer.

Other factors influencing the progression towards cervical cancer are immunosuppression, long-term use of oral contraceptives, multiple sexual partners, early onset of sexual activity, and smoking.

6.2 Tests for HPV Detection

Detection of HPV in human cells has been strenuous because of two main reasons: the early proteins being expressed in low amounts and lack of specific antibodies against the viral proteins. Since HPV cannot be cultured, diagnostics rely mainly on the detection of viral nucleic acids in cervical smear samples. There has been constant evolution in detecting the presence of HPV in cervical smears. These techniques evolved from scoring of koilocytes to indicate the presence of HPV in the specimen to the most recently advanced signal and target-amplified nuclide acid hybridization tests.

For genome analysis, non-amplified nuclide acid hybridization tests, such as *Southern blot* for DNA molecules and *Northern blot* for RNA molecules, were used, but these tests are time-consuming and require well-preserved and full-sized molecules and hence cannot be done with specimens particularly those derived from fixed tissues containing degraded nucleic acid. Therefore, these tests cannot be used for large population studies.

6.2.1 In Situ Hybridization

It is based on the complementary pairing of a labeled probe to HPV antigens or nucleic acids in cells of cervical smear sample [4]. It demonstrates the localization of viral genome in individual cells by using chromogenic or fluorescence technique. The INFORM HPV [5] assay includes a low-risk (6, 11, 42, 43, and 44) and high-risk HPV types (16, 18, 31, 33, 35, 39, 45, 51, 52, 56, 58, 59, 66) assay. The advantage of ISH is that it can be applied to tissues that have been fixed and processed. However, the clinical sensitivity of this technique is limited due to probe cross-hybridization.

6.2.2 Polymerase Chain Reaction (PCR)

It can detect HPV in samples with few cells containing few viral copies with poor DNA quality. PCR can produce one billion copies from a single dsDNA molecule after 30 cycles of amplification. Also the reaction mix includes internal controls to decrease false-positive and false-negative results. Since integration of the HPV genome into the human chromosomes may result in loss of the L1 region, PCR tests can have false-negative results. Furthermore, as PCR can produce millions of copies of a DNA target from a single molecule, hence the environment is extremely vulnerable to contamination with HPV sequences from aerosolized reaction mixtures [6]. The size of the amplified product remains the same regardless of the HPV type; therefore, electrophoresis cannot detect the actual type of HPV. Studies have shown the sensitivity and specificity for detecting CIN 3 or higher with PCR testing to be 88.2 % (78.9–93.8 %) and 78.8 % (77.9–79.7 %), respectively [7]. Recently Roche Diagnostics developed the AMPLICOR HPV kit test that amplifies a smaller fragment of the L1 gene; this short PCR fragment (SPF)-PCR can discriminate a broad spectrum of HPV types and is considered to be more sensitive and usable for less-preserved specimens.

6.2.3 Hybrid Capture

Digene Corporation (now known as Qiagen Corporation) developed signal amplification technique that detects nucleic acid targets directly [8]. It has developed two tests:

- Hybrid capture tube (HCT) test: It is a US Food and Drug Administration (FDA)-approved semiquantitative measure of viral load relative to 10 pg/ml and uses RNA probes that react with nine high-risk HPV types (16, 18, 31, 33, 35, 45, 51, 52, and 56).
- HPV hybrid capture test (HCII): In 1999, FDA approved the second generation of HCT. It detects viral load up to 1 pg/ml and four additional hrHPV (39, 58, 59, 68). The test is based on hybridization, in a solution of long synthetic RNA probes complementary to the genomic sequence of 13 high-risk (types 16, 18, 31, 33, 35, 39, 45, 51, 52, 56, 58, 59, and 68) and 5 low-risk (6, 11, 42, 43, 44) HPV types. It takes around 6–7 hours for detection of HPV; about 90 patients' samples can be processed simultaneously on one microtiter plate. The test result is expressed as relative light units (RLU). The FDA recommended the cutoff value for test-positive results to be 1.0 RLU (equivalent to 1 pg of HPV DNA per 1 ml of sampling buffer). As HCII is based upon signal amplification, it is less prone to cross specimen contamination as compared to PCR. However, there are false-negative and false-positive results because of the absence of internal control for the amount of input of DNA and inability to identify specific HPV types.

6.2.4 RNA-Based Amplification Techniques

Of late, HPV RNA is considered as an important target for molecular diagnosis of HPV infections. Unlike HPV DNA assays that detect only the presence of viral genomes, testing for viral RNA evaluates the HPV genome expression and viral activity in the infected cells. Detection of HPV E6/E7 mRNA in cervical smear samples can be performed by reverse transcription (RT)-PCR or by nucleic acid sequence-based amplification (NASBA) [9] (PreTect HPV-Proofer; Norchip). It detects E6/E7 transcripts from the five common hrHPV types in cervical carcinoma (16, 18, 31, 33, and 45). In this, single-stranded nucleic acids (viral genomic RNA, mRNA, or rRNA) are amplified in a background of dsDNA.

Gen-Probe has developed the APTIMA HPV [10] Assay, targeting E6/E7 mRNA from 14 carcinogenic HPV genotypes. A prototype of this assay was evaluated in 536 women with histological outcomes. Detection of E6/E7 mRNA was strongly correlated with severity of the lesion; all five carcinomas and 90 % of CIN 3 cases revealed E6/E7 mRNA [10].

A Norwegian hospital-based, cross-sectional study has shown that PreTect HPV-Proofer [11] is positive in 89 % of cervical cancer and in 77 % of high-grade precursor lesions. High-grade histology (CIN 2+) was found in 83 % of women with normal cytology and positive PreTect HPV-Proofer. Though the predictive value of HPV testing was not calculated in this study, the specificity of mRNA testing seems to be better compared to HPV DNA testing.

6.2.5 Newer Tests

Khan et al. [12] reported that 21 % of cytology-negative, HPV 16-positive women developed CIN 3+ over a period of 10 years, while 18 % who were cytology negative and HPV 18 positive developed CIN 3+ during this period; for all other high-risk HPV types combined, only 1.5 % developed CIN 3+, reinstating the importance of HPV genotyping. The FDA has approved two tests for HPV genotyping: Cervista HPV 16/HPV 18 (Hologic, Bedford, MA) and cobas HPV Test (Roche Diagnostics).

Cervista HPV 16/HPV 18 [13] is a qualitative, in vitro diagnostic test for the detection of DNA from high-risk HPV types: 16 and 18. The CervistaTM HPV 16/HPV 18 test uses signal amplification method for detection of specific nucleic acid sequences. It uses two types of isothermal reactions: a primary reaction that occurs on the targeted DNA sequence and a secondary reaction that produces a fluorescent signal. A final positive, negative, or indeterminate result for any particular sample is generated based on the analysis of two separate reaction wells.

The cobas® HPV Test [14] is based on automated specimen preparation to simultaneously extract HPV and cellular DNA followed by PCR amplification of target DNA sequences using both HPV and beta-globin-specific complementary primer pairs. The amplified signal from 12 high-risk HPV types (31, 33, 35, 39, 45, 51, 52, 56, 58, 59, 66, and 68) is detected using a common fluorescent dye, while HPV 16, HPV 18, and beta-globin signals are each detected with their own dedicated fluorescent dye. The results are determined as "positive," "negative," or "invalid" in each channel based on predefined parameters and Ct ranges. The ultimate result is determined as a combination of results from all four detection channels according to a predefined table.

careHPV test [15]*:* This is a new test which has been developed by Qiagen to detect high-risk HPV DNA. It is a screening test that is accurate and affordable. It can detect DNA from 14 high-risk types of HPV with the test results being available in about 2.5 hours. The test is based on the same principle of signal amplification as hybrid capture 2 and is only slightly less sensitive than it. As the test requires no electricity, no running water, and only 2.5 h to conduct, it is cheap and is a promising option in the low-resource settings.

6.3 Sample Collection

Studies have shown that HPV testing of self-collected vaginal swabs is less sensitive but as specific as HPV DNA for detecting high-grade cervical disease [16], with provider-collected cervical sample resulting in highest HPV DNA sensitivity of

84–100 % and sensitivity of 66–88 %. A cross-sectional mixed method study was conducted within the context of a cervical cancer screening demonstration project, the Screening Technologies to Advance Rapid Testing-Utility and Program Planning (START-UP) [17] project in India, Nicaragua, and Uganda, with the objective to generate evidence comparing screening options implemented by public health systems in regionally representative developing country settings. The studies show that self-sampling was highly acceptable and that a majority of women preferred self-sampling because it was more comfortable and less painful.

6.4 Clinical Application of HPV Testing

Initially in 1999, FDA approved HCII to be used as an adjunctive test for the triage of patients with equivocal cytology results (ASCUS) so as to determine the need for referral to colposcopy and later in 2003 approved it as primary screening together with cytology in women aged 30 years and older. Presently there are three clear indications for HPV testing:

1. Primary screening modality
   (a) Co-testing with cytology
   (b) hrHPV DNA testing alone
2. Triage of minor cytological abnormalities
3. Follow-up after treatment of CIN

6.4.1 Primary Screening Modality

Strategies of HPV testing for primary screening include:

6.4.1.1 Co-testing with Both HPV and Pap Smear

This is the most acceptable screening method at present. If both tests are negative, there is a very strong negative predictive value, and the tests need to be repeated after 5 years. As more data becomes available, this testing interval might be increased to 10 years.

The International Agency on Research on Cancer (IARC) recommends that the age at which screening begins should aim to maximize the detection of cervical precancer cases while avoiding the large number of transient HPV infections. ACOG and ASCCP both reinforce the same and recommend the following (level A evidence):

- Cervical cancer screening should begin at age 21 years.
- Pap cytology screening is recommended every 3 years for women between the ages of 21 years and 29 years.
- For women aged 30–65 years, co-testing with cervical cytology screening and HPV testing is preferred and should be performed every 5 years.

Pap smear has been the gold standard for screening of cervical cancer for half a century. Its greatest advantage lies in its simplicity and ease of sample collection. But the advantage of the HPV test in comparison to the Pap smear lies in greater sensitivity. This difference allows the screening interval to be increased. However, specificity is an important parameter in screening because it involves healthy women and positive results require a follow-up colposcopy which is costly and time-consuming. Specificity takes on more importance in low-resource settings where colposcopy is not available, and women who are screen positive would be treated in a "screen and treat" approach. Cuzick et al. [18] found HPV testing to be on average 25 % more sensitive than cytology (at an ASCUS threshold) but 6 % less specific for the identification of high-grade CIN. Agorastos et al. also found that HCII is 23 % more sensitive and 6 % less specific than cytology [19].

However, testing for high-risk types of HPV DNA has a very high negative predictive value. In a number of cross-sectional studies, the NPV of HPV DNA testing was consistently greater than 97 % using either the HCII or PCR-based assays, with most studies reporting values around 99 % and some even reporting 100 %. Castle and colleagues [20] analyzed a subcohort of 2020 women with negative results on cytologic evaluation but positive results with HC II assay who were followed up for a period of 57 months. It was found that 15 % of these women had an abnormal cervical smear within 5 years. Thus, HPV DNA testing identifies women who require closer surveillance, and over time the specificity of HPV DNA tests increases. The longest follow-up is for the Hammersmith Study, where only 0.42 % of women who were HPV negative developed CIN 2 or worse after 5 years compared to 0.83 % for women with negative cytology results.

6.4.1.2 Primary Screening with HPV Testing Followed by Triage of the Positive HPV Test by the Pap Smear

There is now growing evidence that cervical cancer screening needs to move away from cytology as a first-line screening test. A number of prospective follow-up studies have clearly shown that co-testing offers minimal benefit over HPV alone as the first-line screening test. For example, a review of co-testing results from over 300,000 women enrolled in Kaiser Permanente [21] found a minimal difference in the cumulative incidence of ≥CIN 3 after 5 years of follow-up among women who were co-test negative (incidence of 0.16 %) compared to women who were HPV negative (incidence of 0.17 %). After 6 years of follow-up, the cumulative incidence of >CIN 3 in HPV-negative women was 0.28 % compared to 0.27 % for women who were co-test negative.

A number of clinical trials have clearly documented the potential of using HPV for primary screening. One of the first studies, Canadian study, demonstrated the superior sensitivity of HPV as a primary screening test over cytology [22]. The study enrolled over 10,000 women, and it found that the sensitivity of HPV testing for ≥CIN 2 was 94.6 %, whereas it was only 55.4 % for cytology. Two additional large studies from Scandinavia found similar findings when they compared HPV alone versus cytology.

The NTCC [23] trial from Italy has also proven the safety and effectiveness of using HPV alone as the first-line screening test. This randomized screening trial included nearly 100,000 women with median age of 41 years and compared a cytology only arm with an HPV only arm and followed for up to 6 years with an additional round of screening. In the first round of screening, the relative detection of CIN 3 for HPV alone versus cytology alone was 2.08 in women 35–60 years.

Although there were a similar number of invasive cancers detected in the first round of screening in both arms, in the second round, nine additional women were diagnosed with cervical cancer women in the cytology arm versus none in the HPV arm; this difference presumably was because HPV testing identified more women at risk for developing invasive cancer in the first round of screening than did cytology.

In the ATHENA trial [24] that included more than 47,000 women, results showed that the HPV test used in the study performed better than the Pap test at identifying women at risk of developing cervical cancer precursor lesions. The greater assurance against future cervical cancer risk with HPV testing has also been demonstrated by a cohort study of more than a million women, which found that after 3 years women who tested negative on the HPV test had an extremely low risk of developing cervical cancer.

The ARTISTIC trial (A randomized trial of HPV testing in primary cervical screening) which involved 8873 women and median follow-up for 72 months also concluded that HPV testing as an initial screen was significantly more protective than cytology and the use of primary HPV screening could allow a safe prolongation of the screening interval. Following negative cytology at entry into the study, the cumulative rate of CIN 2+ was significantly higher than women who were HPV negative at baseline (1.41 % vs. 0.87 %) at 6 years. HPV as the sole primary test was also found to be cost-effective in both the vaccinated and non-vaccinated cohort [25].

Therefore, the Society of Gynecologic Oncology (SGO) and ASCCP issued an Interim Guidance Report in 2014 after the US FDA approved the cobas HPV test as a "primary" or first test performed for cervical cancer screening.

The Interim Guidance Report recommends [26]:

- Primary HPV testing can be considered for women starting at age 25.
- Women under age 25 should continue to follow current guidelines that recommend cytology alone beginning at age 21.
- Women with a negative primary HPV test result should not be retested again for 3 years. This is the same screening interval recommended under current guidelines for a normal cytology test result.
- An HPV test positive for HPV 16 and HPV 18 types should be followed with colposcopy.
- A test that is positive for HPV types other than 16 and 18 should be followed by reflex cytology testing.

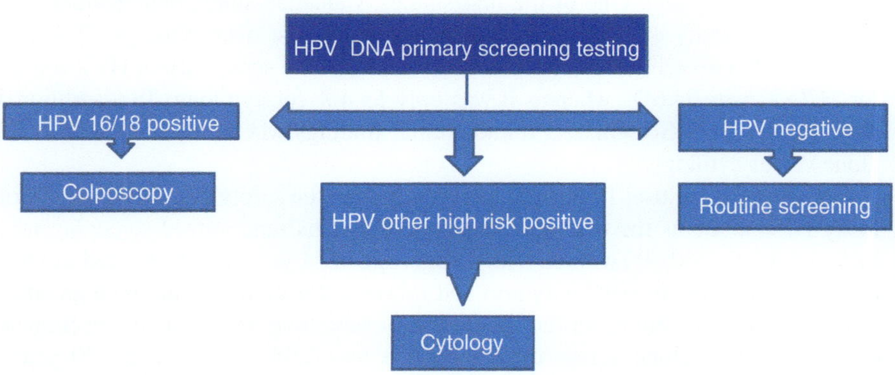

Table 6.1 Comparison of HPV testing, co-test, and cytology alone for primary screening [8]

	Sensitivity (%)	Specificity (%)
HPV	71.7	87.5
Co-testing	72.5	96.5
Cytology	63.8	97.4

Using a highly sensitive test such as HPV test as the primary test helps in picking up the suspicious cases, and applying a more specific cytology test reduces the number of referrals to colposcopy and biopsy. Women found to be HPV positive, but, with a negative or ASCUS cytology result, can be safely managed with repeated testing 12 months later.

Co-testing and LBC had higher positive predictive values for CIN 2+ (97.8 and 98.9 %) than primary HPV screening alone (91 %), whereas primary screening alone and co-testing demonstrated higher negative predictive values (63.6 and 62.5 %) than LBC alone (43.2 %) (Table 6.1).

Also the greater sensitivity of HPV DNA testing allows it to be used as a primary screening test followed by immediate "screen and treat" algorithm based on visual inspection tests in those who are HPV positive.

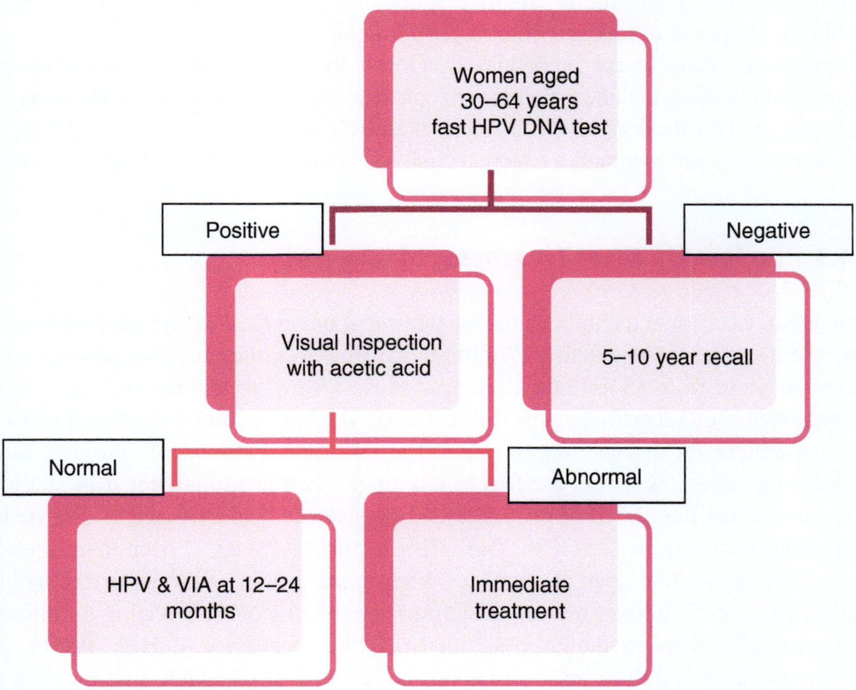

6.4.2 Triage of Minor Cytological Abnormalities

Initially, the US FDA accepted clinical use of HPV DNA testing only for the triage of women found to have ASCUS. Studies have shown that 5–20 % of cases with low-grade cytologic findings (ASCUS or LSIL) may have undetected high-grade lesions. Thus, management of low-grade cytologic has been controversial, and options have included immediate colposcopy or repeated cytologic assessment at 6–12-month intervals. The ASCUS/LSIL Triage Study (ALTS) trial [27] is a large, randomized trial specifically designed to evaluate three methods of managing women with cytologic findings of ASCUS and LSIL. The three methods compared were immediate colposcopy, HPV testing, and referral for colposcopy if the results were positive and repeated cytologic assessment with referral for colposcopy if the smear showed the presence of HSIL. The study concluded that HPV testing was not useful in the management of women with LSIL on cytologic evaluation, and ASCCP recommends that these women should undergo colposcopy instead of HPV testing. With regard to ASCUS on cytologic evaluation, the trial found that HPV triage was at least as sensitive as immediate colposcopy for detecting grade 3 CIN and it also helped to decrease the number of colposcopy referals by 50 %.

The Cochrane Review (2013) also recommends triage with HCII for women with ASCUS as it yields higher accuracy, significantly higher sensitivity; relative sensitivity of 1.27 (95 % CI 1.16 to 1.39; *P* value <0.0001), and similar specificity; relative specificity: 0.99 (95 % CI 0.97 to 1.03; *P* value 0.98) than repeat cytology. When triaging women with LSIL, HCII gives a significantly higher sensitivity but a significantly lower specificity (relative specificity 0.66; 95 % CI 0.58 to 0.75, *P* <0.0001) compared to repeat cytology [28].

Consensus management guidelines developed by ASCCP for the follow-up of women with ASCUS include repeated cytologic assessment or HPV testing. However, if LBC was used for the cervical smear, then reflex HPV testing using the residual fluid is the preferred option, as it makes a second clinic visit unnecessary (Flow Chart 6.1) [29].

6.4.3 Follow-Up After Treatment of CIN

Ablative or excisional techniques for the treatment of cervical cancer precursors are reported to achieve more than 90 % cure rates. However, the precursor lesions will persist or recur in 5–15 %; thus, they need close follow-up and re-treatment once lesions have been identified again. Also, treated women remain at increased risk of cervical cancer for at least next 8 years. Earlier, a combination of cytologic and colposcopic assessment was used to follow up women posttreatment. But studies have shown that likelihood of posttreatment persistence or recurrence of disease is negligible in the absence of HPV DNA; HPV testing has recently been investigated as an alternative for “test of cure” of high-grade lesions following treatment. Paraskevaidis et al. in their review of literature on the role of HPV testing in follow-up period after CIN treatment concluded that the sensitivity of HPV testing in detecting treatment failures was very good and reached 100 % in few studies, but the specificity ranged from 44 to 95 % in various studies. Also in women who were treated successfully, 84.2 % had a negative postoperative HPV DNA test as compared to 17.2 % in treatment failures [29]. Zielinski et al. combined the result of 11 studies and estimated the NPV of hrHPV testing for recurrent/residual disease as 98 % and that of cytology as 93 %. When HPV was combined with cytology, the sensitivity was 96 % and NPV was 99 % [30]. The information gathered so far suggests HPV testing to be significantly more reliable than colposcopy and cytology.

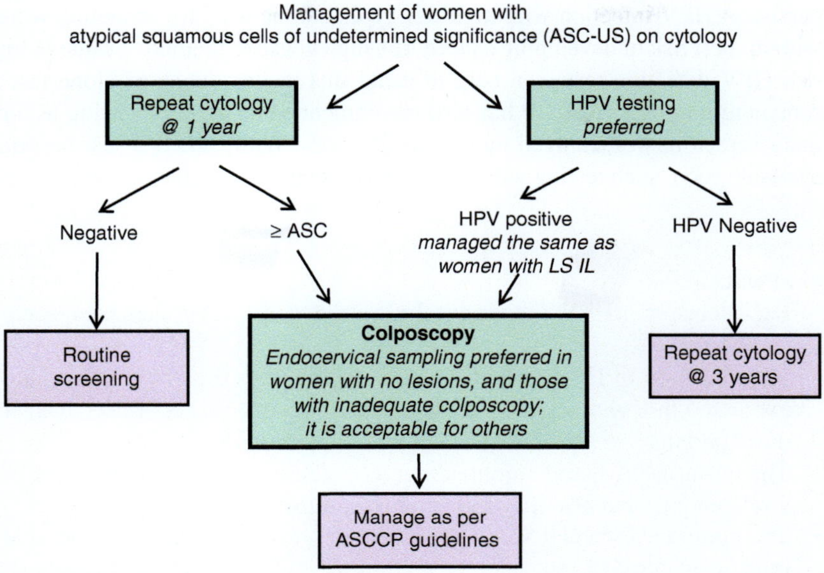

Flow Chart 6.1 ASCCP recommendation (2013) for management of ASCUS

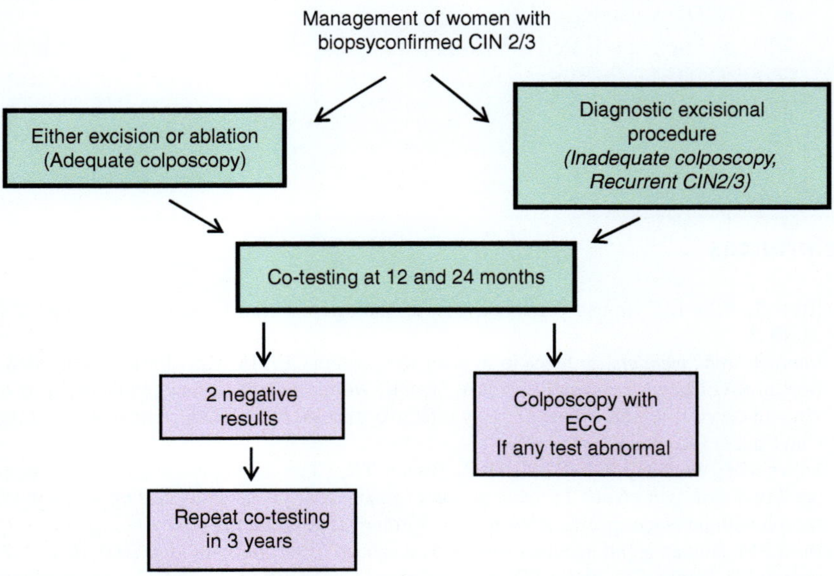

Flow Chart 6.2 ASCCP recommendation (2013) for management of biopsy-proven CIN 2/CIN 3

ASCCP also recommends co-testing at 12 and 24 months following excision or ablative procedure for CIN 2/CIN 3 as described in Flow Chart 6.2 [31].

Conclusion

HPV infection is necessary for development of cervical cancer, and HPV 16 and HPV 18 are responsible for 70 % of cervical precancers and cancers. Detection of persistent HPV infection with high-risk types can be used for screening women with highest risk of developing cancer. The high negative predictive value of high-risk HPV detection tests can help in using this test as the stand-alone test for screening purposes. ASCCP has also recommended using HPV testing as a primary screen in women aged more than 25 years. With careHPV test becoming available soon, such testing will become a commercially viable option.

Key Points

- Persistence of hrHPV infection is the primary cause of cervical precancers and cancer.
- The detection of HPV in human cells is difficult as the viral proteins are expressed in low amounts and there is lack of specific antibodies against these proteins.
- The newer RNA-based amplification tests detect not only the presence of viral genomes but also the viral activity in infected cells.
- The addition of careHPV test for detection of hrHPV DNA will provide impetus to cervical cancer screening in low-resource settings. It is affordable and accurate, and the results are available in 2.5 h.
- Self-sampling for HPV testing is preferred by women, and it is as specific as HPV DNA testing.
- HPV testing is indicated as primary screening modality, for triage of minor cytological abnormalities and for follow-up of women treated for cervical dysplasia.

References

1. Iftner T, Villa LL. Human papillomavirus technologies. J Natl Cancer Inst Monogr. 2003; 31:80–5.
2. Internet: *web2.mendelu.cz;* prace je spojena's projektum CEITEC CZ.1.05/1.1.00/02.0068.
3. Begum S, Gillison ML, Ansari-Lari MA, Shah K, Westra WH. Detection of human papillomavirus in cervical lymph nodes: a highly effective strategy for localizing site of tumor origin. Clin Cancer Res. 2003;9:6469–75.
4. Stoler MH, Wolinsky SM, Whitbeck A, Broker TR, Chow L. Differentiation linked human papillomavirus types 6 and 11 transcription in genital condylomata revealed by in situ hybridization with message specific RNA probes. Virology. 1997;172:331–40.
5. Burd EM. Human papillomavirus and cervical cancer. Clin Microbiol Rev. 2003;16(1):1–17.
6. Gravitt PE, Peyton CL, Alessi TQ, et al. Improved amplification of genital human papillomaviruses. J Clin Microbiol. 2000;38:357–61.
7. Kulasingam SL, Hughes JP, Kiviat NB, et al. Evaluation of human papillomavirus testing in primary screening for cervical abnormalities. JAMA. 2002;14:1749–59.
8. Lorincz A, Anthony J. Advances in HPV detection by hybrid capture [letter]. Papillomavirus Rep. 2001;145:54–8.
9. Molden T, Kraus I, Skomedal H, Nygard JF, Hagmar B. Comparison of human papillomavirus messenger RNA and DNA detection. Cancer Epidemiol Biomarkers Prev. 2005;14(2):367–73.

10. Dockter J, Schroder A, Hill C, et al. Clinical performance of the APTIMA HPV assay for the detection of high-risk HPV and high-grade cervical lesions. J Clin Virol. 2009;45(S1): S55–61.
11. Molden T, Nygard JF, Kraus I, et al. Predicting CIN 2+ when detecting HPV mRNA and DNA by PreTect HPV –proofer and consensus PCR: a 2 year follow up of women with ASCUS or LSIL pap smear. Int J Cancer. 2005;114(6):973–6.
12. Khan MJ, Castle P, Sherman M, et al. The elevated 10-year risk of cervical precancer and cancer in women with human papillomavirus (HPV) type 16 or 18 and the possible utility of type- specific HPV testing in clinical practice. J Natl Cancer Inst. 2005;97(14):1072–9.
13. Boehmer G, et al. A population-based observational study comparing cervista and hybrid capture 2 methods: improved relative specificity of the Cervista assay by increasing its cut-off. BMC Infect Dis. 2014;14:674–80.
14. Internet: http://molecular.roche.com/assays/pages/cobasHPVTest.aspx.
15. Qiao YL, Sellors JW, Eder PS, Bao YP, et al. Anew HPV –DNA test for cervical cancer screening in developing regions: a cross sectional study of clinical accuracy in rural China. Lancet Oncol. 2008;9:929–36.
16. Gravitt PE, Belinson JL, Salmeron J, et al. Looking ahead: a case of human papillomavirus testing of self -sampled vaginal specimens as a cervical cancer screening strategy. Intl Cancer. 2011;129(3):517–27.
17. Jeronimo J, Bansil P, Lim J, et al. A multi –country evaluation of care HPV testing, visual inspection with acetic acid and pap testing for the detection of cervical pre cancer and cancer. Int J Gynecol Cancer. 2014;24(3):576–85.
18. Cuzick J, Clavel C, Petry KU. Overview of the European and North American studies on HPV testing in primary cervical cancer screening. Int J Cancer. 2006;119:1095–101.
19. Agorastos T, Chatzistamatiou K, Katsamagkas T, Koliopoulas G, Daponte A, et al. Primary screening for cervical cancer based on high-risk HPV detection and HPV 16 and HPV 18 genotyping in comparison to cytology. PLoS One. 2015;10(3):e0119755. doi:10.1371/journal.pone.0119755.
20. Castle PE, Lorinez AT, Scott DR, et al. Comparison between prototype hybrid capture 3 and hybrid capture 2 human papillomavirus DNA assays for detection of high –grade cervical intraepithelial neoplasia and cancer. J Clin Microbiol. 2003;41:4022–30.
21. Katki HA, Kinney WK, Fetterman B, Lorey T, Poitras NE, Cheung L, et al. Cervical cancer risk for women undergoing concurrent testing for human papillomavirus and cervical cytology: a population based study in routine clinical practice. Lancet Oncol. 2011;12(7):663–72.
22. Ogilive GS, Krajden M, Niekerk DJ, et al. Primary cervical cancer screening with HPV testing compared with liquid based cytology: result of randomized control trial. Br J Cancer. 2012;107(12):1917–24.
23. Bergeron C, Giorgi-Rossi P, Cas F, Schiboni ML, et al. Informed cytology for triaging HPV-positive women: substudy nested in the NTCC randomized controlled trial. J Natl Cancer Inst. 2015;107(2). pii: dju423.
24. Stoler MH, Wright TC, Sharma A, et al. High risk human papillomavirus testing in women with ASCUS cytology: results from the ATHENA HPV study. Am J Clin Pathol. 2011; 135(3):468–75.
25. Kitchener H, Canfell K, Gilham C, Sargent A, Roberts C, Desai M, Peto J. The clinical effectiveness and cost-effectiveness of primary human papillomavirus cervical screening in England: extended follow-up of the ARTISTIC randomised trial cohort through three screening rounds. Health Technol Assess. 2014;18(23):1–196.
26. Huh WK, Ault KA, Chelmow D, Davey DD, et al. Use of primary high risk human papillomavirus testing for cervical cancer screening: interim clinical guidance. Gynecol Oncol. 2015;125(2):330–7.
27. Schiffman M, Solomon D. Findings to date from the ASCUS-LSIL Triage Study (ALTS). Arch Pathol Lab Med. 2003;127(8):946–9.
28. Arbyn M, Roelens J, Simoens C, Buntinx F, Paraskevaidis E, Martin-Hirsch PP, Prendiville WJ. Human papillomavirus testing versus repeat cytology for triage of minor cytological

cervical lesions. Cochrane Database Syst Rev. 2013;3:CD008054. doi:10.1002/14651858.CD008054.pub2.

29. Paraskevaidis E, Abryn M, Sotiriadis A, Diakomanolis E, et al. The role of HPV DNA testing in the follow-up period after treatment for CIN: a systematic review of the literature. Cancer Treat Rev. 2004;30(2):205–11.
30. Zielinski GD, Bais AG, Helmerhorst TJ, Erheijen RH, et al. HPV testing and monitoring of women after treatment of CIN 3: review of the literature and meta-analysis. Obstet Gynecol. 2004;59:543–53.
31. Massad S, Einstein M, Huh WK, Katki HA, Kinney WK, et al. 2012 updated Consensus guidelines for the management of abnormal cervical screening tests and cancer precursors. J Low Genit Tract Dis. 2013;17:S1–7.

HPV Vaccination

7

Saritha Shamsunder and Deepika Pannu

7.1 Introduction

Human papilloma viruses are small non-enveloped DNA viruses that belong to the *Papovaviridae* family. The viral capsid is composed of two proteins: L1 and L2. Of more than 100 different HPV types identified, 40 of these infect the genital tract [1]. These mucosal HPV types are classified as low-risk and high-risk types based on the prevalence ratio in cervical cancer and its precursors. HPV infections are highly transient and mostly clear within 2 years. The small proportion of HPV infection that persists can cause neoplastic change. Various modes of transmission of HPV are documented, viz. physical contact via autoinoculation or fomites, sexual contact and vertically from the HPV-positive mother to her newborn, causing subclinical or clinical infections.

Oncogenic types of HPV are known to cause 100% of cervical cancer, 90% of anal cancer, 40% of cancers of the vulva, vagina and penis and 12% of head and neck cancers [2]. Approximately, 70% of all cases of cervical cancer are associated with HPV genotypes 16 and 18, and 90% of cases of genital warts are associated with HPV genotypes 6 and 11 [2].

India has the highest incidence of cervical cancer in the world with an age-standardised incidence of 22 per 10,000 females and 67,477 deaths reported in 2013 due to cervical cancer, falling just behind breast cancer [3]. It has been estimated that there will be around 2,05,496 new cases and 1,19,097 deaths due to cervical carcinoma by 2020 in India [4]. Primary prevention by HPV vaccination can prevent most cases of cervical cancer in females, if given before exposure to the virus prior to first sexual debut. In addition, it can prevent vaginal and vulvar cancer in females, and genital warts and anal cancer in both males and females.

S. Shamsunder (✉) • D. Pannu
Department of Obstetrics and Gynecology, Vardhman Mahavir Medical College and Safdarjung Hospital, Delhi, India
e-mail: shamsundersaritha@gmail.com

S. Mehta, P. Sachdeva (eds.), *Colposcopy of Female Genital Tract*,
DOI 10.1007/978-981-10-1705-6_7

7.2 Development

The vaccine development was initiated in parallel, by researchers at Georgetown University Medical Center and the University of Rochester in the USA, the University of Queensland in Australia and the US National Cancer Institute.

The US Food and Drug Administration approved Gardasil (HPV4) manufactured by Merck against four types of HPV, in 2006, and Cervarix (HPV2) manufactured by GlaxoSmithKline against two high-risk types of HPV in 2009 [5], both of which are commercially available in India and approved by the Drug Controller General of India (DCGI).

7.3 HPV Vaccine

Recombinant DNA technology is used to express the L1 major capsid protein of HPV in yeasts, which self-assemble to form empty shells resembling a virus, called virus-like particles (VLPs). The VLPs have the same outer L1 protein coat as HPV but contain no genetic material. The vaccine uses these VLPs as antigens to induce a strong protective immune response [6, 7].

If an exposure occurs, the vaccinated person's IgG antibodies against the L1 protein coat of the virus prevent it from releasing its genetic material.

7.4 Types of Vaccine

Two prophylactic HPV vaccines are being marketed.

Gardasil® the quadrivalent vaccine is manufactured by Merck. It contains VLP antigens for HPV6, 11, 16 and 18, reassembled from L1 proteins of HPV6 (20 μg), 11 (20 μg), 16 (40 μg) and 18 (40 μg), and is designed to protect against infection and disease due to these types. It is produced using yeast substrate, and contains the adjuvant amorphous aluminium hydroxyl phosphate sulphate [6–8].

Cervarix®, the bivalent vaccine, is manufactured by GlaxoSmithKline (GSK). It contains VLP antigens for HPV16 and 18 reassembled from L1 proteins of HPV16 (20 μg) and HPV18 (20 μg) and is designed to protect against infection and disease due to these types. It is produced using a novel recombinant baculovirus expression system and a cell line derived from *Trichoplusia ni* cells. It contains the adjuvant AS04, which includes monophosphoryl lipid A (MPL).

7.5 Immunogenicity

Natural immune response: HPV infections are cleared from the body by the action of two different pathways of immune response.

Firstly, the humoral response leads to the production of neutralising antibodies, which will prevent the virus from entering the epithelial cell. These antibodies, although useful in the prevention of primary infection of basal keratinocytes, are insufficient to prevent new infections [9].

Secondly, the HPV enters the cell through contact with the basal membrane and gets internalised. After internalisation, the epithelial cell sheds the capsid, losing L1 and L2. The cytotoxic T cells then react with infected cells through the recognition of expressed viral proteins for the cellular clearance of HPV [9]. This mechanism is less understood.

Immune response by vaccination: Protection against infection by vaccines is believed to be achieved from neutralising serum immunoglobulin (IgG) antibody, which transudates from capillaries to the genital epithelial mucosa, and binds to viral particles. This serological response is much stronger than the response towards a natural infection, which is likely due to the use of specific adjuvants, the strong immunogenicity of the VLPs themselves as well as the route of administration.

Both vaccines induce serum antibodies for all vaccine-related types in more than 99 % of females after three doses (month 7), and antibody levels for all vaccine-related types are several times higher than those seen after natural infection in all ages [10].

Titres peak after the third dose, gradually decline and level off by 24 months after the first dose; they then remain stable at levels as high as, or higher than, levels seen after natural infection.

The quality of the antibody response is best for HPV16 for both vaccines. The quality of the antibody response to HPV6/11/18 for Gardasil is much poorer than its response to HPV16. Cervarix induces an equally high and sustained antibody response to HPV16/18 [1].

There is some evidence from clinical trials that vaccination might result in some cross protection against other HPV types not included in the vaccine possibly explained by phylogenetic similarities between L1 genes from vaccine and non-vaccine types. It is still not known how long cross protection lasts [1].

HPV16 is most closely related to HPV31 and HPV18 is most closely related to HPV45. The bivalent vaccine gives cross protection against both of them in addition to HPV16 and 18. The quadrivalent vaccine gives 40.3 % cross protection against HPV31 and 45 and 32 % cross protection against HPV31, 33, 45 and 52 [6].

HPV4 vaccine has also demonstrated, together with the protection against cervical cancer, high efficacy against genital warts due to HPV types 6 and 11, vaginal and vulvar precancerous lesions, re-infection, persistent infection and anal precancerous lesions [6].

The bivalent and quadrivalent vaccines available are prophylactic, not therapeutic. Participants who were already positive to any vaccine HPV types before vaccination acquired protection against disease caused by other vaccine types [11].

The immune response may be less robust in the immune-compromised patients like those with HIV-positive or patients with organ transplantation. In a phase I/II study in South Africa, the bivalent HPV vaccine was shown to be immunogenic and well tolerated in HIV-infected women up to 12 months after vaccination [12].

7.6 Efficacy

Both vaccines are highly immunogenic with the highest immune responses being observed in young girls aged 9–15 years. Two phase III studies, FUTURE I and FUTURE II, have evaluated the efficacy of quadrivalent vaccine. The bivalent vaccine also has been evaluated in two phase III studies, PATRICIA and the Costa Rica HPV vaccine trial. Clinical efficacy against infection and cervical lesions associated with HPV16 and HPV18 has been demonstrated up *to 8.4 years* with the bivalent vaccine, and up *to 5 years* with the quadrivalent vaccine [1, 13].

Studies of the quadrivalent HPV vaccine have shown that in participants naive to the vaccine genotypes who followed protocol, the vaccine was almost 100 % effective in preventing high-grade cervical intraepithelial neoplasia CIN 2 and CIN 3 and condylomatous vulvar disease related to the HPV genotypes covered by the vaccine [1, 10]. It was shown to have nearly 100 % protection against genital warts associated with HPV6 and 11, and an efficacy of about 83 % for all genital warts.

For the bivalent vaccine, the efficacy shown by the PATRICIA trial is 95 % for CIN 2 and 100 % for AIS [1, 10]. Results of the studies of this bivalent vaccine indicate that it offers protection similar to the quadrivalent vaccine against HPV infections caused by genotypes 16 and 18 [6–8]. The bivalent vaccine does not protect against lower genital tract condyloma caused by low-risk HPV types 6 and 11 [1].

One study reported that in men who have sex with men, the quadrivalent vaccine was 77.5 % effective in preventing anal intraepithelial neoplasia related to HPV genotypes 6, 11, 16 and 18 [14]. US FDA has approved the quadrivalent vaccine for the prevention of anal cancer and associated precancerous lesions that are caused by these genotypes [15].

The need for booster doses remains to be demonstrated.

7.7 Dosage and Administration

They are available as 0.5-mL suspension for intramuscular injection.

Both of the vaccines are currently marketed as single-dose vials or prefilled syringes which require storage and transport in a cold-chain system [14].

7.8 Method of Administration

The vaccines are for intramuscular use only. Thorough shaking immediately before administration is necessary to maintain suspension of the vaccine. After thorough agitation, this vaccine is a white, cloudy liquid. Vaccine should not be diluted or mixed with other vaccines.

The vaccine should be administered intramuscularly in the deltoid region of the upper arm or in the higher anterolateral area of the thigh.

Observation for 15 min after administration is recommended. Syncope has been reported following vaccination.

7.9 Storage

Both formulations should be stored at 2–8 °C and should not be frozen.

7.10 Schedule

Cervarix: It is given as three intramuscular injections at 0, 1 and 6 months.

Gardasil: It is given as three intramuscular injections at 0, 2 and 6 months.

Minimum interval between first and second dose is 4 weeks. Between second and third dose is 12 weeks. Interval between first and third dose is 24 weeks. If the vaccine schedule is interrupted, the series does not need to be restarted, regardless of the length of time between the doses [15].

At present, there is no data to support the use of boosters.

In March 2014, the Joint Committee on Vaccination and Immunisation (JCVI) of the United Kingdom revised its existing recommendation to change from a three- to a two-dose schedule [16]. Recent research shows that antibody response to two doses in adolescent girls is as good as a three dose course in this age group. Two doses schedule of HPV vaccine has also been recommended by Indian academy of Pediatrics.

Testing for HPV DNA is currently not recommended for adolescents or adults before vaccination. However if the patient is tested and the results are positive, vaccination is still recommended [15].

7.11 Recommended Target Population

Target age: The Advisory Committee on Immunisation Practices has recommended that HPV vaccination should routinely be given to girls when they are 11 or 12 years old. The vaccine can be given to individuals as young as 9 years; catch-up vaccination is recommended in females aged 13 years through 26 years. ACOG also endorses the same [15, 17].

The Indian Academy of Pediatrics Committee on Immunisation (IAPCOI) recommends offering HPV vaccine to all females who can afford the vaccine (Category 2 of IAP categorisation of vaccines) [14].

Women aged 19–26 years are more likely to have been exposed to HPV; the American Cancer Society therefore suggests that the decision to vaccinate women in this age range should be made on an individual basis.

Data available are insufficient to make recommendations for women older than 26 years.

7.12 Specific Issues

Sexually active adolescent: Sexually active adolescents and young women can receive either of the vaccine. However, they need to be counselled that the vaccine may be less effective if they have been exposed to HPV before vaccination [15].

Young women with previous CIN or warts: Vaccination can be given to patients with previous CIN or genital warts. This need to be emphasised to the patients that benefits may be limited and cervical cytology screening should continue afterwards as per protocols [15].

Women older than 26 years: HPV vaccines are currently not licensed for women older than 26 years [15].

Vaccination of pregnant and lactating women: Both the quadrivalent and bivalent HPV vaccines have been classified by the FDA as pregnancy category B. However, HPV vaccination in pregnancy is not recommended. Getting the HPV vaccine when pregnant is not a reason to consider terminating a pregnancy [15].

Lactating women can receive either HPV vaccine because these are inactivated vaccines and do not affect the safety of breastfeeding for mothers or infants.

Vaccination in males: US FDA has approved the quadrivalent vaccine for boys and men aged 9 years through 26 years for the prevention of genital warts. Bivalent vaccine is not recommended for use in males [15].

7.13 Screening After Vaccination

The vaccines do not protect against all HPV types; hence, they will not prevent all cases of cervical cancer. About 30 % of cervical cancers will not be prevented by the vaccines, so it will be important that women continue to get screened for cervical cancer [1, 15].

7.14 Safety

WHO Global Advisory Committee on Vaccine, FIGO Committee on Gynecologic Oncology and the FIGO sub-committee for Cervical Cancer Prevention reviewed all the data available on the safety of vaccine and concluded that both HPV vaccines are generally safe and well tolerated [18]. This conclusion was based on 4 or more years of trial data and 1 year of passive, post-marketing surveillance data on the quadrivalent vaccine in the United States. No safety concerns were reported in a study on bivalent vaccine for up to 9.4 years and with quadrivalent vaccine up to 5 years of follow-up post vaccination. Safety of the vaccines has not been established in pregnant women [6, 19].

7.15 Contraindications

Hypersensitivity, including severe allergic reactions to yeast (a vaccine component), or after a previous dose of vaccine, has been reported [15].

7.16 Adverse Reactions

Headache, fever, nausea, and dizziness and local injection site reactions (pain, swelling, erythema, pruritus and bruising) have occurred after administration of vaccine [15, 17].

Syncope, sometimes associated with tonic-clonic movements and other seizure-like activities, has been reported following vaccination and may result in a fall leading to injury; observation for 15 min after administration is recommended.

Anaphylaxis has also been reported (0.1 %). Reported rates of anaphylaxis following HPV vaccination have been consistent in both national passive surveillance and population-based studies and found to be 1–10 cases per million doses, which compares favourably with other vaccines [18].

Guillain-Barre syndrome (GBS): Population based studies have not provided any evidence that GBS is significantly greater than that expected in the adolescent and young females [18].

Venous thromboembolism (VTE): Studies reported this to be unlikely due to vaccination [18].

7.17 New Developments

7.17.1 Nine-Valent Vaccine

The currently registered vaccines cover only HPV6, HPV11, HPV16 and HPV18. It is estimated that this would protect against 70 % of all squamous cell cancers. To increase the protection, studies are on-going to increase the number of HPV types to nine by adding HPV31/33/45/52 and 58 to the quadrivalent vaccine.

This vaccine, code named V503, is tested in eight trials registered at clinicaltrials.gov. The results of the trials are still unpublished. From mathematical modelling, it was calculated however that this vaccine could raise the protection to 90 % of all SCC cases worldwide [1, 20].

7.17.2 Prophylactic L2 Vaccines

Recently, success has been reported in mice by the use of bacteriophage VLPs and orally administered *Lactobacillus casei* expressing L2 on their surface. The latter induced a significant vaginal mucosal immunity with production of broadly protective IgA, which could be effective in early phases of the viral infection, suggesting that this type of oral immunisation may be a promising strategy for prophylactic vaccination of humans [1].

7.17.3 Therapeutic Vaccines

A lot of trials have been conducted to develop therapeutic vaccines against HPV infection. Most HPV therapeutic vaccines target carcinoma-associated HPV proteins, particularly E6 and E7, to generate the T cell-mediated response. Various forms of HPV vaccines, such as peptide-based vaccines, protein based vaccines, DNA-based vaccines, live vector-based vaccines, chimeric VLP-based vaccines and cell-based vaccines have been tested targeting HPV16 E6 and/or E7 proteins. Recently, phase 1 trial using recombinant E7 protein of HPV16 and 18 concluded it to be safe [1].

7.18 Summary

Two types of prophylactic vaccines have been approved. Both vaccines are based on VLPs of the L1 capsid protein, and are highly immunogenic and efficacious. The vaccine if given before exposure can protect against 70% of the cervical cancers. HPV vaccine should be routinely targeted to females aged 11–12 years. Vaccine is given as three doses of intramuscular injections. Safety data for both of the vaccines is reassuring. Cervical cytology screening should continue as per protocol. Quadrivalent vaccine has also been recently approved for use in males.

Key Points

- Two prophylactic vaccines Cervarix which is bivalent and Gardasil which is quadrivalent are approved.
- Screening should continue as per recommendations after immunisation.
- Recommendations are to give vaccination routinely to girls 11–12 years (can be started as early as 9 years).
- Catch-up vaccination can be given from age 13 through 26 years.
- Nine-valent and prophylactic L2 vaccine are newer developments.
- Clinical efficacy is demonstrated up *to 8.4 years* with the bivalent vaccine, and up *to 5 years* with the quadrivalent vaccine.
- Cross protection is demonstrated with HPV types 31, 33, 45 and 52.

Suggested Reading

1. Docheza C, Bogers JJ, Verhelst R, Rees H. HPV vaccines to prevent cervical cancer and genital warts: an update. Vaccine. 2014;32:1595–601.
2. Parkin DM, Bray F. Chapter 2: the burden of HPV-related cancers. Vaccine. 2006;24:S3/11–25.
3. http://www.hpvcentre.net/dataquery.php.
4. International Agency for Research on Cancer (IARC). Human papillomaviruses. IARC monographs on the evaluation of carcinogenic risks to humans, vol 90, Human Papillomavirus. Lyon: IARC.
5. Kim KS, Park SA, Ko K-N, Yi S, Cho YJ. Current status of human papillomavirus vaccines. Clin Exp Vaccine Res. 2014;3(2):168–75.
6. World Health Organization. Human papillomavirus vaccines. WHO position paper. Wkly Epidemiol Rec. 2009;84(15):118–31.
7. World Health Organization. The immunological basis for immunization series. Module 19: human papillomavirus infection. WHO, Department of Immunization, Vaccines and Biologicals; 2011.

8. Romanowski B. Long-term protection against cervical cancer infection with the human papillomavirus. Hum Vaccin. 2011;7(2):161–9.
9. Stanley M, Pinto LA, Trimble C. Human papillomavirus vaccines -immune responses. Vaccine. 2012;30 Suppl 5:F83–7.
10. Schiller JT, Castellsagué X, Garland SM. A review of clinical trials of human papillomavirus prophylactic vaccines. Vaccine. 2012;30S:F123–38.
11. Kaarthigeyan K. Cervical cancer in India and HPV vaccination. Indian J Med Paediatr Oncol. 2012;33(1):7–12.
12. Denny L, Hendricks B, Gordon C, Hervé C, Thomas F, Hezareh M, et al. Safety and immunogenicity of the HPV16/18 ASO4-adjuvanted vaccine in HIV-positive women in South Africa up to 12 months after vaccination. Int J Gynecol Obstetrics. 2012;119(Supp 3):S323–4.
13. Dillner J, Kjaer SK, Wheeler CM, Sigurdsson K, Iversen OE, Hernandez-Avila M, et al. On behalf of FUTURE I/II Study Group. Four years efficacy of prophylactic human papillomavirus quadrivalent vaccine against low grade cervical, vulvar, and vaginal intraepithelial neoplasia and anogenital warts: randomized controlled trial. BMJ. 2010; 341:3493.
14. Singhal T. Indian Academy of Pediatrics Committee on Immunisation (IAPCOI) – consensus recommendations on immunization 2008. Indian Pediatr. 2008;45:635–48.
15. Committee opinion. The American college of obstetricians and gynecologists. Number 588, Mar 2014.
16. https://www.gov.uk/government/publications/schedule-change-from-3-to-2-doses-in-the-hpv-vaccination-programme.
17. Markowitz LE, Dunne EF, Saraiya M, Lawson HW, Chesson H, Unger ER. Quadrivalent human papillomavirus vaccine: recommendations of the Advisory Committee on Immunization Practices (ACIP).Available from: http://www.cdc.gov/mmwr/preview/mmwrhtml/rr5602a1.htm.
18. Safety of HPV vaccination: a FIGO statement. International Federation of Gynaecology Obstetrics. Int J Gynaecol Obstetrics. 2013;123(3):187–8.
19. Centers for Disease Control and Prevention. Vaccine safety: human papillomavirus (HPV) vaccine. Available at: http://www.cdc.gov/vaccinesafety/vaccines/HPV/index.html.
20. Petrosky E, Bocchini JA Jr, Hariri S, Chesson H, Curtis CR, Saraiya M, et al. Use of 9-valent human papillomavirus (HPV) vaccine: updated HPV vaccination recommendations of the advisory committee on immunization practices. Centers for Disease Control and Prevention (CDC). MMWR Morb Mortal Wkly Rep 2015;64:300–4.

Part III

Colposcopy

Colposcopy: The Scientific Basis

8

Raksha Arora and Sheenam Jain

Colposcopy is the systematic evaluation of the lower genital tract using magnification from a colposcope with a good light source. Introduced in 1925 by Hinselmann, it has become an integral part of modern gynaecologic practice.

8.1 Tissue Basis of Colposcopy

The surface epithelium of the lower genital tract acts as a filtering membrane, through which both the incident and reflected light passes [1]. The epithelium lacks blood vessels and is therefore colourless, while the underlying stroma is red owing to the presence of blood vessels. It is the redness of this subepithelial stroma which is transmitted through the overlying surface epithelium and is visible through the colposcope. The intensity of colour depends on the amount of reflected and absorbed light [2].

During colposcopy, it is important to identify the following to make a colposcopic diagnosis:

- Original squamous epithelium
- Metaplastic squamous epithelium (transformation zone, TZ)
- Columnar epithelium
- Active or new squamocolumnar junction
- Old squamocolumnar junction
- Any abnormal acetowhite areas in the transformation zone with abnormal vascular patterns.

R. Arora (✉) • S. Jain
Department of Obstetrics and Gynecology, Santosh Medical College, Ghaziabad, UP, India
e-mail: rakshaarora47@gmail.com

S. Mehta, P. Sachdeva (eds.), *Colposcopy of Female Genital Tract*,
DOI 10.1007/978-981-10-1705-6_8

Fig. 8.1 Thickness of normal epithelium and CIN

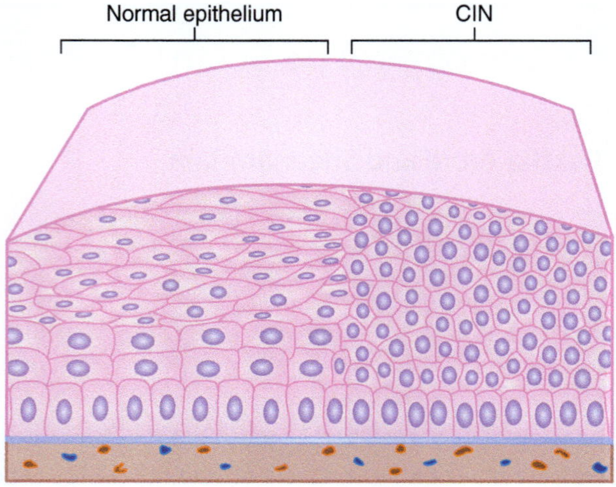

The image seen through the colposcope is based on the reciprocal relationship between the three morphological characteristics:

- Architecture of the epithelium and possible variations in its thickness
- Composition of underlying stroma
- Surface configuration of the tissue.

8.1.1 Architecture of the Epithelium

Squamous epithelium of the ectocervix is multilayered and acts as a filter through which both the reflected and the incident light must pass to produce the final picture. The epithelium is colourless and the stroma is coloured by the blood vessels it contains. The redness of stroma is transmitted back to the observer with modifications depending on the characteristics and thickness of the epithelium.

Squamous epithelium of the normal cervix is thick, multilayered and glycogenated and acts as an effective filter and appears pinkish to red in colour when seen through the colposcope. On the other hand, if it is abnormal as in cases of preclinical cancer, it is much thicker with altered architectures, and the reflected light imparts an opaque appearance especially after acetic acid (Fig. 8.1).

Action of acetic acid: It clears the mucus, induces intracellular dehydration and reacts with nucleoproteins and cytokeratins resulting in coagulation thus causing loss of translucency [acetowhite]. The effect of acetic acid depends on the amount of nuclear proteins and cytokeratins in the epithelium. The acetowhitening is faint and appears slowly in preinvasive lesions because acid takes some time to penetrate up to the atypical cells in the lower third of the epithelium.

Columnar epithelium is thin and single layered, contains mucus and is highly translucent, thus appearing red in colour when seen colposcopically. It is important to identify a thin white line between the pinkish squamous epithelium and reddish columnar epithelium which represents the new or active squamocolumnar junction (Fig. 8.2).

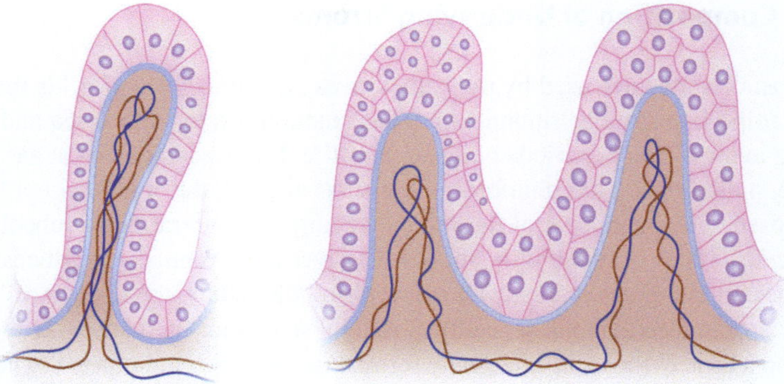

Fig. 8.2 Columnar epithelium

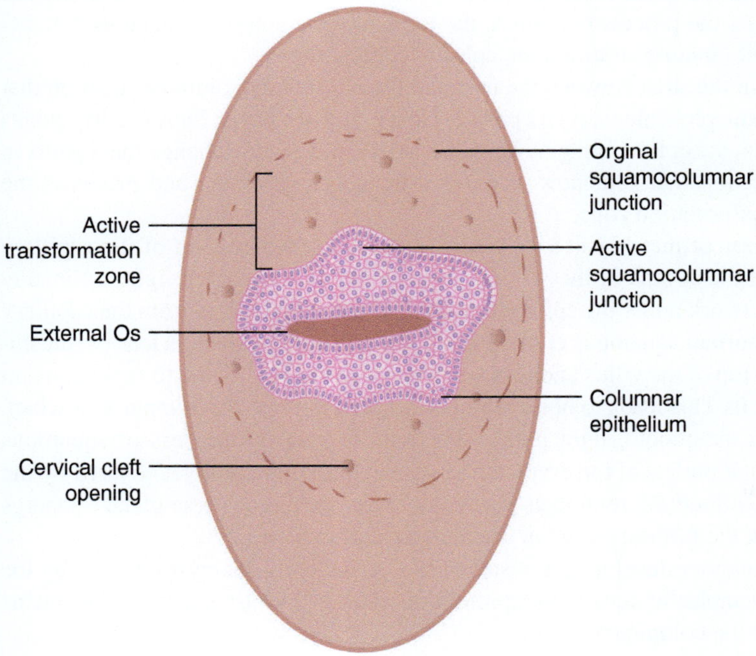

Fig. 8.3 Transformation zone

Next most important area to identify is the transformation zone (Fig. 8.3). This is the area where the physiological process of metaplasia or transformation of columnar to squamous epithelium has occurred. The process of carcinogenesis might have taken place during the phase of metaplasia. The outer boundary of this TZ is the old squamocolumnar junction which is identified by the presence of small hollow areas of gland openings. Within the boundaries of TZ, metaplastic epithelium at various stages of development is found. It may be thinner than the original squamous epithelium, devoid of glycogen and appear reddish. Very rapidly regenerating metaplastic epithelium as seen in immature metaplasia may adopt an opaque appearance.

8.1.2 Composition of Underlying Stroma

"Metaplasia" is the term used by the pathologists and "transformation" is the word used by colposcopists. The squamocolumnar junction is a dynamic area and keeps changing in the different periods of a women's life. It moves outwards at early neonatal life, puberty and after childbirth trauma. As a result, the columnar epithelium gets exposed to the acidic pH of the vagina leading to proliferation of subcolumnar reserve cells. These cells multiply and form a layer that eventually produces a normally differentiating squamous epithelium. Morphologically, the reserve cells have a similar appearance to the basal cells of original squamous epithelium, with round nuclei and a little cytoplasm. The newly formed metaplastic epithelium has no stratification and is called immature metaplasia. It does not contain glycogen and appears faint white after acetic acid application; it also does not take up a brown stain after Lugol's iodine. Squamous metaplasia usually begins at the original squamocolumnar junction at the distal limit of the ectopy, but it may also occur in the columnar epithelium. As the process continues, the immature metaplastic squamous cell differentiates into mature stratified metaplastic epithelium.

It is within this area between the new and the old squamocolumnar junction that all the dynamic physiological and pathological processes occur. During early stages of metaplasia, the epithelium may be vulnerable to the genetic change that results in a cell population that somehow acquires a neoplastic potential and produces the atypical transformation zone.

The process of metaplasia is also associated with compression of the capillary structures of the stroma in the villi leading to reduction in their height, ultimately forming a network under the epithelium. This is indistinguishable from the capillary network of normal squamous epithelium. In the early stage, there is loss of translucency of the top of the villus and later on there is fusion of villi due to rapid division of reserve cells This leads to obliteration of original humps of columnar villi which now appears as smooth, light pink epithelium. During the process of squamous metaplasia, the outlets of the crypts of columnar epithelium, not yet covered by the metaplastic epithelium, remain as persistent crypt openings. These gland openings usually mark the farthest extent of the transformation zone.

Nabothian cysts develop as a result of the occlusion of the cyst opening by the overlying metaplastic squamous epithelium leading to entrapment of the mucus produced by the columnar cells.

8.1.3 Transformation Zone

The original squamous epithelium is derived from the epithelium of urogenital sinus and begins at the vulvovaginal line. It lines the vagina and the ectocervix, whereas the endocervix is lined by the columnar epithelium. The location of squamocolumnar junction in relation to the external os depends on the age, hormonal status, oral contraceptive use, pregnancy and birth trauma. Prior to puberty, the original squamocolumnar junction is located at or very close to the external os. During the

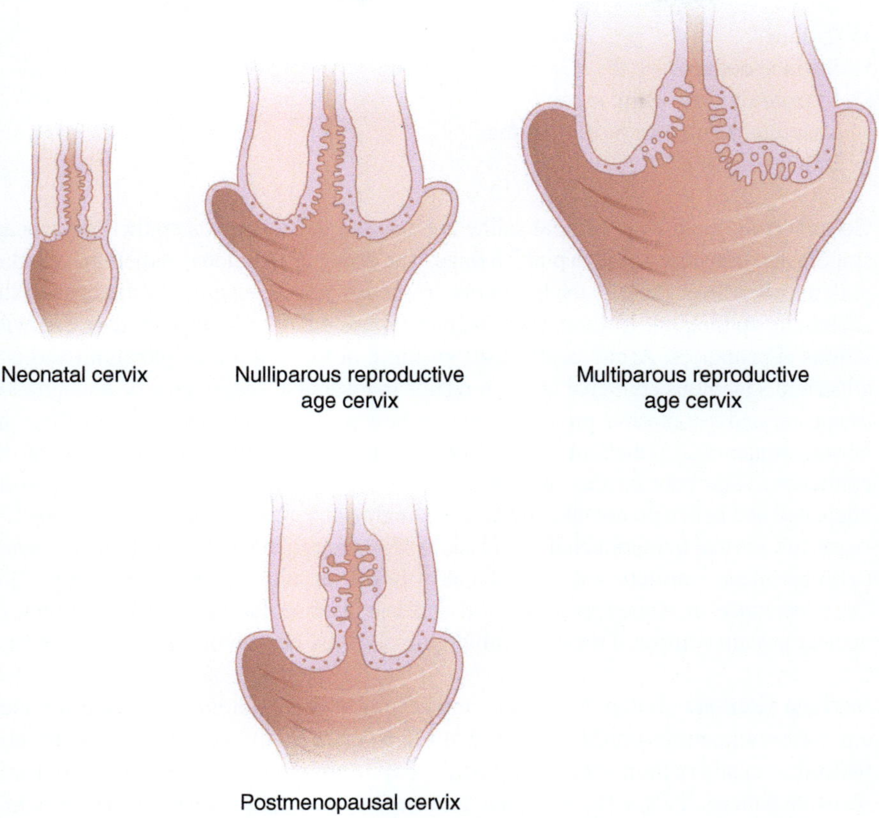

Fig. 8.4 Location of new squamocolumnar junction according to age

reproductive years, the female genital tract remains under the influence of oestrogen resulting in elongation of the endocervical canal thereby everting the columnar lining of the endocervical canal on to the ectocervix. This shifts the original squamocolumnar junction away from the external os. The everted columnar epithelium under the influence of vaginal acidity eventually gets destroyed and is replaced by the metaplastic squamous epithelium. Thus, a new squamocolumnar junction is formed between the newly formed metaplastic squamous epithelium and the columnar epithelium. As the women progresses towards menopause, the location of new squamocolumnar epithelium moves on the ectocervix towards the external os (Fig. 8.4). The area between the original and new squamocolumnar junction is known as the transformation zone.

It is within this area that all the dynamic physiological and pathological processes occur. During early stages of metaplasia, the epithelium may be vulnerable to the genetic change that results in a cell population that somehow acquires a neoplastic potential and produces the atypical transformation zone.

The colposcopic findings are described keeping in mind the following criteria:

- Colour
- Surface contour
- Margin of acetowhite areas
- Vasculature pattern of the stroma
- Iodine staining

Colour Tone Following normal saline application, the squamous epithelium appears smooth and translucent with a pinkish tinge. The original squamous epithelium is darker pink in colour in contrast to the light pink or whitish pink appearance of the metaplastic squamous epithelium. Columnar epithelium on the other hand appears dark red with villous appearances. Acetic acid causes swelling of the columnar epithelium and any abnormal squamous epithelial areas. It results in reversible coagulation or precipitation of nuclear and cytoplasmic proteins in the epithelium. The acetic acid does not affect the normal squamous epithelium as it cannot penetrate below the outer one-third of the epithelium. The cells in the superficial layers of squamous epithelium are sparsely nucleated and hence do not take the acetowhitening and appear pink on colposcopy [3]. Areas of Cervical Intraepithelial Neoplasia (CIN) undergo maximum coagulation owing to higher nuclear protein content and appear opaque/acetowhite. With low-grade CIN, the appearance of whiteness is delayed and less intense due to a smaller amount of nuclear protein compared to areas with high-grade CIN or preclinical invasive cancer.

Surface Contour It may be smooth, uneven, granulated, papillomatous or nodular, e.g. native squamous epithelium has a smooth surface, while ectopic columnar epithelium is easily recognisable by grapelike papillomatous excrescences (villi). Early invasive cancer or CIN III may have an uneven or slightly elevated surface, while frank invasive cancer is characterised by a nodular or polypoidal surface.

Clarity of Demarcation The sharpness of the boundary between high-grade lesions and the adjacent normal tissue is much better appreciated than in inflammatory lesions or mild dysplasia. The junctional zone also presents a sharp border between squamous and columnar epithelium.

Vasculature Pattern of the Stroma Normal vasculature pattern in the original squamous epithelium can be seen under higher magnification with green filter after normal saline application. They can be seen as fine network of terminal capillaries, treelike branching vessels or small end on points of hairpin capillaries seen as dots (Fig. 8.5). But in an atypical epithelium, the vascular elements may take characteristic appearances to which the term such as mosaic or punctations are given.

Inter-capillary Distance It refers to the space between corresponding parts of two adjacent vessels or to the diameter of fields delineated by network or mosaic vessels. On colposcopy, inter-capillary distance can be estimated by comparison with that of capillaries in the adjacent normal epithelium. In the preinvasive and invasive carcinoma, inter-capillary distance increases.

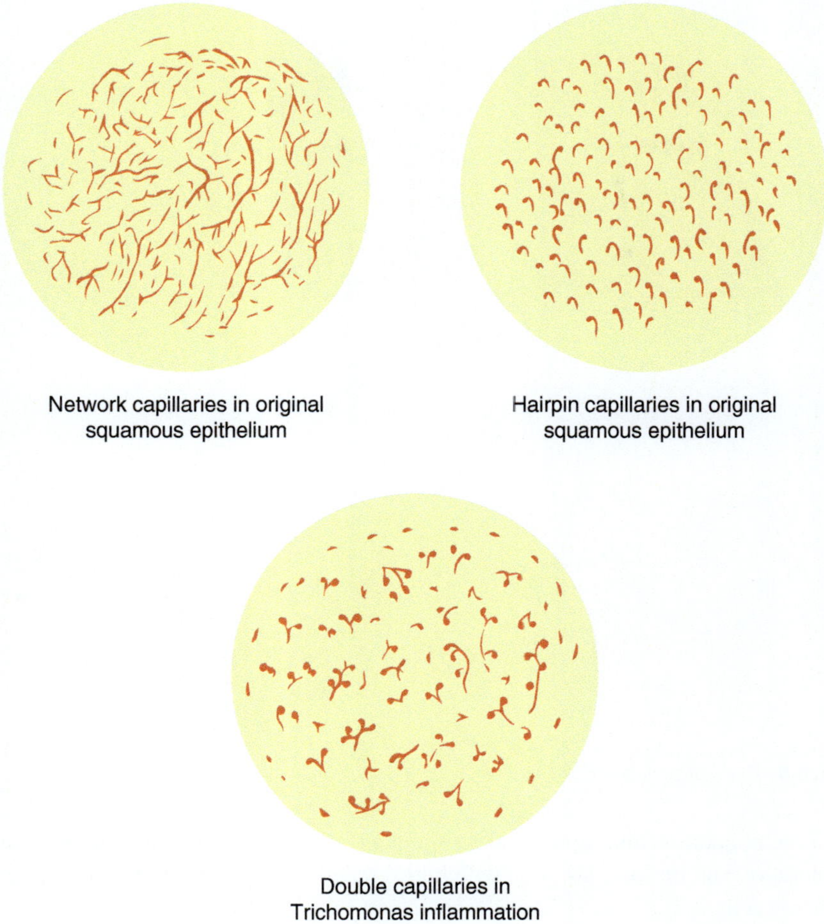

Fig. 8.5 Vascular pattern of stroma

Punctation The central vascular network of previously grapelike papillae of the columnar epithelium remains as thick stromal papillae surrounded by metaplastic epithelium (Fig. 8.6). Acetic acid application will show the stromal papillae as red fields seen as dots surrounded by white areas of atypical epithelium. This is also called stripling.

Mosaicism As atypical metaplasia proceeds, proliferative activity of epithelium within the clefts leads to compression of stromal papillae. Vessels within these papillae undergo dilatation and proliferation near the surface or tend to form a basketlike vascular network around the buds of abnormal epithelium. These capillaries lying parallel to the surface form a quasi pavement-like appearance. The interconnecting blood vessels in the stromal papillae surrounding the rete pegs of epithelium appear colposcopically as cobblestone or mosaic pattern [3].

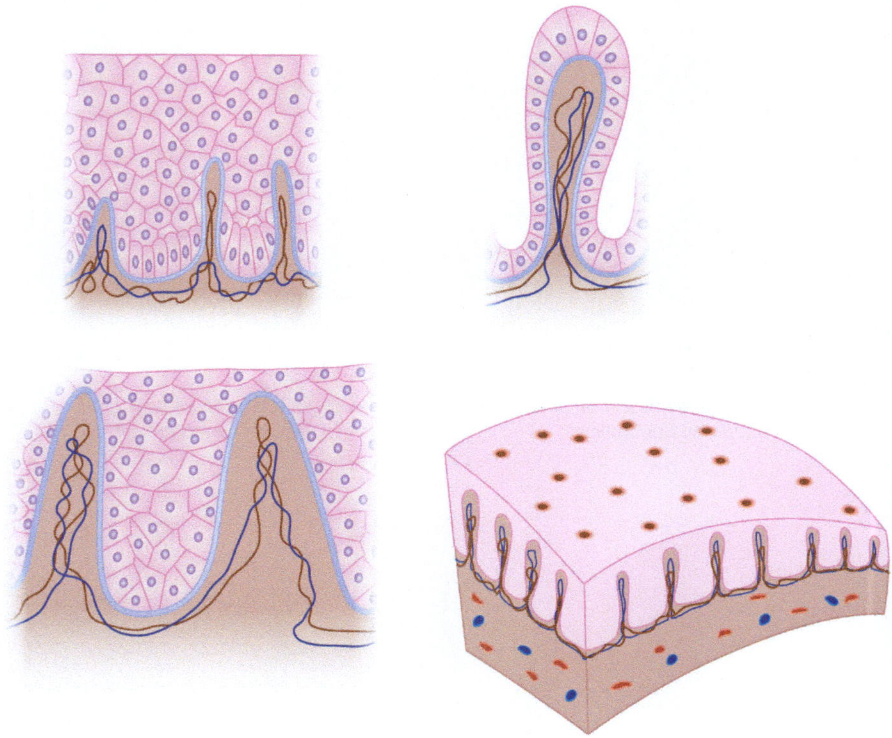

Fig. 8.6 Basis of punctation

Fine punctation and mosaics are associated with low-grade CIN, whereas coarse punctation and mosaics are seen with high-grade CIN and early preclinical invasive cancers (Fig. 8.7).

Hairpin or Looped Vessels These vessels originate from vessels of punctations and mosaic. As the neoplastic epithelium grows, it crowds out the punctate and mosaic vessels. In order to maintain the blood supply, the vessels begin to tuft at the top and then usually spread out along the surface in cases of early cancer. Their course over the surface is usually short (2–3 mm) and they do not branch; instead they spiral or loop and end abruptly. After acetic acid application, they maintain their surface position and appear visible.

Branching Vessels These originate from the stroma. Normal cervical stromal vessels can be seen over nabothian cyst as cyst pushes the stromal vessels to the surface. When cancer develops, the surface epithelium is so thinned out that stromal vessels are more visible. The underlying cancer stimulates the growth of vessels and they become more bizarre. Instead of becoming smaller as the vessels branch, these vessels become larger. The branches may be at right angles or even obtuse angles instead of acute angles, frequent sharp turns, dilatations and narrowing. These vessels are close to the surface, bleed easily on contact and lead to postcoital bleeding (Fig. 8.8).

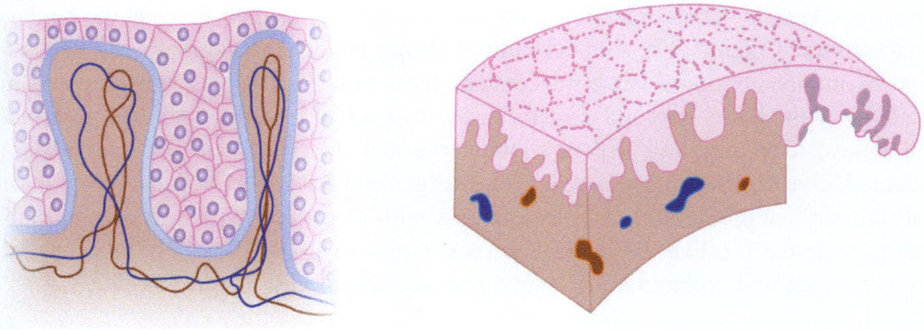

Fig. 8.7 Basis of mosaicism

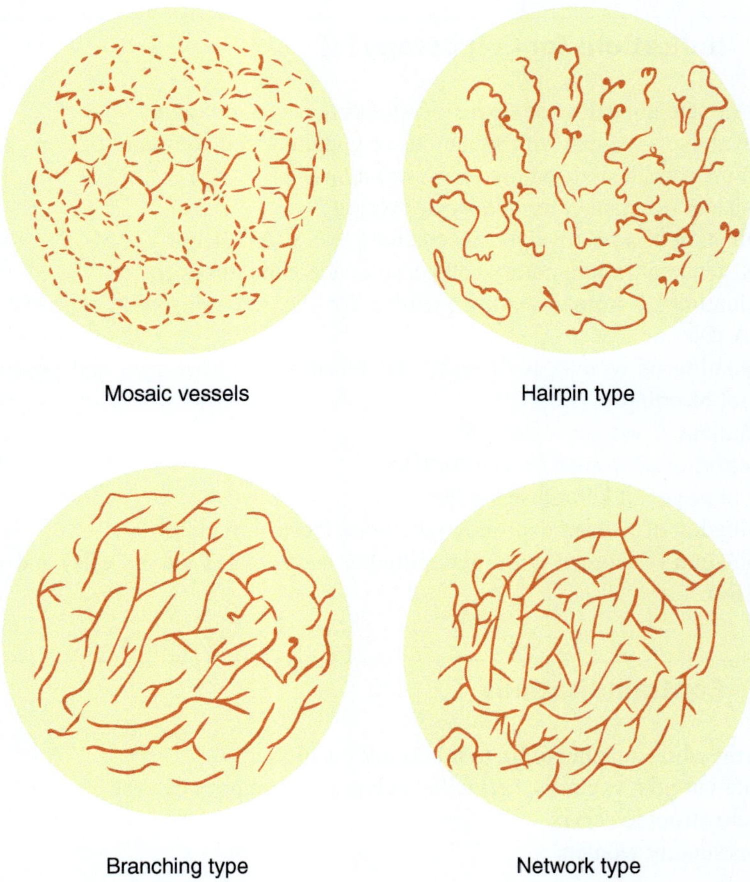

Fig. 8.8 Vasculature in CIN

Network Vessels These arise from the network of terminal capillaries at the epithelial stromal junction. The thin epithelium allows underlying capillaries to be seen easily and the abnormal vessels accentuate these vessels. They become irregular in calibre with dilatations and constrictions. Instead of ending with fine terminal branches, they may end with a slight curve and dilatation and become comma shaped. Overall pattern is collection of disorganised fine, short vessels with thin or absent surface epithelium. Atypical vessels with comma, irregular branching patterns, wide hairpin-like vessels and corkscrew pattern are a hallmark of invasion but may be seen with inflammation condylomas and post radiotherapy [4].

Iodine Staining Iodine is glycophillic, and hence the application of iodine solution results in the uptake of iodine in the glycogen-containing epithelium. Normal glycogen-containing squamous epithelium stains mahogany brown or black, whereas CIN, invasive cancers and columnar epithelium do not take up the stain and remain unstained and appear as thick mustard yellow or saffron-coloured areas.

8.2 Indications for Colposcopy [5]

- To evaluate unhealthy or suspicious-looking cervix or vagina
- To evaluate a woman with squamous or glandular cell abnormalities on cytology with no gross lesions on the cervix or vagina
- Persistent unsatisfactory quality of cytology
- Evaluation of a positive visual screening test-VIA/VILI or VIAM
- Persistence of inflammatory cells despite adequate treatment
- Evaluation of woman testing positive for the screening with high-risk HPV DNA test
- Evaluation of woman with postcoital bleeding, metrorrhagia and post menopausal bleeding
- Treatment of women with CIN
- Monitoring of women treated for CIN
- The presence of keratinised cells
- Evaluation of women exposed to diethylstilbestrol in utero
- Evaluation of women with intraepithelial neoplasia of vulva (VIN) and vagina (VAIN).

8.3 Contraindications

- Patient who is unable to lie in lithotomy position
- Acute vulvitis, vaginitis, cervicitis, pelvic inflammatory disease
- Severe atrophic cervix
- Menstruating women.

Conclusion

The aim of colposcopy is to detect high-grade CIN and microinvasive cancer. The image which is seen through colposcopy is based on morphological characteristics of epithelium, composition of underlying stroma and surface configuration. Transformation zone is the area where carcinogenesis generally takes place as it is the zone of maximum mitotic activity. This is the area which is inspected during colposcopy and a note is made on colour tone, contour, margins, vasculature pattern and iodine staining. Whenever a suspicious area is demarcated, it is biopsied for histopathological confirmation of CIN.

Key Points

1. Transformation zone is the area between the old and new squamocolumnar junction.
2. TZ is dynamic with maximum mitotic activity and dysplasia usually starts in the transformation zone.
3. Well-demarcated, dense opaque white area in the transformation zone close to or abutting the squamocolumnar junction is the hallmark of colposcopic diagnosis of CIN.
4. Low-grade CIN is often seen as thin, smooth acetowhite lesion with well-demarcated but irregularly feathery margins.
5. High-grade CIN is associated with thick, dense, opaque or greyish white acetowhite area with well-demarcated, regular margins which sometimes may be raised and rolled out or the lesions may be outgoing towards the endocervical canal.
6. Vascular features such as fine punctations and fine mosaic in acetowhite areas indicate low-grade lesions, while coarse punctations and mosaic indicate high-grade lesion.
7. CIN lesions do not take up brown colour after Lugol's iodine application.

References

1. Burghardt E, Pickel H, Girardi F. Colposcopy-cervical pathology. Textbook and atlas. 3rd ed. New York: Thieme; 1998. p. 62–98.
2. Hatch KD. Handbook of colposcopy: diagnosis and treatment of lower genital tract neoplasia and HPV infections. Boston: Little Brown; 1989.
3. Coppleson M, Pixleyb E, Reid B. Colposcopy. Springfield: Charles C Thomas; 1971. p. 14–6, 53–110, 155–92.
4. Kolstad P. The development of the vascular bed in tumors as seen in squamous-cell carcinoma of the cervix uteri. Br J Radiol. 1965;38:216–23.
5. Baliga BS. Step by step colposcopy cryosurgery and LEEP. New Delhi: Jaypee Brothers Medical Publishers (P) Ltd; 2008.

Colposcopic Technique, Scoring and Documentation

9

Pakhee Aggarwal

9.1 Introduction

The practice of colposcopy dates back nearly a century, when Hans Hinselmann first described the use of a basic colposcope in 1925. Since then, colposcopy has come a long way in terms of refinement of optics, stereoscopic vision and image quality. However, the basic principles of the colposcopic technique have stood the test of time and remain the same to this day. Briefly, the current colposcope is a low-power (4–40×), binocular, stereoscopic microscope with a powerful light source which helps to illuminate and magnify the genital tract (cervix, vagina and vulva) to aid identification of precancerous lesions.

9.2 Indications for Colposcopy

It must be borne in mind that colposcopy is not a screening technique for precancerous lesions. Instead, its use should be restricted to the confirmation of positive screening test results, be it Pap smear or visual tests and to guide the site of biopsy. The various indications for a colposcopic examination are [1, 2]

1. Clinically suspicious cervix
2. Abnormal Pap smear (ASCUS, LSIL, HSIL, AGUS, ASC-H, invasive cancer)
3. Persistent unsatisfactory smear with HPV positive, or borderline cytology with HPV positive
4. Infection with oncogenic HPV types

P. Aggarwal, MS (O&G), MICOG, MRCOG (London)
Commonwealth Fellow in Gyne Oncology Delhi, India

Department of Obstetrics and Gynecology, Fortis Healthcare (Fortis Memorial Hosp, Gurgaon, Flt Lt Rajan Dhall Hospital and Aashlok Hospital Delhi) Delhi, India
e-mail: pakh_ag@yahoo.com

S. Mehta, P. Sachdeva (eds.), *Colposcopy of Female Genital Tract*,
DOI 10.1007/978-981-10-1705-6_9

5. Visual inspection with acetic acid (VIA) positive
6. Visual inspection with acetic acid and magnification (VIAM) positive
7. Visual inspection with Lugol's iodine (VILI) positive
8. Treatment planning and posttreatment surveillance of CIN – either abnormal cytology or HPV positive during follow-up
9. DES exposure in utero
10. Forensic examination

9.3 Principles of Colposcopic Examination

Colposcopic examination carried out in a systematic manner is very informative in identifying precancerous lesions and quantifying their grade. The key examination steps are

- Application of normal saline and observation with green filter
- Application of 5 % acetic acid and observation with normal filter after 1 min (repeat applications as required)
- Application of Lugol's iodine

Application of Normal Saline After swabbing the cervix of any excessive mucus, cotton swab dipped in normal saline is generously dabbed on the cervix. The light filter is changed to green/blue and magnification increased to 15×. This makes the vascular pattern stand out and any abnormal vessels easy to identify. The study of this subepithelial pattern becomes more difficult after the application of acetic acid due to tissue swelling; hence saline examination is the first step of colposcopic examination.

Application of Acetic Acid The next step is application of freshly prepared dilute acetic acid (5 %) made by mixing glacial acetic acid (5 cc) with normal saline (95 cc). This is applied using cotton swabs as before or can even be filled in a syringe to spray on the cervix. The acetic acid serves a dual purpose. It causes a reversible coagulation of the nuclear protein and cytokeratins in the epithelial layer. The extent of this coagulation depends on the amount of nuclear protein in the cells. Normal squamous epithelium is sparsely nucleated, hence appears pink after application of acetic acid as the subepithelial vasculature is visible through the poorly coagulated epithelium. Precancerous lesions, ranging from CIN1 to CIN3 not only have increasing amounts of nuclear protein (increased nuclear to cytoplasmic ratio at cellular level) but also the extent of involvement above the basement membrane increases as grade of lesion increases. In colposcopic terms, when acetic acid is applied to such lesions, they undergo more coagulation due to their higher nuclear protein content and prevent light from passing through the epithelium. As a result, the colour of the underlying stroma and the subepithelial vessel pattern is obliterated and the epithelium appears white. This reaction is called acetowhitening. With low-grade CIN, the appearance of acetowhiteness is delayed and less intense compared to high-grade CIN, where the acetowhiteness is immediate and more intensely opaque, due to the larger number of dysplastic cells in superficial layers of the latter.

Cotton swab may be used to reapply the acetic acid pooled in the posterior fornix if required.

The other advantage of using acetic acid is that it helps to coagulate and remove tenacious mucus which in turn helps with better penetration of acetic acid into the epithelium.

However, acetowhite lesions may also be seen with immature squamous metaplasia (translucent white), congenital transformation zone, leukoplakia (white even before application of acetic acid), condyloma and healing and regenerating epithelium (e.g. after a biopsy). These lesions also have increased nuclear protein content compared to normal squamous epithelium and hence the false positive reaction. Training and expertise in colposcopy is necessary to distinguish which lesions need biopsy and which can be followed up. Indeed in many centres, like the UK, the colposcopist's visual impression and its correlation with final histology form a part of regular appraisal of colposcopic skills.

Application of Lugol's Iodine After removing any excess acetic acid from the posterior fornix where it usually tends to pool as copious amounts are used in the previous test, Lugol's iodine is applied. Iodine is glycophillic, and application of iodine-containing solution results in uptake of this iodine within glycogen-rich epithelium which turns a distinct dark (mahogany) brown or black colour. Both original squamous and mature metaplastic epithelium contain glycogen and stain this colour. The degree of differentiation in precancerous lesions determines the amount of intracellular glycogen and the degree of staining. Therefore, high-grade CIN cells, which do not contain glycogen, appear as mustard yellow or saffron-coloured areas, while low-grade CIN appears as partially brown. In high-grade CIN, repeated application of iodine can sometimes peel off the abnormal epithelium and the underlying stroma then appears pale as it lacks glycogen. Columnar epithelium does not contain glycogen and remains unstained. Immature metaplasia stains patchily, while leukoplakia, condyloma and inflammatory lesions do not take up iodine and remain unstained and colourless in a dark background.

The final colposcopic impression of normal cervix or low- or high-grade lesion is made on the combined findings of all three tests and never on a single test.

Step by step colposcopy examination also includes some prerequisites and post-procedure components to complete the examination.

1. Explain the procedure to the woman and take written informed consent: Every effort should be made to put the woman at ease and maintain privacy during the examination. Prior explanation of the procedure is essential to ensure patient cooperation during the procedure. A written informed consent which contains information about the colposcopic examination and any subsequent procedures like cryotherapy, biopsy or Loop electrosurgical excision procedure (LEEP) should be obtained. This should include any complications and side effects of treatment, or if 'see-and-treat' is being followed, the chances and risks of overtreatment (appendix of consent form).

Fig. 9.1 Instrument tray for colposcopy

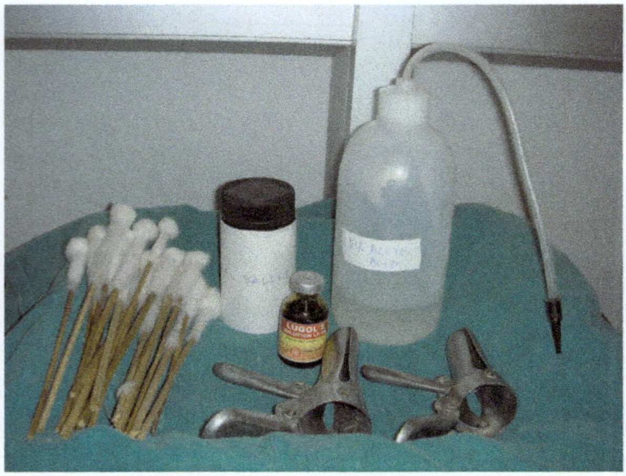

2. Take relevant gynaecological history and elicit any comorbidities: This includes last menstrual period, any intermenstrual or postcoital bleeding, number of previous pregnancies, the use of oral contraceptive pills or hormonal supplements, STIs, any medical disorders like high blood pressure or diabetes. Screening smear report should be at hand while doing colposcopy if she has been referred because of an abnormal smear.
3. Insert the self-retaining speculum and inspect the cervix: After the woman lies in modified lithotomy position (legs in stirrups), the widest speculum that can comfortably fit in the vagina is used to have optimal visualisation. Overhanging vaginal walls can be kept away by the use of lateral retractors or using a latex condom (with its tip cut off) on the speculum. The instruments needed are placed at hand in a small trolley or tray beside the examination table. The instrument tray is shown in Figs. 9.1 and 9.2 and includes the following: Cusco's speculum, vaginal side wall retractor, cotton swabs, sponge-holding forceps, endocervical speculum, punch biopsy forceps/loops, endocervical curette, normal saline, freshly prepared 5 % acetic acid and Lugol's iodine. If cryotherapy or LEEP is planned, additional instruments are required.

   Once the speculum is inserted and the blades separated, a good view of the cervix and vaginal fornices is obtained. A note is made of any cervicovaginal secretions, ectropion, polyp, nabothian follicles, leukoplakia, ulcer, growth, atrophy, inflammation and obvious lesions on the vaginal fornices. If a Pap smear needs to be taken it should be done now, before any saline is applied. Swabs to test for STIs or HPV are also taken at this point if required.
4. Follow the examination protocol in sequence (normal saline, acetic acid, Lugol's iodine) to avoid diagnostic errors (Figs. 9.3, 9.4, 9.5 and 9.6 showing colposcopic images after each).
5. Examine the squamocolumnar junction (SCJ) in its entirety and the transformation zone (TZ) up to its distal margin. The proximal margin of the TZ is formed by the SCJ, while the distal margin is demarcated by the most distal nabothian follicles or crypt openings. Sometimes the inner margin of TZ recedes into the

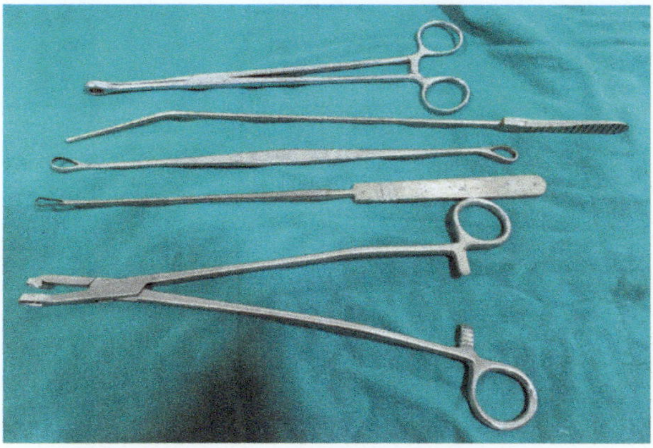

Fig. 9.2 Instrument tray for colposcopic biopsy

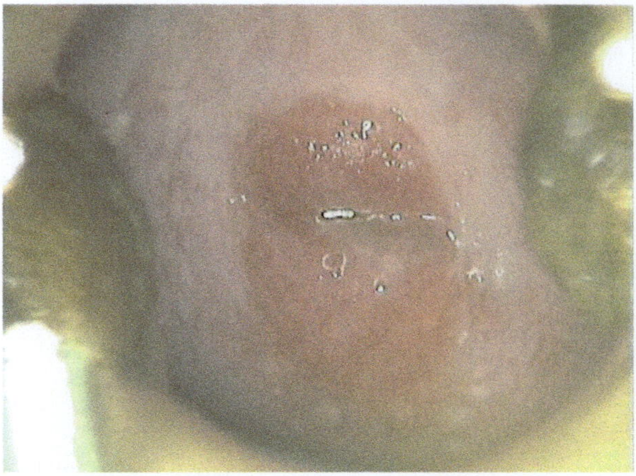

Fig. 9.3 Cervix after application of normal saline

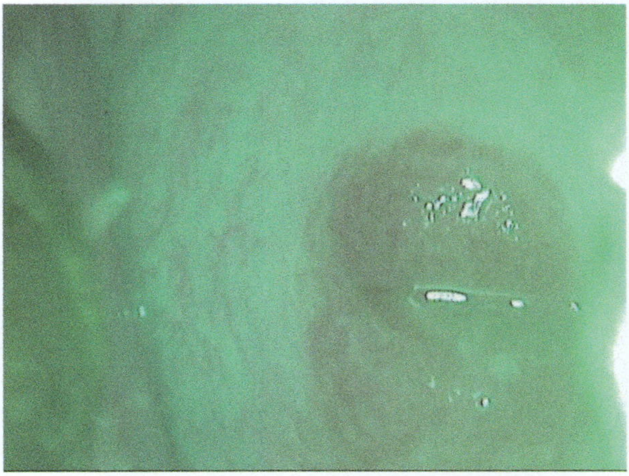

Fig. 9.4 Application of normal saline with green filter

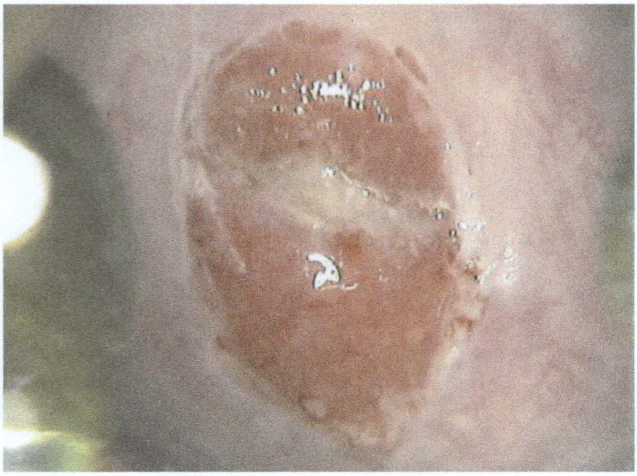

Fig. 9.5 Application of acetic acid on cervix

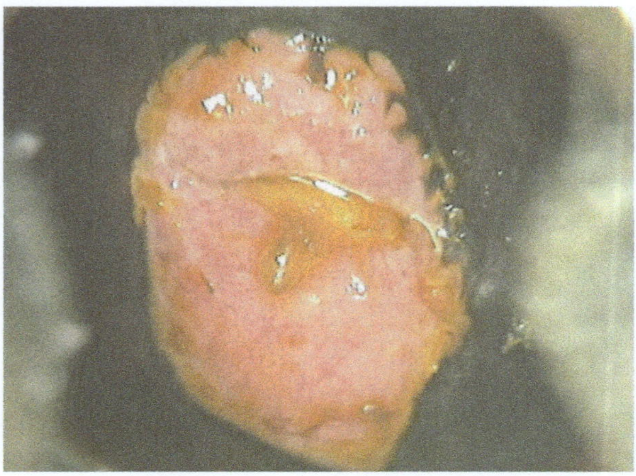

Fig. 9.6 Application of Lugol's iodine

cervical canal and may require additional manoeuvres to visualise, like using an endocervical speculum or opening the vaginal speculum wider and using a long dissecting forceps to try opening the canal. Based on the extent of TZ visible, it is classified into three types. Type 1 TZ is completely ectocervical, Type 2 TZ is partially endocervical but the upper limit can be visualised by manipulating the cervix or inserting an endocervical speculum, whereas a Type 3 TZ is predominantly endocervical and its upper limit cannot be visualised.

The previously used terms satisfactory and unsatisfactory have been replaced by new terminology by the IFCPC in 2011, and one must be familiar with these terms for adequate colposcopic reporting [3] (Annexure 5).

6. Document and score any lesions within the TZ or abutting the SCJ: Documentation of findings is as important as the practice of colposcopy itself and serves as a tool for follow-up after treatment. This may be done electronically or in paper form. Usually a structured proforma is used to document results. Two formats (Hammond graph and Odell diagram) are shown to document results in paper

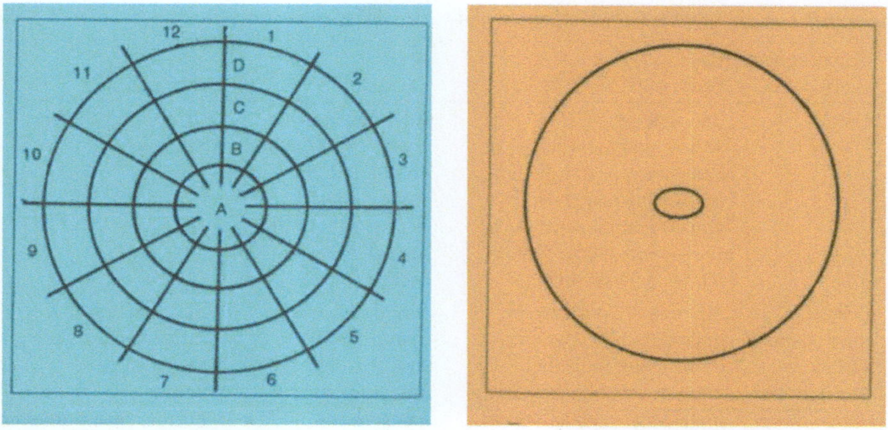

Hammond's Graph *Odell's diagram*

Fig. 9.7 Documentation charts

form (Fig. 9.7). Most colposcopes have image management systems which store images and patient data electronically using a computer with custom software. This has a capacity for recording video and also selective image enhancement and annotation. In addition, a report can be accessed as a drop-down menu thereby enabling procedure documentation and image retrieval. The obvious advantages of documentation in following up changes in lesion location, size and volume, objective response to treatment and monitoring remote colposcopy practice in clinical trials cannot be over emphasised.

The second part of documenting findings is scoring the lesion to know whether it is high grade or low grade so that appropriate treatment and follow-up can be advised. This is done with the help of one of the many scoring systems in use. These include two-tier system, Coppelson's grading, Reid's Colposcopic Index and the two most commonly used ones: Modified Reid's Combined Colposcopic Index and Swede Score [4, 5]. The latter two are described in detail in Tables 9.1 and 9.2, respectively.

It is a good idea to keep one of these scoring systems at hand every time a colposcopic examination is done so that the lesion can immediately be scored and managed appropriately.

7. The completion of colposcopic examination requires biopsy to be taken from any abnormal areas as highlighted. Biopsy is taken with punch biopsy forceps (Kevorkian, Tischler-Morgan) with sharp jaws using a sharp quick motion, taking care to include the stroma (Fig. 9.8). Biopsy should be done under colposcopic guidance and from the area/s with worse features and those abutting the SCJ. Endocervical curettage (ECC) is also done at the same time. Post-biopsy bleeding is controlled by using Monsel's paste or packing. The biopsy and ECC are sent in 10 % formalin for histopathological evaluation. In a 'see-and-treat' protocol, the abnormal lesion may be dealt with cryotherapy or LEEP in the same sitting.

Table 9.1 Reid score and its interpretation [4]

Colposcopic signs	Zero point	One point	Two points
Colour	Low-intensity acetowhitening; (indistinct transparent or translucent), beyond the margin of transformation zone, pure snow-white colour with intense surface shine	Intermediate shade – grey/white colour and shiny surface (most lesions should be scored in this category)	Dull, opaque, oyster white; grey
Lesion margin and surface configuration	Microcondylomatous or micropapillary contour, flat lesions with indistinct margins (feathered or finely scalloped), angular, jagged lesions, satellite lesions beyond the margin of the transformation zone	Regular-shaped, symmetrical lesions with smooth, straight outlines	Rolled, peeling edges, internal demarcations between areas of differing colposcopic appearance – a central area of high-grade change and peripheral area of low-grade change
Vessels	Fine/uniform-calibre vessels, closely and uniformly placed, vessels beyond the margin of transformation zone, vessels within microcondylomatous or micropapillary lesions, poorly formed patterns of fine punctation/mosaic	Absent vessels	Well-defined coarse punctation or mosaic, sharply demarcated – and randomly and widely placed
Iodine staining	Positive iodine uptake (mahogany-brown). Negative uptake of insignificant lesion, i.e. yellow staining by a lesion scoring three points or less. Negative areas beyond the margin of transformation zone (parakeratosis)	Partial iodine uptake – variegated, speckled appearance	Negative iodine uptake of significant lesion, i.e. yellow staining by a lesion already scoring four points or more on the first three criteria

Score: *0–2* likely to be CIN 1; *3–4 overlapping lesion* likely to be CIN 1 or 2; *5–8* likely to be CIN 2–3

Table 9.2 Swede score and its interpretation [5]

S. no	Original model	Level 'A'	Level 'B'	Level 'C'
1.	Aceto uptake	0 or transparent	Shady, milk	Distinct
2.	Margins and surface	0 or diffuse	Sharp but irregular, jagged, 'geographical' satellites	Sharp and even, difference in surface level, including 'cutting'
3.	Vessels	Fine, regular	Absent	Coarse or atypical vessels
4.	Lesion size	<5 mm	5–15 mm or 2 quadrants	>15 mm or 3–4 quadrants or endocervically defined
5.	Iodine staining	Brown	Faintly or patchy yellow	Distinct yellow

Score: *<5* likely benign, no need for biopsy, *5–7* high grade, biopsy confirmation, *>8* see and treat diagnostic excision

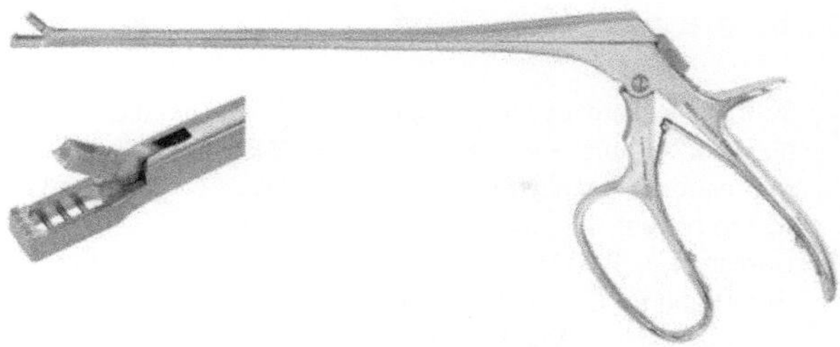

Fig. 9.8 Kevorkian biopsy forceps

8. As the speculum is withdrawn, it is prudent to examine the vaginal walls, vulva and perineum and record any abnormal findings. Acetic acid can also be applied to look for any abnormal areas.
9. Explain the findings to the woman and proposed management and follow-up plan after she is dressed.
10. What to do differently if the woman is pregnant: Pregnancy causes tissue oedema, vaginal wall laxity, increased cervical mucus, increased vascularity and eversion of os. As a result, CIN may appear as a worse grade than it truly is and the blood vessel pattern tends to mimic invasive cancer. The protocol followed in colposcopic examination is same as nonpregnant, taking care to avoid injury during speculum insertion and withdrawal. Thus, considerable skill and experience is required to conduct colposcopy in pregnancy. Cervical biopsy should only be considered if invasive cancer is suspected, as bleeding can be severe and difficult to control.

Thus colposcopy is a highly specialised examination that requires skill (both at microscopic and endoscopic level) and experience to successfully demarcate high-grade from low-grade lesions and treat accordingly. If step by step colposcopic examination is followed, the procedure becomes easy to learn and teach.

Key Points

1. Colposcopy and guided biopsy is considered as a diagnostic (not screening) test for diagnosing precancerous lesions of the cervix.
2. Systematic colposcopic examination is necessary to arrive at accurate diagnosis.
3. The application of normal saline followed by green filter, acetic acid and Lugol's iodine should be in a sequential manner giving adequate time to each step.
4. The final colposcopic impression should incorporate a scoring system (Reid's or Swede's) so that objectivity is maintained.
5. Accurate documentation is useful not only in deciding appropriate treatment but also in follow-up.
6. One must keep up to date with the changes in terminology.

References

1. Sellors JW, Sankaranarayanan R. Colposcopy and the treatment of cervical intraepithelial neoplasia: a beginner's manual. Lyon: IARC Press; 2003. p. 30.
2. International Agency for Research on Cancer. Handbook of cancer prevention, Cervical cancer screening, vol. 10. Lyon: IARC Press; 2005.
3. Bornstein J, Bentley J, Bosze P, et al. 2011 colposcopic terminology of the International Federation for Cervical Pathology and Colposcopy. Obstet Gynecol. 2012;120:166–72.
4. Hong DG, Seong WJ, Kim SY. Prediction of high-grade squamous intraepithelial lesions using the modified Reid index. Int J Clin Oncol. 2010;15(1):65–9.
5. Strander B, Ellström-Andersson A, Franzén S, et al. The performance of a new scoring system for colposcopy in detecting high-grade dysplasia in the uterine cervix. Acta Obstet Gynecol Scand. 2005;84(10):1013–7.

Colposcopic Appearance of Normal Cervix

10

Kavita N. Singh and Poorva Badkur

10.1 Normal Anatomy of the Cervix

10.1.1 Gross Anatomy

The uterine cervix is the lowest part of the uterus protruding in the vagina. The cervix has two sections, the portio vaginalis or ectocervix and the supravaginal portion. The portio vaginalis cervix is clearly marked with an opening, the external os which roughly marks the junction between the ectocervix and the endocervix (Figs. 10.1 and 10.2). The gross and microscopic anatomy of cervix is discussed in detail in Chap. 1.

10.2 IFCPC Classification (2011)

Normal colposcopic findings include:

1. Original squamous epithelium
2. Columnar epithelium
3. Ectopy
4. Transformation zone 1,2,3
5. Deciduosis of pregnancy
6. Atrophic epithelium
7. Nabothian cyst
8. Gland openings

The original squamous and columnar epithelium have been discussed in Chap. 1.

K.N. Singh (✉) • P. Badkur
Department of Obstetrics and Gynecology, NSCB Govt. Medical College, Jabalpur, MP, India
e-mail: drkavitasingh@rediffmail.com

S. Mehta, P. Sachdeva (eds.), *Colposcopy of Female Genital Tract*,
DOI 10.1007/978-981-10-1705-6_10

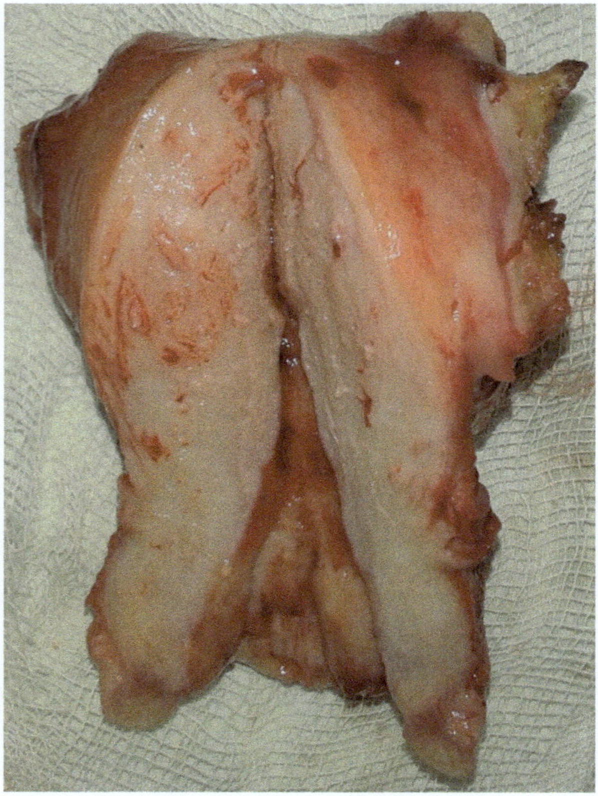

Fig. 10.1 Hysterectomy specimen of the uterus and cervix

10.3 Ectopy

It is the presence of glandular epithelium on the portio of the cervix. It refers to the presence of endocervical tissue or mucus-secreting epithelium, on the portio vaginalis of the uterine cervix (Fig. 10.3). Erosion is a misnomer.

10.4 Transformation Zone

An imaginary line drawn connecting the most distal crypt openings and/or nabothian follicles that one can see in the cervical lips colposcopically defines the original squamocolumnar junction (the junction between the original or native squamous epithelium and the metaplastic squamous epithelium). The new squamocolumnar junction is the line of demarcation where the metaplastic squamous and columnar epithelia meet.

The area between the old and new squamocolumnar junction is the transformation zone.

The vast majority of CIN changes occur in the transformation zone, and the most severe changes tend to abut, rather than farther from, the new squamocolumnar junction.

A variable zone of young squamous cells lies at the area of transformation between multilayered squamous epithelium of ectocervix and the single-layered, mucus-secreting columnar epithelium of endocervical canal.

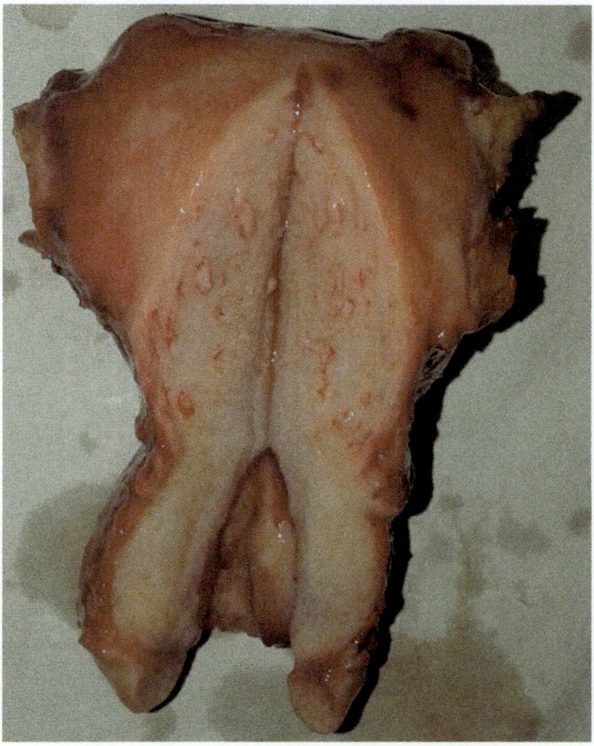

Fig. 10.2 Specimen showing internal and external os

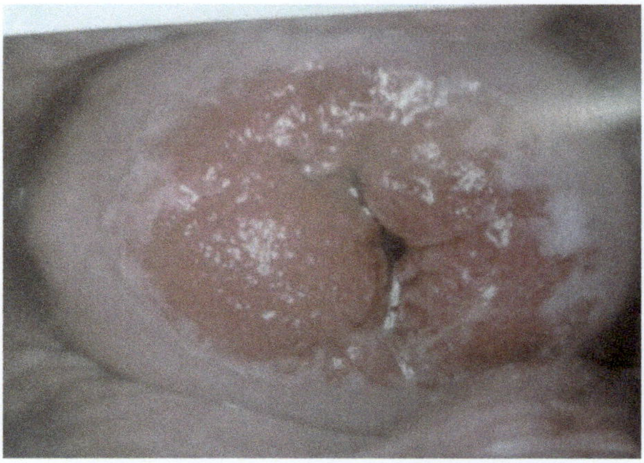

Fig. 10.3 Ectopy with peripheral area of immature squamous metaplasia

There are three types of transformation zones (Figs. 10.4, 10.5, and 10.6):

1. TZ-1

   This zone is completely ectocervical and is fully visible on examination. It can be small or large depending upon the size and shape of the cervix.
2. TZ-2

   This zone has endocervical component as well as ectocervical component which are visible on colposcopic examination.

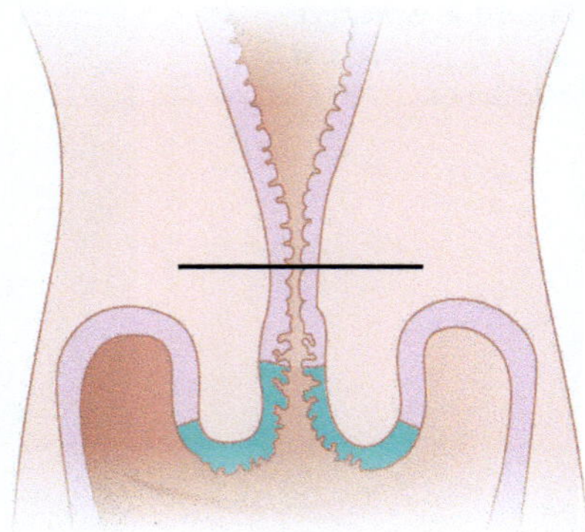

Fig. 10.4 Diagrammatic representation of TZ-1

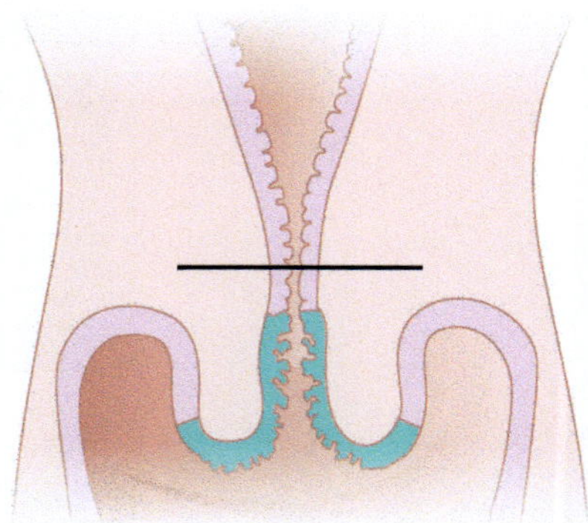

Fig. 10.5 Diagrammatic representation of TZ-2

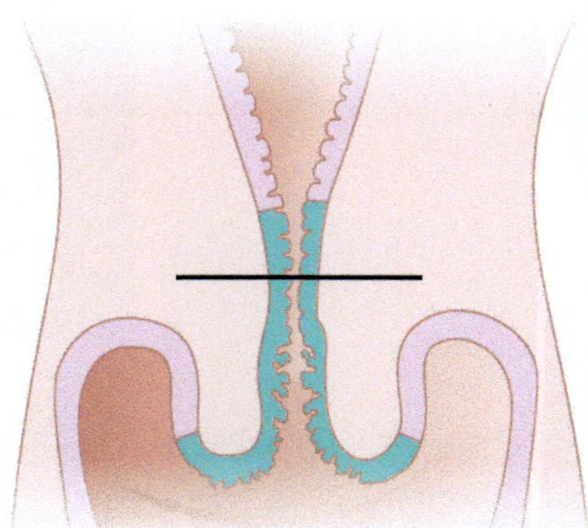

Fig. 10.6 Diagrammatic representation of TZ-3

3. TZ-3

   This zone has endocervical component which is not fully visible and lies in the endocervical canal. This may have an ectocervical component.

10.5 Squamous Metaplasia

During the different stages of the development of metaplasia, a vast range of colposcopic appearances may be seen. In the earliest stage, the translucence of the columnar epithelial villi is lost, and the villi become opaque at their tips; the villi widen and flatten, and successive villi fuse in clusters and sheets with a pale pink color. Consequently the metaplastic epithelium looks like a patchily distributed pale cluster, or sheetlike areas, in the ectopic columnar epithelium (Fig. 10.7).

Squamous metaplasis is classified into five types or stages (Figs. 10.8 and 10.9):

Stage 1: It consists of squamous differentiation of subepithelial reserve cells.
Stage 2: Immature cells divide and create a layer of 5–6 rows of red staining polyhedral cells that lift the columnar cells away from the basement membrane.

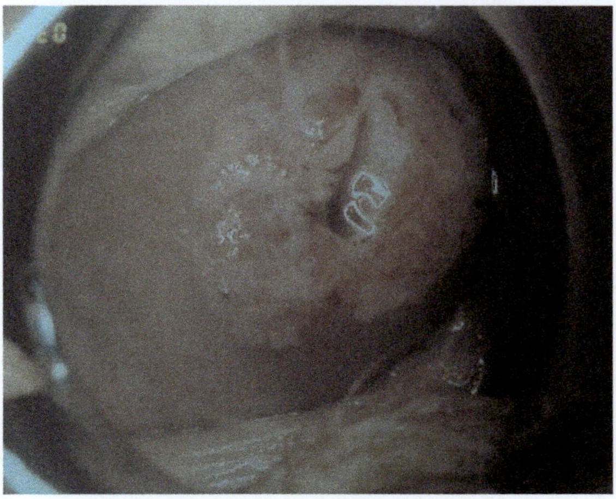

Fig. 10.7 Squamous metaplasia of the entire transformation zone

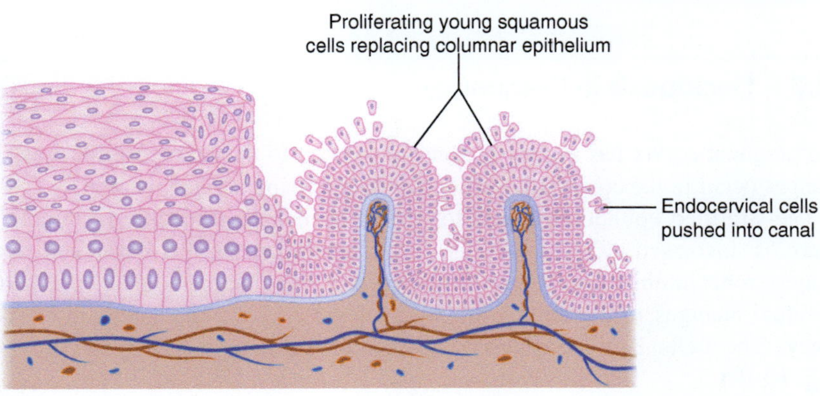

Fig. 10.8 Diagrammatic representation of immature squamous cells 5–6 layers thick

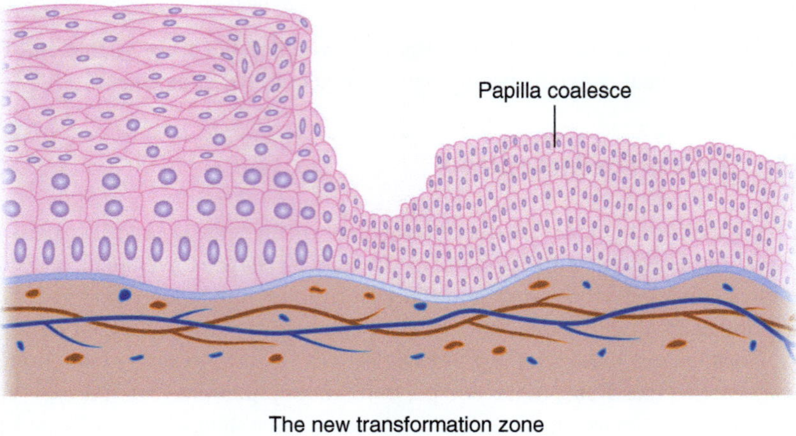

Fig. 10.9 Diagrammatic representation of formation of new transformation zone

Stage 3: The young squamous cells are 8–12 layers thick, and they begin to differentiate. Glandular epithelium casts off.

Stage 4: In this stage differentiation continues.

Stage 5: This culminates in the formation of 20–30-layered mature squamous epithelia that contain previously described 5 cell types.

10.6 Gland Openings

Cervical Stroma: It contains collagen-interspersed arterioles, venules, and lymphatic vascular channels. Deep within the stroma are glandular structures that are lined by low, cuboidal cells. The large structure is the mesonephric duct, and the smaller spaces may be remnants of the mesonephric tubules or outpouches of the duct.

10.7 Deciduosis in Pregnancy

The pregnant cervix has a great propensity to react to the hormonal changes. The changes occur in the columnar, stratified epithelium and cervical stroma.

The stratified epithelium reacts to the estrogen with a specific hyperactivity. There is increased DNA synthesis and metabolism in the basal cell layer. Progesterone inhibits the mitosis but increases the thickness of all the layers. Decidual changes in the stroma are well known and are characteristic of pregnancy. The cells become bizarre and appear similar to the dysplastic cells (Fig. 10.10).

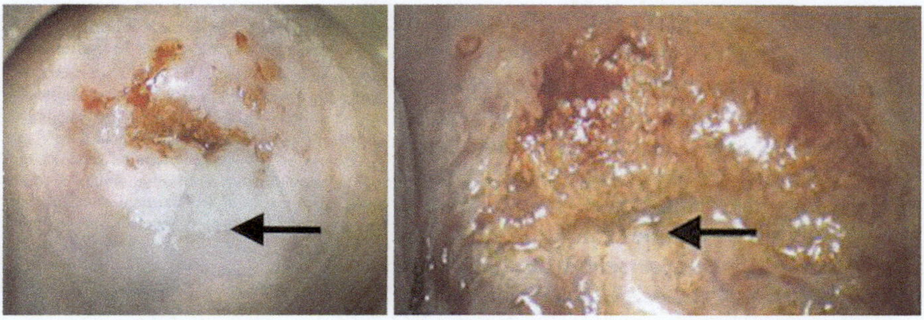

Fig. 10.10 Colposcopic findings of deciduosis in pregnancy

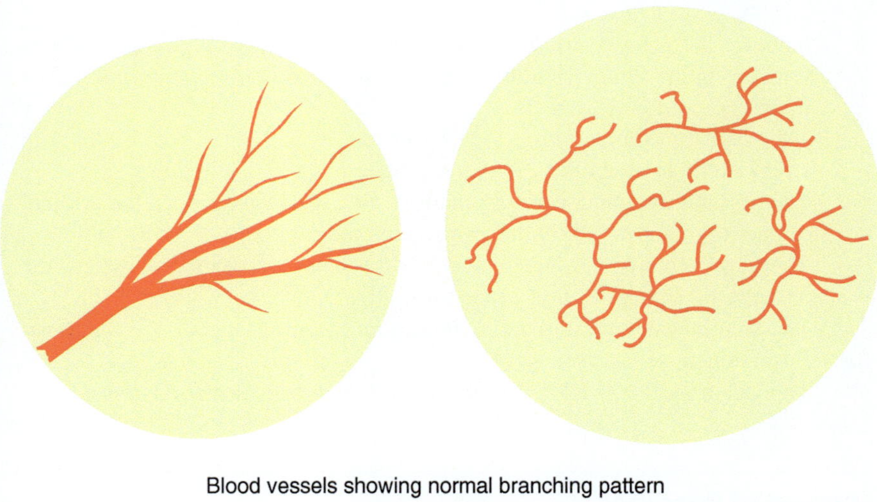

Fig. 10.11 Diagrammatic representation of normal vasculature

10.8 Vasculature

The examination of vessels is facilitated by applying normal saline and using green filter. Depending on the thickness and opacity of the overlying epithelium small vessels may or may not be visible. The smaller vessels may be visible in the stroma below epithelium.

There are two types of vessels in the native squamous epithelium:

1. Reticular pattern: This is seen in women taking oral contraceptive pills and in postmenopausal women.
2. Hairpin-shaped capillary-loop appearance of vessels: These are commonly seen more prominently toward the original squamocolumnar junction. Near new squamocolumnar junction, there is presence of the tree-branching-like pattern.

The regular structure and decrease in the caliber of the vessels toward the ends of the branches suggest benign (normal) nature (Fig. 10.11).

Key Points

- The uterine cervix is the lowest part of the uterus protruding in the vagina.
- The cervix is a cylindrical and measures approximately 3–4 cm in height and ranges between 1 and 3 cm in diameter.
- The portio vaginalis is covered by stratified squamous epithelium, and essentially mucous membrane, which is five layered having basal cell layer, prickle cell layer, glycogenated cell layer, non-vacuolated flattened cell layer, and stratum corneum.
- Endocervix is composed of a single layer of tall, columnar cells.
- The cervical stroma consists of collagen interspersed with the arterioles, venules, and lymphatic vascular channels.
- According to new 2011 IFCPC classification, normal colposcopic finding includes the original squamous epithelium, columnar epithelium, ectopy, transformation zone, deciduosis of pregnancy, atrophic epithelium, nabothian cyst, and gland openings.
- The squamous epithelium is seen as a translucent smooth epithelium with a pinkish tinge, and the columnar epithelium is reddish in color.
- The original squamocolumnar junction is the junction between the original or native squamous epithelium and the metaplastic squamous epithelium.
- The new squamocolumnar junction is the line of demarcation where the metaplastic squamous and columnar epithelia meet.
- The area between the old and new squamocolumnar junction is the transformation zone.
- The vast majority of CIN changes occur in the transformation zone.

Suggested Reading

1. Baggish MS. Colposcopy of the cervix, vagina and vulva, a comprehensive textbook, 1st ed, section 2. Philadelphia: Mosby; 2003. p. 25–38.
2. Waxman AG, Diaz ML. HPV, colposcopy and prevention of squamous anogenital tract malignancy. Obstetrics & Gynecology Clinics of North America 2013; 40(2):235–51.
3. Sankaranarayanan R, Sellors JW. Colposcopy and treatment of cervical intraepithelial neoplasia, a beginner's manual, chap. 6. Lyon: International Agency for Research on Cancer; 2003. p. 45–54.

Colposcopic Evaluation of Preinvasive and Early Cervical Cancer

11

Sruthi Bhaskaran

Colposcopic assessment of the grade of abnormality and therefore the risk of progression is the key to the process of managing a screen-positive woman. In the presence of cytologic suspicion of low-grade or borderline smear reports, the decision to treat poses a dilemma to the colposcopist, and the ability to discriminate between low-grade from high-grade disease becomes of paramount importance, particularly in young women. To this end several attempts have been made to make colposcopic examination more objective and reproducible over the last decade, by introduction of new scoring systems and nomenclatures [1–5].

11.1 Atypical Transformation Zone (ATZ)

Normal transformation zone contains mature stratified squamous epithelium, squamous metaplasia, nabothian cysts, gland openings and normal arborising or fine reticular cells. Under the influence of HPV and oncogenic cofactors, the normal metaplastic epithelial cells are transformed to atypical metaplastic cells and result in an abnormal transformation zone. Abnormal transformation zone is characterised by blocks of epithelium exhibiting pleomorphism, nuclear atypia and disorganisation. These abnormal cells stimulate the capillary endothelial cells of adjacent capillaries, thus initiating an alteration of the vascular network. So, ATZ is manifested as a wide spectrum of epithelial and vascular findings. On ultrastructural level, the abnormal epithelial cells exhibit decreased glycogen and disruption of desmosomes.

In majority of cases, cervical neoplasia progresses through various stages of CIN to invasion over a period of time [6]. Colposcopically, the cellular transformation from metaplasia to atypia, then to intraepithelial neoplasia and invasion, results in

S. Bhaskaran
Department of Obstetrics and Gynecology, University College of Medical Sciences and Guru Teg Bahadur Hospital, Delhi, India
e-mail: sruthi_bhaskaran@yahoo.co.in

S. Mehta, P. Sachdeva (eds.), *Colposcopy of Female Genital Tract*,
DOI 10.1007/978-981-10-1705-6_11

characteristic features including leukoplakia, acetowhite epithelium, abnormal blood vessels (mosaic and punctation), atypical blood vessels and ulceration.

Accurate identification of the entire TZ and appropriate recognition of the colposcopic signs of CIN and invasive cancer are essential steps in the colposcopic examination.

Grade of lesion is assessed by evaluation of the transformation zone in terms of acetowhite epithelium, location, margins, vascular pattern (punctate, mosaic), atypical vessels and iodine negativity.

Lesion is assessed according to [7]

1. General principles: These include the location and size of the lesion.
2. Grade of the lesion: This is further assessed according to:
   (a) Acetowhiteness
   (b) Margins
   (c) Vascular pattern
3. Nonspecific changes: These include:
   (a) Leukoplakia
   (b) Erosion
   (c) Colour changes after application of Lugol's iodine
4. Suspicious for invasion:
   (a) Atypical vessels
   (b) Exophytic with irregular surface
   (c) Necrosis and ulceration
   (d) Tumour or gross neoplasm

11.2 General Principles

11.2.1 Location of the Lesion

A lesion within the transformation zone, as opposed to the one outside, has been shown to be an independent predictor of a high-grade lesion or carcinoma (odds ratio 8.60, 95 % confidence interval 1.2–63.4) [8].

The presence within transformation zone with proximity to the squamocolumnar junction (SCJ) is indicator of a higher-grade lesion. It is suggested that CIN2 or 3 begins as a small focus of highly dysplastic epithelium near SCJ, probably in an area of immature metaplasia, and eventually expands peripherally.

Also, it is important to determine whether the acetowhite epithelium is present on the squamous or columnar epithelium. If acetowhite epithelium is present on the columnar epithelium, it may represent metaplasia or glandular epithelial abnormality.

11.2.2 Size of Lesion

It can be measured as:

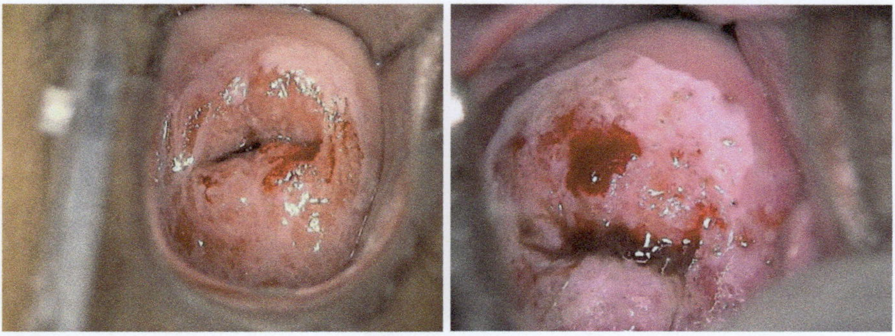

Fig. 11.1 and 11.2 Acetowhite epithelium

Percentage of the cervix involved – depending on the surface area of the cervix occupied by the lesion; it can be categorised as small (occupying <25 % of the cervix), medium (26–50 % of the cervix) or large (>50 % of the cervix).

Both large and medium lesions show an independent increased risk with odds ratio of 3.6 (OR, 2.1–6.3) and 2.0 (OR, 1.3–3.0), respectively [9].

Quadrants of the cervix involved – involvement of two or more quadrants of the cervix and a lesion involving both lips of the cervix indicate a high-grade lesion.

11.3 Grade of the Lesion

11.3.1 Acetowhite Epithelium

Epithelium that appears grossly normal but turns white after application of 3–5 % acetic acid is called an acetowhite epithelium (Figs. 11.1 and 11.2). The varying degrees of whiteness depend on whether metaplastic cells or abnormal cells are present. Acetic acid when applied to cells with enlarged nuclei and scanty cytoplasm, as in cervical intraepithelial neoplasia, causes temporary dehydration of the cells. Also, it transiently coagulates the increased amount of proteins present in abnormal cells. Light is reflected back by the dehydrated cells with overlapping enlarged nuclei, producing the acetowhite appearance of CIN.

Colour and duration: The degree to which the epithelium takes up the acetic acid stain is correlated with the colour tone or intensity, the surface shine, and the duration of the effect and, in turn, with the degree of neoplastic change in the lesion. Higher-grade lesions are more likely to turn dense white rapidly and remain visible longer than minor-grade lesions. A direct correlation exists between the intensity of the dull, white colour and the severity of the lesion. Grey white or dull oyster shell white, thickened epithelium indicates higher-grade lesion as compared to thin translucent epithelium of low-grade lesion.

If cytology report suggests glandular abnormality, carefully visualise the columnar epithelium. If intraepithelial neoplasia is present at the mouth of a glandular crypt, it may appear as a white-cuffed gland opening. These cuff gland openings

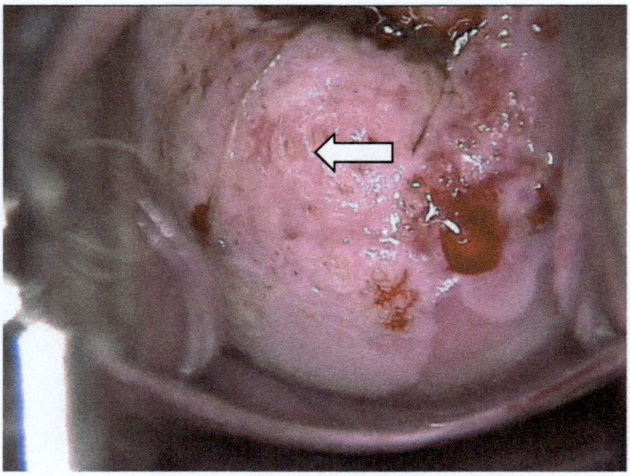

Fig. 11.3 Cuffed gland

should be easily distinguished from the faint rim of metaplastic epithelium surrounding normal gland openings (Fig. 11.3).

Colposcopic classification of gland (crypt) openings: Gland openings of the uterine cervix have been classified into five types for colposcopy [10]:

Type I: Normal gland opening
Type II: Gland opening surrounded by a narrow white ring
Type III: Gland opening surrounded by a rather indistinct white ring
Type IV: Gland opening surrounded by a distinct and mostly thickened white ring (doughnut-like)
Type V: Solid gland opening

In a study by Scheungraber et al., CIN was found to be present in 5 % of cases with Type I/II gland openings and in 46 % of cases with Type III gland openings. The rate of CIN was as high as 96 % in cases with Type IV/V gland openings [11].

11.3.2 Margins of the Lesion

Margins of the lesion are an important predictor of severity of the lesion. Lesions with feathered, finely scalloped, angular, irregular or geographic margin, flat lesions with indistinct borders, satellite lesions not contiguous with SCJ and lesions showing irregular surface that appears condylomatous or micropapillary contour indicate low-grade lesion.

Flat or raised lesion of symmetrical shape, with well-delineated sharp and straight peripheral margin, indicates high-grade lesion. Rolled-out margins due to cell-to-cell fragile cohesiveness leading to epithelial edges detaching from underlying stroma and curling back on themselves are also a sign of high-grade lesion.

It is possible to have varying degrees of acetowhiteness within the same lesion known as inner border.

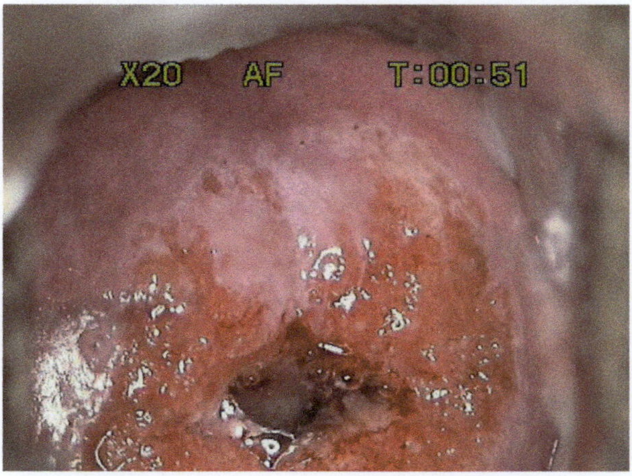

Fig. 11.4 Lesion within a lesion

Inner Border Sign The inner border is a dull, oyster white area, inside a less opaque acetowhite area (Fig. 11.4). The peripheral area represents an earlier, minor-grade change; the central area being the subsequent evolution of a high-grade CIN at the advancing edge of the new squamocolumnar junction with ageing [11]. Its significance lies during cervical biopsy. It is therefore important to sample the central lesion, because the central and peripheral lesions likely represent two different pathological processes in the same lesion.

In a study by Scheungraber et al., in 70 % of women with inner border sign, CIN2 or 3 was confirmed histologically. Though the sensitivity of the sign for detection of CIN2 or 3 was 20 %, the specificity was 97 %. There was a significant association between women younger than 35 years and CIN2 or 3 with inner border sign [12].

11.3.3 Surface Contour

As lesions become more severe, their surfaces tend to be less smooth and less reflective of light, compared to normal squamous epithelium. The surfaces can become irregular, elevated and nodular relative to the surrounding epithelium.

Ridge Sign It is an opaque lesion, adjacent to the squamocolumnar junction, which resembles mountain ridges (Fig. 11.5) [13, 14]. In a study by Scheungraber et al., CIN2 or 3 was diagnosed in 63.8 % of women with ridge sign. Sensitivity of ridge sign was 33.1 %, and specificity was 93.1 %.

11.3.4 Vascular Pattern

The arrangement of the terminal vessels in the stroma underlying squamous epithelium leads to colposcopic vascular findings which can be normal arborising vessels

Fig. 11.5 Ridge sign

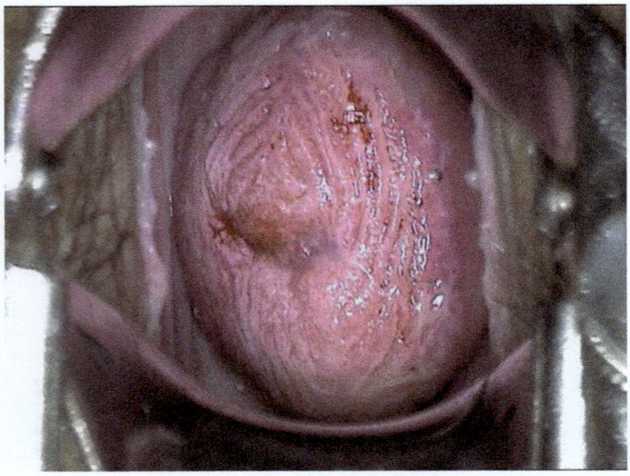

or abnormal vessels called punctate or mosaic [6]. Normal vessels usually run perpendicular to the surface.

Punctation is a colposcopic finding reflecting the capillaries in the stromal papillae that are seen end on and penetrate the epithelium.

When the stroma and accompanying capillaries are pressed between islands of squamous epithelium in a continuous fashion, a cobblestone pattern called *mosaic* is produced [15, 16].

If the punctation or mosaic is not located in the field of acetowhite epithelium, it is unlikely to be associated with CIN. These can be described either as fine or coarse.

Fine If the vessels are fine in calibre, regular and located close together, it is more likely a benign or low-grade CIN.

Coarse If the intercapillary distance of vessels is increased and they are coarser in appearance with larger calibre, it is usually a higher-grade lesion (CIN2, 3 and early preinvasive cancer) (Figs. 11.6 and 11.7).

Sometimes, the two patterns are superimposed in an area so that the capillary loops occur in the centre of each mosaic 'tile'. This appearance is called *umbilication*.

Many preinvasive lesions lack abnormal vessels and are identified only by acetowhite epithelium. So the lack of abnormal vasculature does not imply lack of significance. A high-grade lesion devoid of surface vessels is due to gradual compression and depression of the normal capillary looped vessels within a nuclear dense lesion, preventing them from being visualised. Also as the metabolic rate increases with high-grade lesions, vascular dilatation resists the constrictive effects of epithelial swelling, thus resulting in persistence of mosaic and punctuation patterns after application of acetic acid.

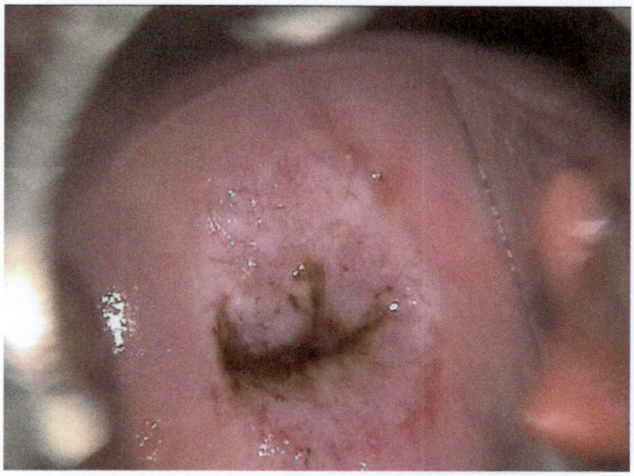

Fig. 11.6 Coarse mosaic

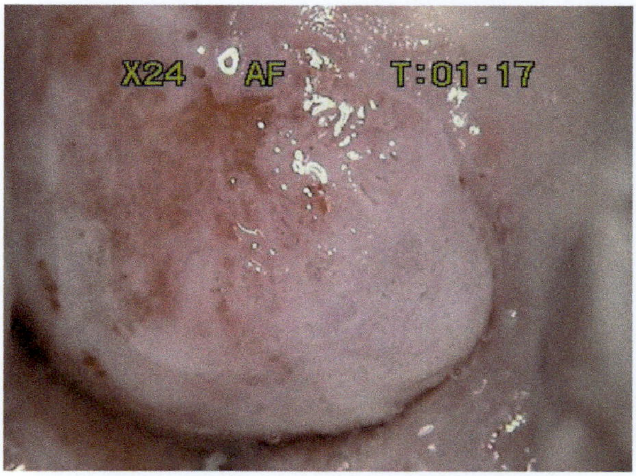

Fig. 11.7 Coarse punctation

Certain non-neoplastic epithelium exhibiting punctation and mosaic includes:

- Inflammatory conditions such as trichomoniasis (leopard skin appearance), gonorrhoea or chlamydial infections
- Active immature metaplasia

11.4 Nonspecific Changes

11.4.1 Uptake or Rejection of Iodine

Normal squamous epithelium cells are glycogenated and appear mahogany brown on application of dilute iodine. Normal columnar epithelium, *condylomata acuminata*, high-grade lesions and many low-grade lesions do not contain glycogen, reject iodine and appear either mustard yellow or a variegated uptake pattern. It is considered as a nonspecific finding in the new IFCPC classification 2011 [7].

11.4.2 Leukoplakia

It is a white plaque visible grossly even without the application of 3–5 % acetic acid. It is often seen as a raised area and is not necessarily confined to the TZ. Cytologically, leukoplakia is represented by hyperkeratosis or parakeratosis. Histologically, it may be represented as thickened, keratinised squamous epithelium. Depending on its adherence to the underlying epithelium, leukoplakia may be dislodged during cytologic sampling or after wiping the cervix with a cotton swab. It occurs as a result of irritation to the epithelium due to trauma, chronic infection or neoplasia. It should be biopsied to rule out neoplasia [17, 18].

11.4.2.1 Colposcopic Features of Low-Grade Lesions (Minor Change) [19]

- A smooth surface with an irregular outer border
- Slight acetowhite change, slow to appear and quick to disappear (Figs. 11.8 and 11.9)
- Fine punctation and fine regular mosaic
- Mild, often speckled iodine partial positivity

11.4.2.2 Colposcopic Features of High-Grade Lesions (Major Change) [7, 10, 19]

- Dense acetowhitening which appears rapidly and is slow to fade (Fig. 11.10 and 11.11)
- Smooth or irregular surface with sharp border, inner border sign or ridge sign
- Coarse mosaic or punctation
- Type IV or V cuffed gland (crypt) openings
- Nonuptake of iodine
- Dense acetowhite change in columnar epithelium

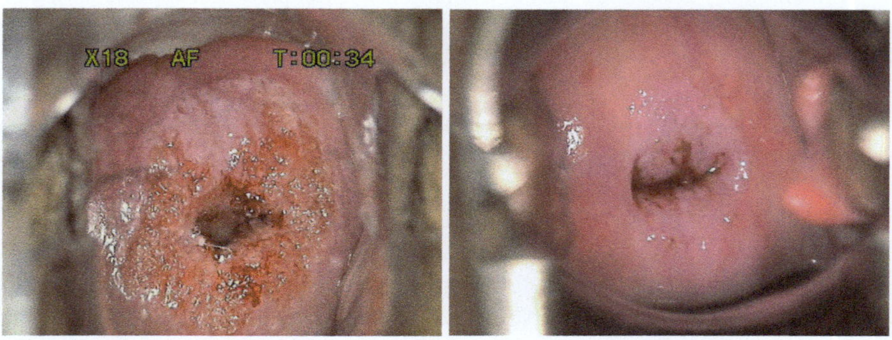

Fig. 11.8 and 11.9 Low-grade lesion

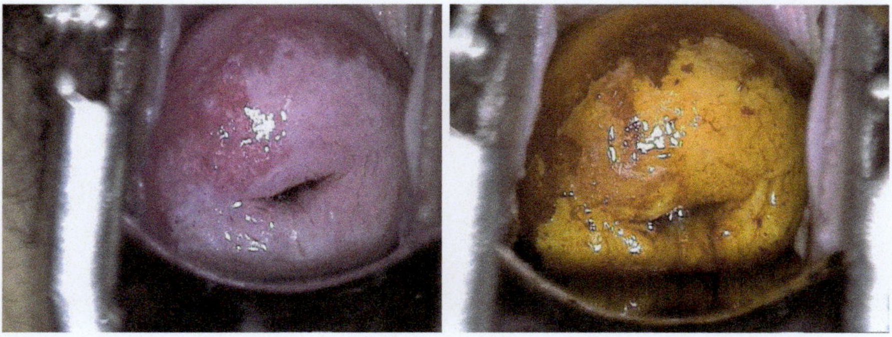

Fig. 11.10 and 11.11 High-grade lesion

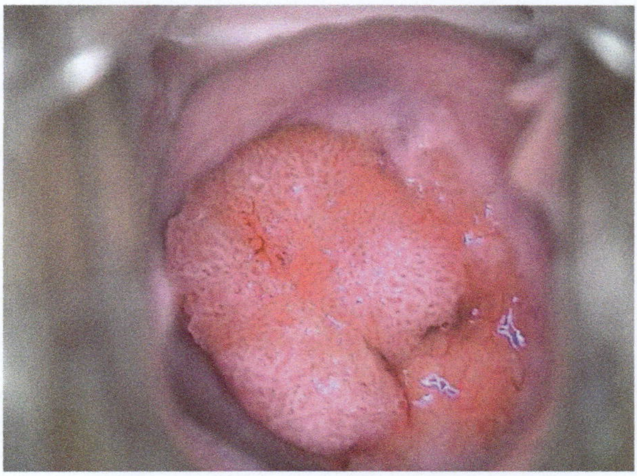

Fig. 11.12 Exophytic growth

11.5 Suspicious for Invasion

Colposcopic assessment of microinvasive or invasive disease can be difficult at times as the most severe lesions do not always demonstrate the most abnormal findings. The abnormal findings on colposcopy in such women are:

11.5.1 Exophytic Lesion

Invasive lesions mostly appear as an irregular exophytic mass (Fig. 11.12) but at times can be endophytic when they can be missed.

11.5.2 Atypical Vessels

Although atypical vessels are a hallmark of invasion, they can be associated with inflammation, post-radiation and condylomas (Fig. 11.13). When intraepithelial

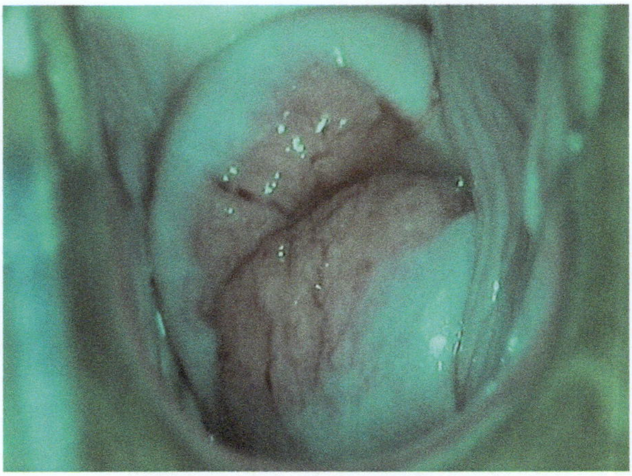

Fig. 11.13 Atypical vessels

lesions progresses to invasive lesion, tumour angiogenic factor (TAF) is released leading to development of aberrant vessels, known as atypical vessels with cork screw, comma or hairpin pattern [17]. As the severity of lesion progresses, the abnormal vessels may undergo transition to atypical vessels seen running bizarrely across the epithelium.

11.5.3 Ulcerations

When a breach of the epithelium occurs, the underlying stromal vessels are revealed, leading to a reddish appearance of the epithelium. These can result from trauma, infection or neoplasia. Careful colposcopic evaluation and directed biopsy is essential.

Following a traumatic event, the edges of the ulcer are usually normal in appearance. With high-grade lesions, there is decrease in the number of desmosomes accounting for finding of peeling of the underlying basement membrane producing erosion or rolled margin [20].

Rag Sign It is an iatrogenic small erosion of the epithelium generally caused when opaque acetowhite area at the squamocolumnar junction is mechanically abraded during either collection of smear for cytology or HPV testing (Fig. 11.14) [14].

Mostly women with invasive disease have a constellation of these findings. Liu et al. found that 40 % of women with microinvasive disease had mosaic, punctation and acetowhite epithelium, 37 % had only two findings and 5 % had no abnormal colposcopic findings. The sensitivity of colposcopy to detect microinvasive disease varies between 50 and 60 %.

11.5.3.1 Scoring the Lesion

There are two scoring systems which are commonly used to grade the severity of the lesion – modified Reid's colposcopic index (RCI) and the Swede System [4]

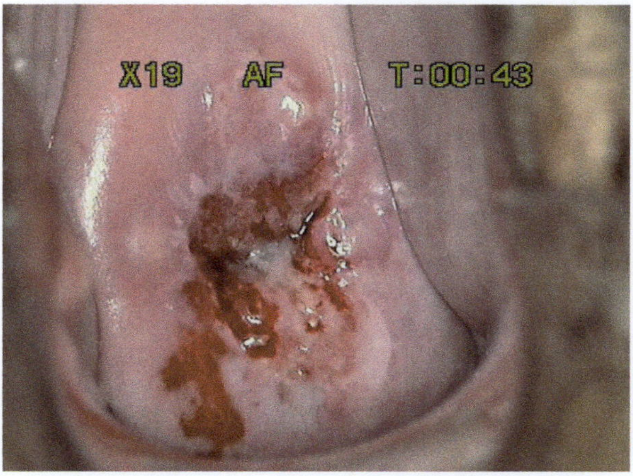

Fig. 11.14 Rag sign

(Annexure 8 and 9). This scoring system differs from the previous ones in that it includes lesion size which is an important predictor of high-grade lesions. It is simple and easy to understand. The details of scoring the lesion are given in Chap. 10.

11.5.3.2 Disadvantages of Colposcopy in Diagnosis of CIN

- Low specificity – though colposcopy is more sensitive than cytology in the presence of high-grade lesions, but this is at the cost-reduced specificity. Even changes induced by HPV infection or immature metaplasia can mimic CIN on colposcopy.
- Inadequate colposcopy – when the transformation zone is Type 2/3, the lesion may be partly or completely in the endocervical canal, and colposcopy for grading such cases is unreliable.
- Colposcopy is a subjective technique with results depending on the skill of the colposcopist. There is a high intra-observer variability among colposcopists in the diagnosis of CIN.

11.5.3.3 Accuracy of Colposcopy as a Diagnostic Modality

The diagnostic accuracy of colposcopy depends upon the competence of the examiner which, in turn, is dependent upon appropriate training and experience. Overall, there is only moderate correlation between colposcopic assessment and histological diagnosis [21–23]. Despite reporting of high variation in colposcopic performance, the sensitivity to distinguish normal from abnormal is relatively high. However, the sensitivity to distinguish low-grade lesions from high-grade lesions remains low and hence risk of overtreatment. Also, a substantial number of women with high-grade lesions may fail to be identified on colposcopy. Hence, new approaches continue to be evaluated to minimise the interobserver and intra-observer variability and improve colposcopic practice. This includes new grading systems such as the Swede score [4], Shafi–Nazeer index [24], etc. which incorporate new features to improve diagnosis, also new technologies such as digital imaging colposcopy, electric impedance spectroscopy, LUMA cervical imaging system, TruScreen, etc.

In a meta-analysis, colposcopy was found to be sensitive (96 %) for the detection of CIN2 with a specificity of 48 % [25]. Systematic review showed a positive predictive value of a colposcopic impression of CIN3 of 78 % [21]. The positive predictive value declined as severity of CIN decreased. In the ASCUS–LSIL Triage Study, immediate baseline colposcopy only identified 54 % to 56 % of cumulative CIN3 cases diagnosed over 2 years in women with atypical cells of undetermined significance or low-grade squamous intraepithelial lesions, respectively. In HPV vaccine trials, colposcopy underestimated CIN3+ in 57 % of cases [26, 27].

Conclusion

Colposcopic assessment of the grade of abnormality and therefore the risk of progression is the key to the process of managing the screen-positive women. It still remains an important tool in identification of atypical transformation zone, for defining the grade of the underlying lesion, for targeted biopsies and for excisional therapy.

Key Points

- Accurate identification of the entire TZ and appropriate recognition of the colposcopic signs of CIN and invasive cancer are essential steps in the colposcopic examination.
- Grade of lesion is assessed by evaluation of the transformation zone in terms of acetowhite epithelium, location, margins, vascular pattern (punctate, mosaic) and atypical vessels.
- A lesion within the transformation zone, as opposed to the one outside, has been shown to be an independent predictor of a high-grade lesion or carcinoma.
- Size of lesion can be assessed according to the percentage or quadrants of the cervix involved.
- The degree to which the epithelium takes up the acetic acid stain is correlated with the colour tone or intensity, the surface shine, and the duration of the effect and, in turn, with the degree of neoplastic change in the lesion.
- Low-grade lesions are characterised by a smooth surface with an irregular outer border and slight acetowhite change, slow to appear and quick to disappear, fine punctation and fine regular mosaic and mild, often speckled iodine partial positivity.
- High-grade lesion is characterised by dense acetowhitening, which appears rapidly and is slow to fade, smooth or irregular surface with sharp border, inner border sign or ridge sign, coarse mosaic or punctuation, Type IV or V cuffed gland (crypt) openings, nonuptake of iodine and dense acetowhite change in columnar epithelium.

References

1. Reid R, Scalzi P. Genital warts and cervical cancer. An improved colposcopic index for differentiating benign papillomavirus infections from high grade cervical intraepithelial neoplasia. Am J Obstet Gynecol. 1985;153:611–8.
2. Mousani AS, Fakour F, Giliani MM, et al. A prospective study to evaluate the correlation between Reid colposcopic index impression and biopsy histology. J Low Genit Tract Dis. 2007;11:147–50.
3. Seidl S. Reflection on the international colposcopic nomenclature. Geburstshilfe Frauenheilkd. 2005;65:1028–30.
4. Bowring J, Strander B, Young M, et al. The Swede score: evaluation of a scoring system designed to improve the predictive value of colposcopy. J Low Genit Tract Dis. 2010;14:301–5.
5. Strander B, Elstrom-Andeson A, Franzen S, et al. The performance of a new scoring system for colposcopy in detecting high grade dysplasia in the uterine cervix. Acta Obstet Gynecol Scand. 2005;84:1013–7.
6. Coppleson M, Dalrymple J, Atkinson K. Colposcopic differentiation of abnormalities arising in the transformation zone. Obstet Gynecol Clin North Am. 1993;20:83.
7. Bornstein J, Bentley J, Bosze P, et al. Colposcopic terminology of the international federation for cervical pathology and colposcopy. Obstet Gynecol. 2012;120:166–72.
8. Hammes LS, Naud P, Passos EP, et al. Value of the international federation for cervical pathology and colposcopy (IFCPC) terminology in predicting cervical disease. J Low Genit Tract Dis. 2007;11:158–65.
9. Ole K, Byrjalsen C, Hamen K, et al. Association between colposcopic findings and histology in cervical lesion: the significance of the size of the lesion. Gynecol Oncol. 1995;57:66–71.
10. Kishi Y. Colposcopy for gland (Crypt) openings. J Low Genit Tract Dis. 2006;10(2):79–82.
11. Kishi Y, Inui S, Sakamoto Y. Colposcopic findings of gland openings in cervical carcinoma: their histological background. Int J Gynecol Obstet. 1987;25:223–33.
12. Scheungraber C, Glutig K, Fechtel B, et al. Inner border – a specific and significant colposcopic sign for moderate or severe dysplasia. J Low Genit Tract Dis. 2009;13:1–4.
13. Scheungraber C, Koenig V, Fechtel B, et al. The colposcopic features ridge sign is associated with the presence of cervical intraepithelial neoplasia 2/3 and human papillomavirus 16 in young women. J Low Genit Tract Dis. 2009;13:13–6.
14. Vercellino G, Erdemoglu E, Chiantera V, et al. Validity of the colposcopic criteria: inner border sign, ridge sign and rag sign for detection of high grade cervical intraepithelial neoplasia. Obstet Gynecol. 2013;121:624–31.
15. Coppleson M, Pixley E, Reid B. Colposcopy. Springfield: Charles C Thomas; 1971. p. 14–6, 53–110, 155–192.
16. Burghardt E. Premalignant conditions of the cervix. Clin Obstet Gynecol. 1976;3:257.
17. Ferency A, Wright T. Anatomy and histology of the cervix. In: Kurman R, editor. Blaustein's pathology of the female genital tract. 4th ed. New York: Springer; 1994.
18. Gray LA. Colposcopy. In: Dysplasia, carcinoma in-situ and microinvasive cancer of the cervix uteri. Springfield: Charles C Thomas; 1964. p. 246–9.
19. Walker P, DePalo G, Campion M, Jakob C, Ray M. International terminology of colposcopy: an updated report from the International Federation for Cervical Pathology and Colposcopy. Obstet Gynecol. 2003;101:175–7.
20. Richart R. Cervical intraepithelial neoplasia. Pathol Ann. 1973;8:301.
21. Hopman EH, Voorhorst FJ, Kenemans P, et al. Observer agreement on interpreting colposcopic images of CIN. Gynecol Oncol. 1995;58:206–9.
22. Etherington IJ, Dunn J, Shafi MI, et al. Videocolpography: a new technique for secondary cervical screening. Br J Obstet Gynecol. 1997;104:150–3.

23. Etherington IJ, Lusley DM, Shafi MI, et al. Observer validity among colposcopists from the west midlands region. Br J Obstet Gynecol. 1997;104:1380–4.
24. Shafi MI, Nazeer S. Colposcopy: a practical guide. Slisury: Fivepin Publishing; 2006.
25. Mitchell MF, Scottenfeld D, Tortolero-lung G, et al. Colposcopy for the diagnosis of squamous intraepithelial lesions: a meta-analysis. Obstet Gynecol. 1998;91:626–31.
26. Schiffman M, Soloman D. Findings to date from the ASCUS-LSIL triage study (ALTS). Arch Pathol Lab Med. 2003;127:946–9.
27. ALTS group. Results of a randomized trial on the management of cytology interpretation of atypical squamous cells of undetermined significance. Am J Obstet Gynecol. 2003;188: 1383–92.

Preinvasive Lesions in Pregnancy and Menopause

12

Aruna Nigam, Sumedha Sharma, and Pikee Saxena

12.1 Introduction

The incidence of CIN complicating pregnancy is reported to be 2000–8000 per 100,000 pregnancies [1]. Almost 1 % of women in the reproductive age group who are screened annually will be diagnosed with varying degrees of cervical intraepithelial neoplasia (CIN) [2]. The peak incidence of CIN 3 is around the age of 30 which coincides with the age of first pregnancy. The exact incidence of cervical cancer in pregnancy is lacking but is estimated to be 1.5–12 per 100,000 pregnancies [3]. Overall, 3 % of cases of newly diagnosed cervical cancer occur in pregnant women [4].

12.2 Cervical Cancer Screening in Pregnancy

Pregnancy is a unique period for screening and diagnosis of preinvasive and invasive lesions of uterine cervix. On one hand, pregnancy brings women in contact with the health system, thereby providing an opportunity for screening them, but on the other hand, the physiological changes associated with pregnancy make interpretation of various screening tests and performance of diagnostic procedures difficult.

There are no clear guidelines regarding screening for preinvasive lesions during pregnancy. The UK National Health Service Cervical Screening Programme

A. Nigam, MS (✉) • S. Sharma, MS
Department of Obstetrics and Gynecology, Hamdard Institute of Medical Sciences and Research, Jamia Hamdard, Delhi, India
e-mail: prakasharuna@hotmail.com

P. Saxena, MD
Department of Obstetrics and Gynecology, Lady Hardinge Medical College and Associated SSK Hospital, Delhi, India

S. Mehta, P. Sachdeva (eds.), *Colposcopy of Female Genital Tract*,
DOI 10.1007/978-981-10-1705-6_12

(NHSCSP) advises against the routine screening and treatment of CIN during pregnancy [5]. However if women with CIN lesion become pregnant, the follow-up should be done as scheduled. It has been suggested that in countries wherever organized screening programs are not available, screening by cytological examination or by visual screening methods such as VIA or VILI should be encouraged.

12.3 Natural History of CIN in Pregnancy

The risk of progression of preinvasive lesions of cervix during pregnancy is very low [6]. Ilancheran A et al. found spontaneous postpartum regression of CIN 2/CIN 3 in 70 % of pregnant patients and progression to CIN 3 in only 7 % [7]. It has been suggested that regression of CIN during pregnancy may be attributable to cervical trauma from birth or transient ischemic changes in the cervical epithelium leading to activation of inflammation and repair mechanisms thereafter [8]. Many authors have supported this hypothesis of postpartum regression in their studies [9, 10]. Ahdoot et al. reported spontaneous regression of CIN 2/CIN 3 in 60 % of women who delivered vaginally but in none of the patients who delivered by cesarean section [11]. It is still controversial whether the mode of delivery plays a role in regression of CIN in the postpartum period [12, 13].

12.4 Methods for Screening of CIN During Pregnancy

12.4.1 Cervical Cytology (Pap Smear)

Cervical sampling (Pap test) can safely be performed in pregnancy. The ectocervix is sampled using an Ayre's spatula and the endocervix using a Cytobrush.

The interpretation of cytologic smears in pregnancy is difficult due to:

- The hormonal changes affecting the squamous and glandular epithelium.
- Decidual cells which are hypervacuolated cells with large nuclei and variably staining cytoplasm may mimic dysplastic cells.
- The number of inflammatory cells and immature metaplastic cells are more.
- The presence of cytotrophoblasts and syncytiotrophoblasts may mimic moderate to severe dysplasia.
- Hyperplasia and reactive atypia in squamous and glandular epithelial cells combined with the Arias-Stella reaction make it more difficult to identify atypical glandular cells on cytological specimens [14].

In spite of the above difficulties, the accuracy of Pap test in pregnancy is equivalent to the nonpregnant state, and both conventional and liquid-based cytologies demonstrate similar diagnostic features in pregnant and nonpregnant patients [15].

12.4.2 Colposcopy

Colposcopy can be safely performed in pregnancy and is not associated with any adverse fetal outcomes or complications. However, significant experience and expertise is required for interpreting colposcopic findings in pregnancy. The indications for colposcopy in pregnancy are same as for nonpregnant women.

12.4.2.1 Indications

- For follow-up of histologically confirmed CIN in women who became pregnant prior to definitive treatment
- Abnormal cervical cytological results from opportunistic screening at the time of booking visit
- Abnormal cervical cytological results in women who have become pregnant while awaiting referral to colposcopy
- To exclude early cervical cancer in women who have repeated antepartum hemorrhage in the absence of another obvious cause

12.4.2.2 Procedural Difficulties During Colposcopy

- The cervix is hypertrophied, hyperemic, and friable which may lead to traumatic bleeding [16, 17]. The vaginal walls are lax and tend to protrude from the sides, thereby blocking visibility of the cervix. To retract the vaginal walls, a large-sized Cusco's speculum with a condom whose closed end has been removed may be used (Fig. 12.1, 12.2, and 12.3).
- Cervical mucus plug is copious and tenacious in pregnancy (due to hormonal stimulation) and may be difficult to remove.
- The vascular changes and features of squamous metaplasia appear exaggerated during pregnancy and may lead to difficulty in differentiating it from low-grade dysplasia (Fig. 12.4).
- Deciduosis in pregnancy may mimic high-grade lesions or malignancy. It appears colposcopically as dense acetowhite areas around lacy superficial capillaries. Normal capillaries may also have thin acetowhite areas all around due to decidualized stroma called as "starry sky appearance."
- Cervical ectropion (Fig. 12.5) is a normal finding in pregnancy. This makes visualization of the squamocolumnar junction (SCJ) and transformation zone (TZ) easier. If however colposcopy in the first trimester is inadequate, it should be repeated in the second trimester when visualization of SCJ junction and TZ becomes easier.

If a pregnant woman requires colposcopic or cytological examination after treatment for CIN or follow-up of untreated CIN, her review can safely be postponed until after delivery, unless it is the first clinical review following treatment for CIN 2/CIN 3 with involved or uncertain margin status. If repeat cytological examination is due and the woman has defaulted from a follow-up appointment prior to pregnancy, consideration should be given to her undergoing cytological or colposcopic examination during pregnancy.

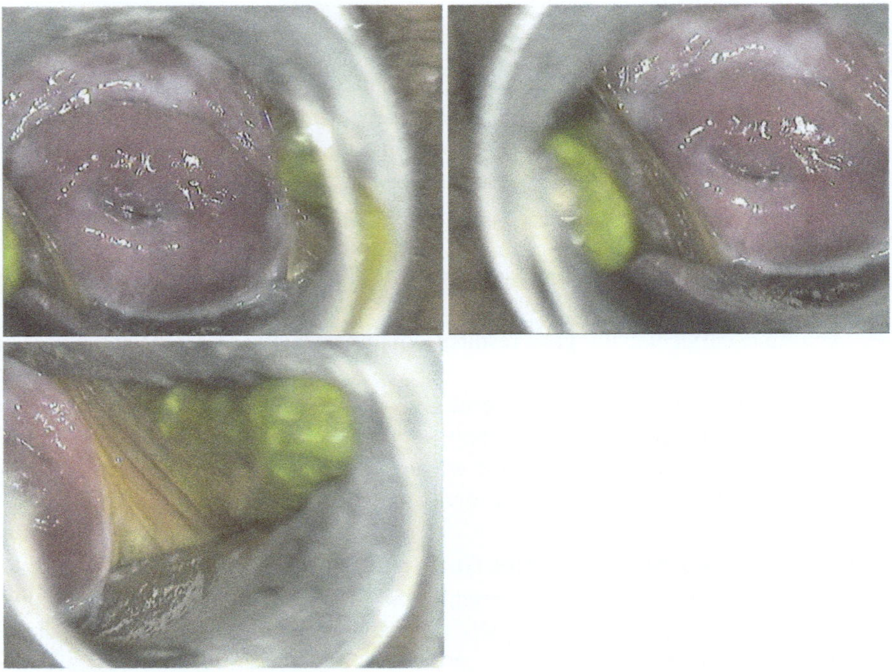

Fig. 12.1, 12.2 and 12.3 Condom over the Cusco's speculum preventing the vaginal walls from coming in the field

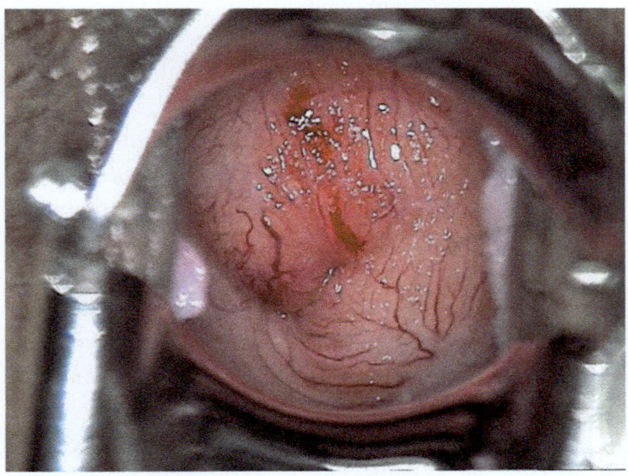

Fig. 12.4 Hyperemia of the cervix showing prominent vessels but maintaining the normal pattern

12.4.3 Cervical Biopsy

Biopsy should only be performed in pregnancy for high-grade CIN or invasive lesions. When invasive disease is suspected, conventional punch biopsies may not be adequate as they may fail to give a representative sample and microinvasion

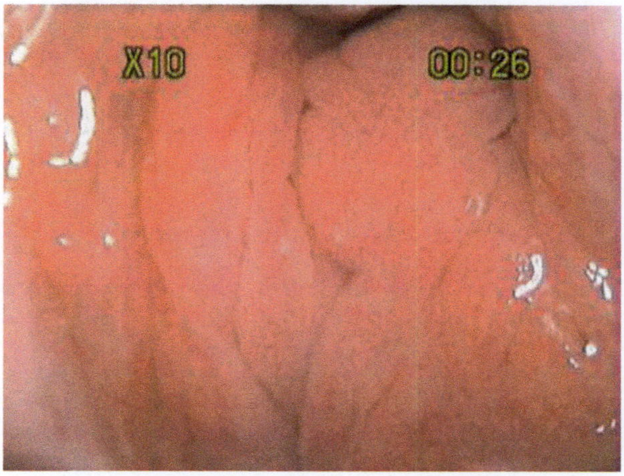

Fig. 12.5 Hypertrophied endocervical mucosa

cannot be ruled out with certainty. Multiple punch biopsies are also not advisable as they may cause trauma and significant bleeding [18]. Therefore, a wedge biopsy from the suspicious area identified colposcopically is taken. This procedure should be done in the operating theater as there is a significant risk of hemorrhage; silver nitrate or Monsel's paste can be applied for hemostasis. In case of excessive bleeding, suturing or vaginal packing may also be done. Endocervical curettage (ECC) is not recommended in pregnancy [19]. Decisions regarding the need for a wedge biopsy and the procedure itself should be performed by an experienced clinician with relevant expertise.

12.5 Management of Abnormal Cytology During Pregnancy

1. *Atypical squamous cells of undetermined significance* (*ASC-US*)

   Management options for pregnant women with ASC-US are identical to those described for nonpregnant women, with the exception that deferring colposcopy until 6 weeks postpartum is acceptable [20]:

   - For young women between 21 and 24 years of age, repeat cytology at 1 year is preferred.
   - For women >24 years of age, HPV testing is preferred, and if HPV is negative, then co-testing at 3 years is recommended. If HPV is positive, then colposcopy is to be performed (this can be deferred until 6 weeks postpartum).
   - For women with ASC-US cytology and no HPV result, repeat cytology at 1 year is acceptable.
   - For pregnant women who have no cytologic, histologic, or colposcopically suspected CIN 2+ at the initial colposcopy, postpartum follow-up is recommended.
   - ECC is not to be performed for inadequate colposcopy.

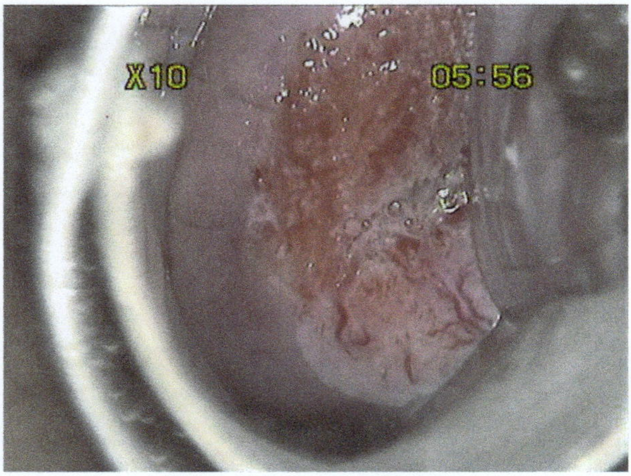

Fig. 12.6 Colposcopy showing mosaic pattern and CIN 2 lesion

2. *Atypical squamous cells-cannot exclude high-grade squamous intraepithelial lesions* (*ASC-H*)

   Women with ASC-H should undergo a colposcopic examination in pregnancy as the risk of CIN 2/CIN 3 on colposcopic-directed biopsy is as high as 50% [21].

3. *Low-grade squamous intraepithelial lesion* (*LSIL*)
   (a) For pregnant women aged 21–24 years with LSIL, follow-up with cytology at 12-month interval is recommended; colposcopy is not recommended. At 12-month follow-up, women with ASC-H or HSIL are recommended for colposcopy. If cytology is ASC-US or LSIL, then repeat cytology at 12 months is recommended. For women with ASC-US or worse at the 24-month follow-up, colposcopy is recommended. For women with two consecutive negative results, return to routine screening is recommended.
   (b) For pregnant women >24 years with LSIL, colposcopy is preferred, but deferring colposcopy till 6 weeks postpartum is acceptable. ECC is not to be performed even if the colposcopy is inadequate or no lesion is identified.

   If there is no cytologic, histologic, or colposcopically suspected CIN 2+ at the initial colposcopy, postpartum follow-up is recommended. Additional colposcopic and cytologic examinations during pregnancy are unacceptable for these women.

4. *High-grade squamous intraepithelial lesions* (*HSIL*)(Fig. 12.6)

   Pregnant women with HSIL should undergo colposcopy with biopsy of any lesion suspicious of CIN 2/CIN 3 or cancer. Women without CIN 2/CIN 3 on biopsy do not require further evaluation during pregnancy; however, ECC is not to be performed in pregnancy.

5. *Atypical glandular cells or cytologic adenocarcinoma in situ* (*AGC or cytologic AIS*)

Pregnant women should be evaluated with colposcopy and biopsy, but endocervical curettage or endometrial sampling is not to be performed because of the risk of pregnancy-related complications. Studies have suggested that 9–38 % of women with a Pap showing AGC have high-grade CIN or adenocarcinoma in situ and an additional 3–17% of women have invasive cancer.

6. *CIN 1*

   Pregnant women with CIN 1 on histology need to be followed up without any treatment.

7. *CIN 2/3*

   In women remote from term and with absence of any invasive disease, follow-up with repeat colposcopy and cytology at an interval of 12 weeks is recommended. Repeat biopsy is to be performed only if the appearance of the lesion worsens or if cytology suggests invasive cancer. However, deferring reevaluation until 6 weeks postpartum is also acceptable. At postpartum follow-up, a repeat cytology and colposcopy should be done to account for any regression of lesions.

12.5.1 Excisional Biopsy and Treatment During Pregnancy

A diagnostic excisional procedure/LEEP is recommended only if invasion is suspected as it leads to increase in preterm births and also increases the risk of cesarean deliveries. If required, it should preferably be performed in the second trimester of pregnancy under general anesthesia.

A recent meta-analysis has estimated twofold increase in risk of preterm deliveries and other pregnancy complications after excisional procedures in pregnancy [22]. There is also an excessively high risk of incomplete excision and disease persistence [23, 24]. Therefore, special consideration should be given to young women between 21 and 24 years age and to women who have not completed childbearing.

12.5.2 Glandular Lesions During Pregnancy

The natural history and implications of glandular atypia in pregnancy are poorly understood. In nonpregnant women, glandular atypia is often associated with squamous lesions; therefore, these women require a close follow-up with colposcopy during pregnancy, and biopsy of suspicious areas should be taken in the postpartum period [20].

Line diagram 1 shows the outline of management of abnormal smear during pregnancy

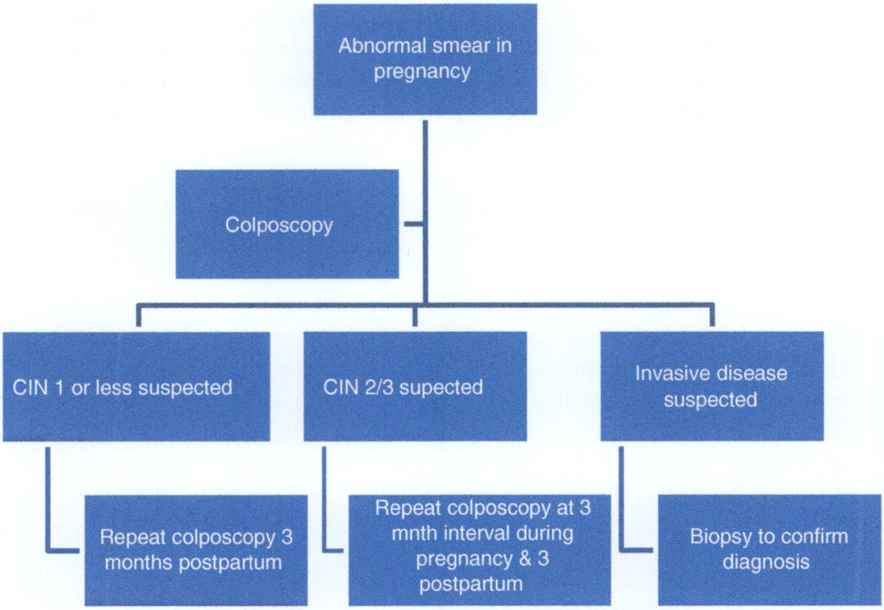

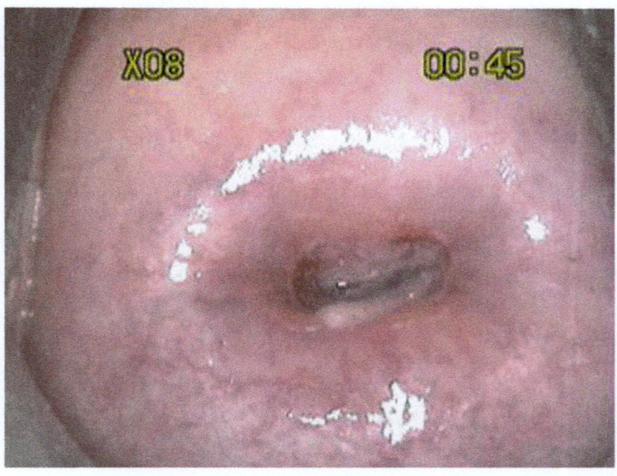

Fig. 12.7 Cervix in a menopausal female showing regression of SC junction into endocervical canal

12.6 CIN and Menopause

The physiological changes affecting the cervix after menopause bring challenges for interpretation of cervical cytology and colposcopy. The decreased estrogen levels result in reduced thickness of squamous epithelium and decrease in cytoplasmic glycogen, stromal vascularity, and cervical mucus. There is a reduction in the size of the cervix and regression of the transformation zone into the endocervical canal (Fig. 12.7).

12.6.1 Cytology Screening

According to ACS and ACOG guidelines, women >65 years of age with normal screening results in last 10 years do not require further screening for cervical cancers and precursors [25].

12.6.2 Cervical Cytology in Postmenopausal Women

The smears are usually dry and atrophic. The cell yield is low because of poor cellular exfoliation and inadequate sampling from the small endocervical canal. The cytoplasm appears eosinophilic with nuclear pyknosis and karyorrhexis. There is a background of senile inflammatory changes. The smears are dominated by basal and parabasal cells with reduced cytoplasm and increased nuclear cytoplasmic ratio. Endocervical glands are often absent. These findings make differentiation from abnormal dysplastic cells difficult. Many times dysplastic glandular cells may be seen which might originate from endocervical canal, endometrium, ovary, or fallopian tubes.

12.6.3 Colposcopy in Postmenopausal Women

Due to senile changes, the introitus is small and the vaginal walls are lax. As the squamous epithelium is thin, speculum insertion may lead to traumatic hemorrhages which appear as petechiae. An appropriate-sized speculum should be used to prevent trauma. The cervix is pale and may be flushed with the vagina. The squamocolumnar junction regresses into the endocervical canal, and as a result it cannot be visualized in its entirety. Toplis et al. reported complete visualization of the transformation zone in only 47 % of postmenopausal women [26]. Similarly, another study reported inversion of the transformation zone in 60 % of women who were more than 50 years of age [27]. These changes can be temporarily reversed by short-term course of exogenous estrogen which leads to better assessment of suspicious lesions. Both ethinyl estradiol and conjugated estrogen can be used for the purpose.

In postmenopausal women, obtaining biopsy from the cervix is also difficult as the cervix is small and tends to slip away from the biopsy forceps. Therefore, biopsy forceps with tooth at both ends of the blades should be used such as Tischler Morgan forceps.

12.7 Abnormal Cytology

1. *ASC-US*

   The management in postmenopausal women is the same as women in general population. They should preferably undergo HPV testing, but follow-up with cytology at 1 year is also acceptable. If the results are ≥ ASC or HPV positive, then colposcopy is required to identify the lesion. If colposcopy is inadequate or no lesion is identified, endocervical sampling is preferred.

For women >65 years considering exit from routine screening, ASC-US with HPV negative is considered abnormal. They require follow-up at 1 year by co-testing, but cytology alone is also acceptable.

2. *LSIL*

   Women with no HPV results can be triaged to either HPV testing, cytology at 6 and 12 months, or colposcopy. If HPV is positive or cytology ≥ ASC-US, then colposcopy is to be performed. If two consecutive cytology results are negative, then these women can return to routine screening.

3. *HSIL/AGC*

   The management of HSIL in menopausal women is the same as the general population with colposcopy (with endocervical assessment) and directed biopsy or LEEP.

   Women with AGC should undergo colposcopy with endocervical sampling and endometrial sampling.

4. *ASC-H*

   Women should undergo colposcopy and directed biopsy irrespective of HPV status.

Key Points

- Pregnancy is a unique period for screening and diagnosis of preinvasive and invasive lesions of the uterine cervix.
- There are no clear guidelines regarding screening for preinvasive lesions during pregnancy.
- It has been suggested that in countries where organized screening programs are not available, screening by cytological examination or by application of acetic acid is a good opportunity to detect the high-risk females who might otherwise not turn up for the checkup.
- There is a reported regression of CIN lesions during pregnancy and postpartum period which may be attributable to cervical trauma from birth or transient ischemic changes in the cervical epithelium and the subsequent activation of inflammation and repair mechanisms.
- The interpretation of cytologic smears in pregnancy is difficult due to the hormonal changes affecting the squamous and glandular epithelium.
- Colposcopy can be safely performed in pregnancy and is not associated with any adverse fetal outcomes or complications. However, significant experience and expertise is required for interpreting colposcopic findings in pregnancy.
- Excisional procedures like LEEP should only be performed in pregnant women with suspected malignancy as it is associated with morbidity such as preterm births and increased risk of cesarean deliveries.

- The decreased estrogen levels result in reduced thickness of squamous epithelium and decreased cytoplasmic glycogen, stromal vascularity, and cervical mucus during menopause.
- The Pap smears are usually dry and atrophic in menopausal females. The cell yield is low because of poor cellular exfoliation and inadequate sampling from the small endocervical canal. The cytoplasm appears eosinophilic with nuclear pyknosis and karyorrhexis.
- Colposcopic examination is many times unsatisfactory in menopausal women because the squamocolumnar junction cannot be visualized in its entirety due to its regression into the endocervical canal.

References

1. Amant F, Brepoel S, Halaaska MJ, et al. Gynaecological cancer complicating pregnancy: an overview. Best Pract Res Clin Obstet Gynaecol. 2010;24:61–79.
2. Insinga RP, Glass AG, Rush BB. Diagnoses and outcomes in cervical cancer screening: a population based study. Am J Obstet Gynecol. 2004;191:105.
3. Hunter MI, Tewari K, Monk BJ. Cervical neoplasia in pregnancy. Part 2: current treatment of invasive disease. Am J Obstet Gynecol. 2008;199:10–8.
4. Mcintyre-Seltman K, Lesnock JL. Cervical cancer screening in pregnancy. Obstet Gynecol Clin North Am. 2008;35:645–58.
5. Luesley D, Leeson S. Colposcopy and programme management. Guidelines for the NHS Cervical Screening Programme. 2nd ed. Sheffield: NHS Cancer Screening Programmes; 2010.
6. Owens GL, Kitchener HC. Premalignant disease in the genital tract in pregnancy. Best Pract Res Clin Obstet Gynaecol. 2015. http://dx.doi.org/10.1016/j.bpobgyn.2015.10.009.
7. Ilancheran A, Low J, Ng JS. Gynaecological cancer in pregnancy. Best Pract Res Clin Obstet Gynaecol. 2012;26:371–7.
8. Paraskevaidis E, Koliopoulos G, Kalantaridou S, et al. Management and evolution of cervical intraepithelial neoplasia during pregnancy and postpartum. Eur J Obstet Gynecol Reprod Biol. 2002;104:67–9.
9. Coppola A, Sorosky J, Casper R, et al. The clinical course of cervical carcinoma in situ diagnosed during pregnancy. Gynecol Oncol. 1997;67:162–5.
10. Kaneshiro BE, Acoba JD, Holzman J, et al. Effect of delivery route on natural history of cervical dysplasia. Am J Obstet Gynecol. 2005;192:1452–4.
11. Ahdoot D, Van Nostrand KM, Nguyen NJ, et al. The effect of route of delivery on regression of abnormal cervical cytologic findings in the postpartum period. Am J Obstet Gynecol. 1998;178:1116–20.
12. Yost NP, Santoso JT, McIntire DD, et al. Postpartum regression rates of antepartum cervical intraepithelial neoplasia II and III lesions. Obstet Gynecol. 1999;93:359–62.
13. Kaplan KJ, Dainty LA, Dolinsky B, et al. Prognosis and recurrence risk for patients with cervical squamous intraepithelial lesions diagnosed during pregnancy. Cancer. 2004;102:228–32.
14. Connolly TP, Evans AC. Atypical Papanicolaou smear in pregnancy. Clin Med Res. 2005;3:13–8.
15. Morimura Y, Fujimori K, Soeda S, et al. Cervical cytology during pregnancy comparison with non-pregnant women and management of pregnant women with abnormal cytology. Fukushima J Med Sci. 2002;48:27–37.
16. Flannelly G. The management of women with abnormal cervical cytology in pregnancy. Best Pract Res Clin Obstet Gynaecol. 2010;24:51–60.

17. Van Calsteren K, Vergote I, Amant F. Cervical neoplasia during pregnancy: diagnosis, management and prognosis. Best Pract Res Clin Obstet Gynaecol. 2005;19:611–30.
18. Freeman-Wang T, Walker P. Colposcopy in special circumstances: pregnancy, immunocompromised, including HIV and transplants, adolescence and menopause. Best Pract Res Clin Obstet Gynaecol. 2011;25:653–65.
19. Wright Jr TC, Massad LS, Dunton CJ, et al. 2006 Consensus guidelines for the management of women with abnormal cervical cancer screening tests. Am J Obstet Gynecol. 2007;197:346–55.
20. Massad LS, Einstein MH, Huh WK, Katki HA, Kinney WK, Schiffman M, Solomon D, Wentzensen N, Lawson HW, 2012 ASCCP Consensus Guidelines Conference. 2012 Updated consensus guidelines for the management of abnormal cervical cancer screening tests and cancer precursors. J Low Genit Tract Dis. 2013;17(5):S1–27.
21. Wetta L, Matthews K, Kemper M. The management of cervical intraepithelial neoplasia in pregnancy: is colposcopy necessary? J Low Genit Tract Dis. 2009;13(3):182–5.
22. Bruinsma FJ, Quinn MA. The risk of preterm birth following treatment for precancerous changes in the cervix: a systematic review and meta-analysis. BJOG. 2011;118:1031–41.
23. LaPolla JP, O'Neill C, Wetrich D. Colposcopic management of abnormal cervical cytology in pregnancy. J Reprod Med. 1988;33:301–6.
24. Robinson WR, Webb S, Tirpack J, et al. Management of cervical intraepithelial neoplasia during pregnancy with LOOP excision. Gynecol Oncol. 1997;64:153–5.
25. Saslow D, Solomon D, Lawson HW, et al. American cancer society, american society for colposcopy and cervical pathology, and american society for clinical pathology screening guidelines for the prevention and early detection of cervical cancer. CA: a cancer journal for clinicians. 2012;62(3):147–72. doi:10.3322/caac.21139.
26. Toplis PJ, Casemore V, Hallam N, Charnock M. Evaluation of colposcopy in postmenopausal women. Br J Obstet Gynaecol. 1986;93:843–51.
27. Cronipron AC. The cervical epithelium during the menopause. In: Jordan J, Singer A, editors. The cervix. London: WB Saunders; 1976. p. 128–33.

Colposcopic Examination in Pregnancy 13

Sumita Mehta and Anshuja Singla

Cervical cancer is the most commonly diagnosed gynecological malignancy during pregnancy with an incidence of 0.5–12/10,000 pregnancies. Pregnancy does not increase the risk for cervical dysplasia or neoplasia with abnormal cytology being seen in 1.26–2.2 % of pregnant women. Histologically diagnosed cervical intraepithelial neoplasia (CIN) is found in 0.19–0.53 % of pregnant women, but cervical carcinoma is rare [1, 2]. Pregnancy also has no effect on progression or prognosis of cervical cancer.

13.1 Cervix and Pregnancy

Pregnancy alters the anatomical, physiologic, cytologic, and histologic milieu of the cervix, thereby changing the colposcopic interpretation. The changes in the cervix during pregnancy have been discussed in detail in Chap. 3. The colposcopist has to have the required expertise and an eye for detecting the difference between the normal and abnormal changes in the pregnant cervix.

13.2 Aims of Colposcopy During Pregnancy

1. To exclude invasive disease
2. To defer biopsy or treatment until the woman has delivered

S. Mehta (✉)
Babu Jagjivan Ram Memorial Hospital, Delhi, India
e-mail: sumitadr@gmail.com

A. Singla
Department of Obstetrics and Gynecology, University College of Medical Sciences and Guru Teg Bahadur Hospital, Delhi, India

S. Mehta, P. Sachdeva (eds.), *Colposcopy of Female Genital Tract*,
DOI 10.1007/978-981-10-1705-6_13

The safety of delaying treatment of pregnant women has been shown in a number of cohort and retrospective uncontrolled studies [3–5]. The incidence of invasive cervical cancer in pregnancy is low, and pregnancy itself has no adverse effect on the prognosis. Of the dysplasia cases diagnosed in pregnancy, 10–70 % regress, persistence of severity is seen in 25–47 %, and progression is reported in only 3–30 % [6].

13.3 Indications for Colposcopy in Pregnancy

The indications for colposcopy in pregnant women are similar to the ones in non-pregnant women:

- Women with cervical abnormalities suggestive of high-grade squamous lesions (to exclude invasive disease).
- All glandular lesions on cytology.
- Persistent postcoital bleeding or suspicious-looking cervix. A woman with unexplained persistent bleeding in pregnancy especially postcoital should have a speculum examination, cytology, and colposcopy [7].

The recommendations of SOGC Joint Clinical Practice Guideline (2012) of managing abnormal cytology in pregnancy are [8]:

1. Women with ASC-US or LSIL test should have repeat cytology testing at 3 months postpartum. This practice is safe as the rate of cancer in this group is low [9].
2. Pregnant women with HSIL, ASC-H, or AGC should be referred for colposcopy within 4 weeks.

13.4 Normal Colposcopic Changes in Pregnancy

The colposcopic appearance of the cervix changes dramatically throughout pregnancy. The most important changes seen are shown in Table 13.1

13.4.1 Increased Vascularity of the Cervix (Figs. 13.1 and 13.2)

Increased vascularity of the cervix and vasodilatation result in prominent vascular patterns of mosaic and punctation which can lead to an overestimation of the degree of atypia.

Table 13.1 Colposcopic changes of the cervix in pregnancy

Increased prominence of vascular patterns
Decreased prominence of acetowhite epithelium
Immature metaplasia difficult to distinguish from low-grade squamous lesion
Decidual changes – atypical vascular pattern, polypoid, less intense acetowhite staining
Fine punctation and mosaic pattern within metaplasia, leading to misdiagnosis of lesion

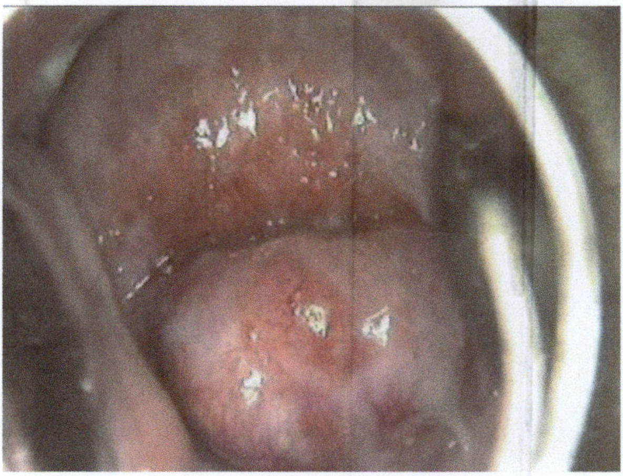

Fig. 13.1 Increased vascularity of pregnant cervix

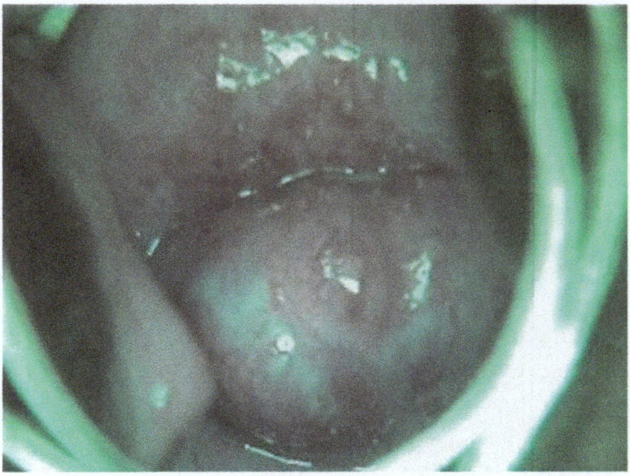

Fig. 13.2 Cervix as seen through *green* filter

Vasodilatation causes intraepithelial blood vessels to be larger so that patterns of mosaic and punctation appear coarser, thereby adding to the confusion.

13.4.2 Increased Prominence of Acetowhite Epithelium

There is progressive eversion of lower endocervical canal epithelium due to increased interstitial fluid. When this everted columnar epithelium is exposed to the acidic milieu of the vagina, it undergoes squamous metaplasia which progresses throughout pregnancy. Towards the end of the first trimester, this produces area of fusion of columnar villi with islands of immature metaplastic epithelium (Fig. 13.3a, b). This process rapidly progresses through the second trimester, producing a layer of smooth, opaque squamous metaplasia that appears acetowhite after application of acetic acid. The acetowhiteness is further exaggerated by the bluish hue of the cervix due to increased vascularity. This immature metaplasia often causes diagnostic difficulty with low-grade lesion.

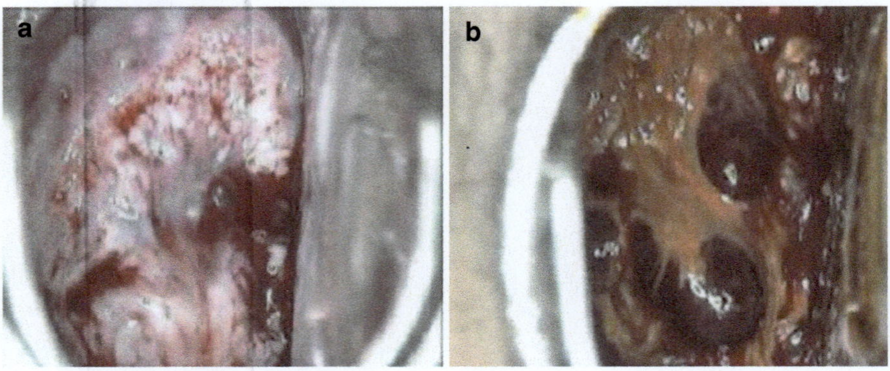

Fig. 13.3 Increased acetowhiteness (**a**) and non-uptake of Lugol's iodine (**b**) at colposcopy

In the third trimester, eversion and progressive metaplasia continue until 36 weeks of gestation and then stops. This area of metaplasia either returns to its endocervical position in the puerperium or matures into squamous epithelium.

In the subsequent pregnancy, the preexisting area of metaplasia may again get everted but not as dramatically as in the first pregnancy.

13.4.3 Diminished Acetowhitening

Edema of the cervix during pregnancy makes acetowhite epithelium look less intense, and the lesions can appear less severe than they actually are.

13.4.4 Cyanosis of Stroma

Cyanosis of stroma causes a dusky appearance (Fig. 13.4), and normal capillaries have a ring of acetowhite decidualized stroma surrounding them, which causes a "starry sky" appearance.

13.4.5 Decidual Changes

These changes are due to high levels of circulating progesterone in pregnancy. They are usually focal and can affect the endo- or ectocervix in the form of cuffing of gland openings or decidual polyps. Decidual polyps can appear as raised plaques or polypoidal with a yellowish appearance and no covering epithelium. They regress spontaneously in the postpartum period.

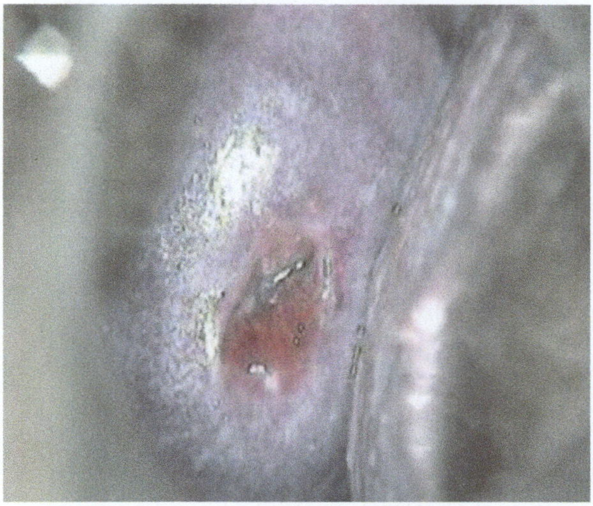

Fig. 13.4 Congested and cyanosed appearance of pregnant cervix

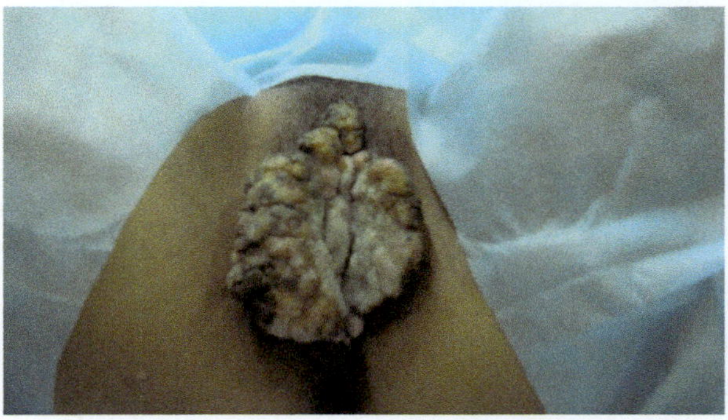

Fig. 13.5 Condyloma in pregnant patient

13.4.6 Condylomas

Condylomas can become extremely florid and enlarged in pregnancy (Fig. 13.5). Their benign nature can be confirmed on colposcopy. Their treatment can be safely postponed until postpartum by which time they would have decreased in size.

13.4.7 Microglandular Endocervical Hyperplasia

It results from stimulation of the columnar epithelium by progesterone. So, it is also seen in women on oral contraceptive pills. Though they are generally microscopic but if florid, can appear polypoidal with covering columnar epithelium.

13.5 Colposcopic Technique in Pregnant Women

Position In early pregnancy, no changes in patient positioning are needed. But as pregnancy progresses, women may develop supine hypotension syndrome during colposcopic examination, and it is helpful to place folded sheets to wedge the hip off the table.

Visualization of the Cervix A large-sized speculum is needed to visualize the cervix in pregnant women owing to cervical hypertrophy and lax vaginal walls. If this does not provide adequate exposure, a condom can be placed on the speculum and opened at the distal end, or lateral vaginal wall retractors can be used. Effacement and dilatation of the cervix which occur late in pregnancy further make visualization difficult. So, colposcopy in late gestation should be limited to women most likely to have invasive cancer.

It is easier to carry out colposcopy after 16–18 weeks of gestation because of the eversion of the endocervical columnar epithelium (Figs. 13.6 and 13.7). As a result of this physiologic eversion, the transformation zone (TZ) becomes more accessible.

Removing Cervical Mucus Cervical mucus during pregnancy is usually thick, opaque, and tenacious (Fig. 13.8). Pulling onto the mucus to remove it is generally not successful. It can be twisted around a dry cotton swab to be mobilized and removed or one can also use a sponge forceps to remove it.

Applying Acetic Acid More liberal application of acetic acid is required for the acetowhitening to take place (Fig. 13.9). As the cervix is friable, care must be taken to spray or dab the acetic acid rather than rubbing it on the cervix and traumatizing it (Fig. 13.10).

Also, pregnant women experience more burning sensation with acetic acid application than nonpregnant women.

13.5.1 Applying Lugol's Iodine

After application of acetic acid, Lugol's iodine is applied to the cervix. The areas of dysplasia do not stain brown and remain unstained or take up iodine patchily.

13.5.2 Colposcopic-Directed Biopsy

Due to increased vascularity and edema of the pregnant cervix and its tendency to bleed excessively, biopsy is generally avoided during pregnancy. Cervical biopsy is

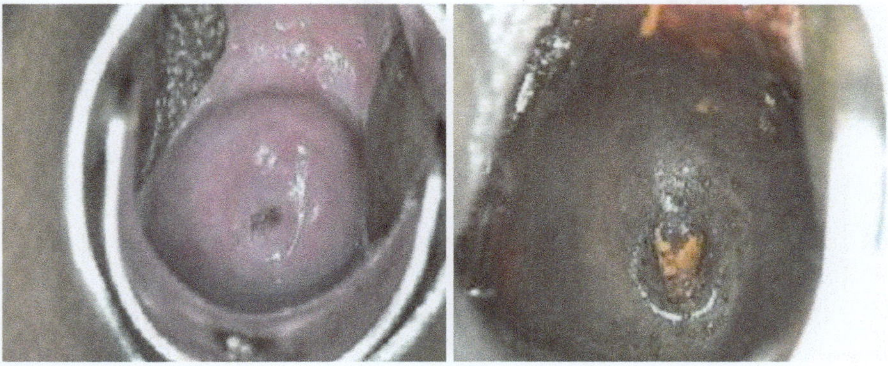

Fig. 13.6 Inadequate colposcopy in early pregnancy

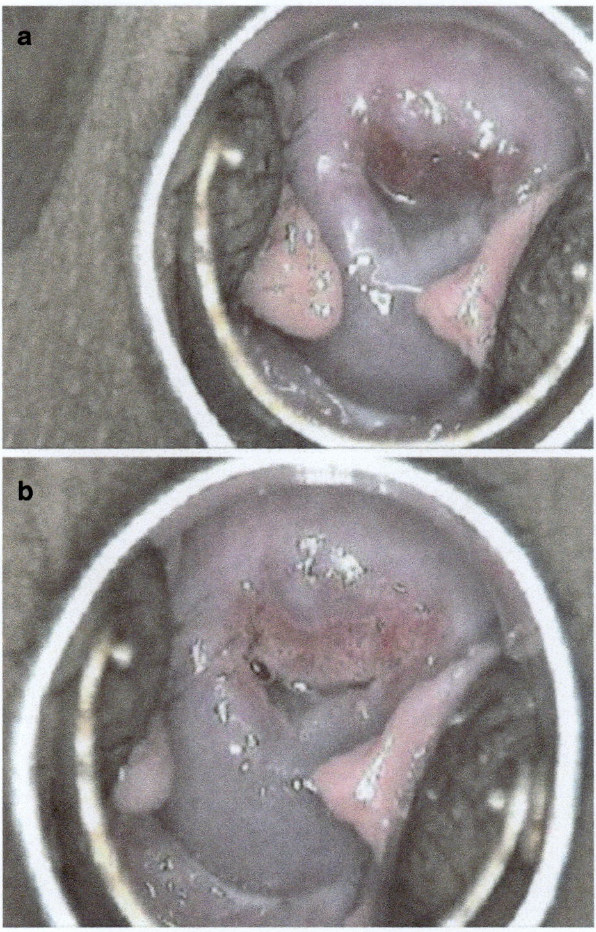

Fig. 13.7 Eversion seen before (**a**) and after acetic acid application (**b**) in late pregnancy

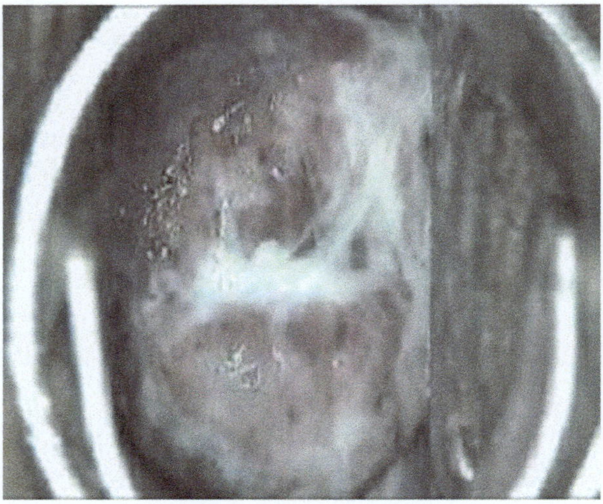

Fig. 13.8 Thick tenacious mucus covering the cervix

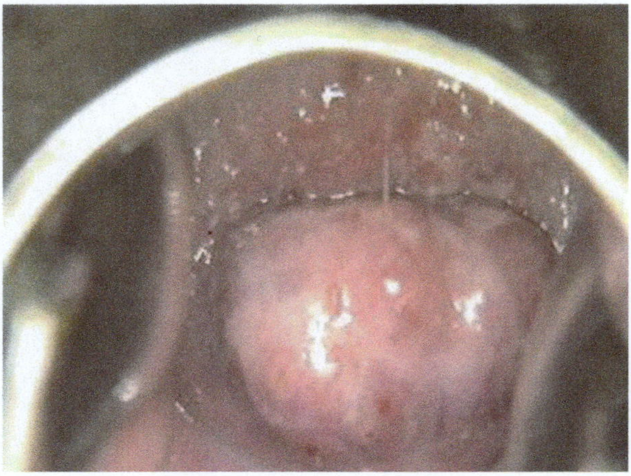

Fig. 13.9 Acetowhitening seen on the posterior lip of the cervix

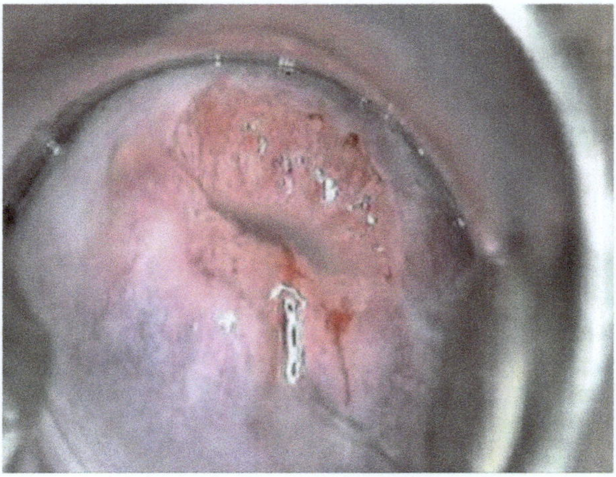

Fig. 13.10 Small bleeding vessels after acetic acid application

indicated when the lesions are suspicious for microinvasion or invasive cancer, and the results can potentially impact management options.

13.5.3 Indications for Biopsy

- Clinical suspicion of high-grade dysplasia or cancer.
- Worsening appearance of the lesion.
- Cytology results suggesting invasive cancer.

Biopsy is relatively safe in pregnancy but is not necessarily part of standard management. Biopsies have a good correlation with the final diagnosis with very minimal risks for both the mother and fetus. The overall risk of cervical biopsy-related complications is approximately 0.6 % [10, 11]. In a retrospective study of 612 pregnant women, no cases of invasive cancer were missed when colposcopy was combined with biopsy. However, 14 % of low-grade lesions on colposcopy revealed to be CIN 3 on histology, and 54 % of normal colposcopies were CIN 1 or CIN 2 on histopathology [11].

Endocervical sampling is contraindicated because of potential for fetal injury.

The diagnosis of a frank malignancy must be confirmed by target biopsy with small, sharp biopsy forceps.

When early invasive disease is suspected, a larger biopsy in the form of a wedge biopsy, cone biopsy, or loop excision is required.

Immediately after obtaining the biopsy specimen, pressure can be applied to the cervix to decrease bleeding. Alternatively Monsel's paste or silver nitrate can be applied. Both of these agents are caustic and so should be applied in minimum quantity. Also, Monsel's solution interferes with histologic interpretation and should not be applied until after the biopsy is completed.

13.6 Conization in Pregnancy

While the complication rate for cervical punch biopsy is low and acceptable, the complication rate for cervical conization is more significant. The indications for conization in pregnant women are different from those in the nonpregnant. There is no apparent role for therapeutic conization in antepartum period. Diagnostic cone should be reserved for those women in whom there is a significant risk of invasive cancer. In younger women, it can be deferred even if there is a lack of correlation between cytology and biopsy results or an inadequate colposcopy.

Case series of biopsies taken by diathermy loop in pregnancy have shown that the risk of hemorrhage is as high as 25 %. Many studies have advocated additional hemostatic sutures or cerclage to reduce risk of hemorrhage and subsequent pregnancy loss [12, 13]. Due to the risks involved, conization during pregnancy should only be done when either the biopsy or cytology is suggestive of invasive cancer and the diagnosis of invasion would result in treatment modification, timing, or mode of delivery.

13.6.1 Indications for Conization in Pregnancy [14]

- Histologic presence of microinvasive or invasive disease
- Histologic presence of adenocarcinoma in situ
- Persistent cytologic impression of invasive cancer (which cannot be ruled out by colposcopic examination)
- Strong colposcopic, cytologic, or histologic suspicion of invasion that cannot be confirmed

13.6.2 Complications of Cone Biopsy

- Hemorrhage: It is dependent on the period of gestation, and the greatest risk of hemorrhage is seen if conization is done in the third trimester. Almost 10% of women having conization in late gestation have blood loss of more than 500 ml [12, 13]. A shallow cone suffices during pregnancy, and only minimum cervical epithelium and stroma should be excised with no attempt to remove all of the dysplastic tissue.
- Pregnancy loss: Overall fetal death due to the procedure has been reported as 5% and is mostly due to chorioamnionitis or prematurity [15].
- Preterm delivery: The rate of preterm delivery following cone biopsy in pregnancy is 10–15% [15].
- Residual disease: Up to 50% of pregnant women have residual CIN after conization.

13.7 Histologic Appearance During Pregnancy

Interpretation of biopsies during pregnancy is challenging because of the normal histologic changes associated with pregnancy. The changes which mimic high-grade lesion are:

- Glandular hyperplasia and atypia
- Decidual reaction
- Arias-Stella reaction
- Immature metaplasia (Fig. 13.11)

Several studies have shown a high correlation between antepartum colposcopic impression and histologic diagnosis [3, 16].

13.8 Postpartum

The cervix undergoes extensive remodeling and repair in the postpartum period. If colposcopy has been performed during pregnancy, postpartum assessment of women with an abnormal colposcopy or biopsy-proven CIN is essential, though this

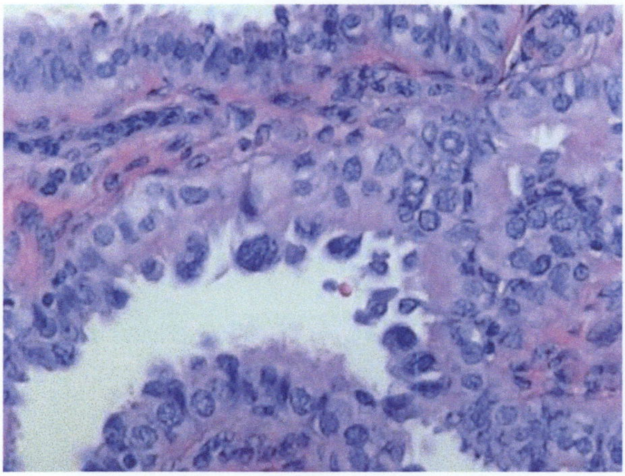

Fig. 13.11 Arias-Stella reaction

can be deferred up to 8–12 weeks after delivery [17]. By this time, any cervical damage would have resolved, and pregnancy-induced colposcopic changes would have reverted. Regression of lesions postpartum may simply reflect the natural history of HPV infection of the cervix. The viral load increases during pregnancy and decreases in the postpartum period. About 11 % of prenatal patients with histologically proven CIN have normal postpartum cytology. The rate of progression of high-grade disease to malignancy is about 0.4 % [18]. Regression rates also do not depend on the mode of delivery [19].

13.9 Management of Colposcopic Findings

13.9.1 Low-Grade Lesion

Pregnant women with low-grade lesion on colposcopy can be managed conservatively, and a repeat examination is done 3 months following delivery [11]. According to 2012 ASCCP guidelines, follow-up without treatment is recommended in pregnant women with low-grade lesion. Treatment of pregnant women for CIN 1 is unacceptable [20].

13.9.2 High-Grade Lesion

If CIN 2 or CIN 3 is suspected, a repeat colposcopy at the end of the second trimester is advocated (Fig. 13.12). If the pregnancy has advanced beyond that point, then colposcopy is repeated 3 months postpartum [11].

According to 2012 ASCCP guidelines:

- In the absence of invasive disease or advanced pregnancy, additional colposcopic and cytologic examinations are acceptable at intervals no more than every 12 weeks.

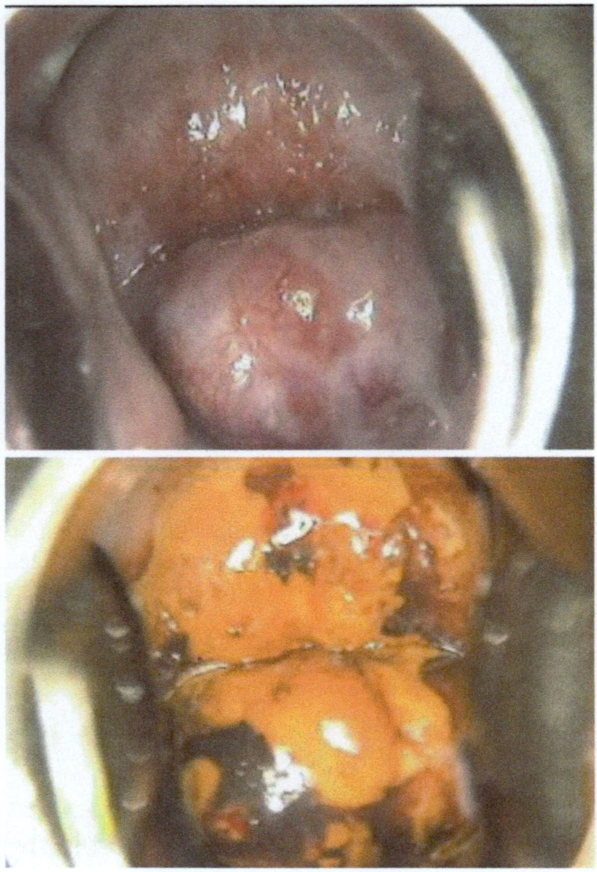

Fig. 13.12 High-grade lesion on colposcopy

- Repeat biopsy is done only if the appearance of the lesion worsens or if cytology suggests invasive cancer.
- Deferring reevaluation until at least 6 weeks postpartum is acceptable.

The regression of antenatal lesions is low averaging from 20 to 45 % in various studies [4, 21, 22]. So, a postnatal assessment is important in all women who have a high-grade colposcopic lesion antenatally.

13.10 Unsatisfactory Colposcopy

In most cases, the colposcopic examination of pregnant women is adequate because of the eversion and gaping of the endocervical epithelium.

If colposcopic examination is inadequate early in gestation, it should be repeated in the second trimester. In almost all women, it becomes satisfactory by the end of the second trimester. If the transformation zone still cannot be visualized completely, then the risk of diagnostic conization must be balanced against the likelihood of malignancy, and in majority it is appropriate to defer further evaluation till postpartum period.

Key Points

- The primary goal of colposcopy in pregnancy is to exclude invasive disease.
- Colposcopic diagnosis is challenging in pregnant women because of pregnancy-related changes in appearance of the cervix and difficulties in visualization of the cervix.
- Conservative management by colposcopic assessment allows deferring of treatment of CIN until after delivery.
- Regression rates of CIN in pregnancy are low, and postpartum assessment is essential.
- Biopsy is generally avoided during pregnancy unless there is suspicion of high-grade dysplasia or invasive cancer; endocervical sampling is contraindicated because of the potential fetal injury.

References

1. Al-Halal H, Kezouh A, Abenhaim HA. Incidence and obstetrical outcomes of cervical intraepithelial neoplasia and cervical cancer in pregnancy: a population-based study on 8.8 million births. Arch Gynecol Obstet. 2013;287(2):245–50.
2. Takushi M, Moromizato H, Sakumoto K, Kanazawa K. Management of invasive carcinoma of the uterine cervix associated with pregnancy: outcome of intentional delay in treatment. Gynecol Oncol. 2002;87(2):185–9.
3. Woodrow N, Permezel M, Butterfield L, Rome R, Tan J, Quinn M. Abnormal cervical cytology in pregnancy: experience of 811 cases. Aust N Z J Obstet Gynaecol. 1998;38(2):161–5.
4. Coppola A, Sorossky J, Casper R, Anderson B, Buller RE. The clinical course of cervical carcinoma in situ diagnosed during pregnancy. Gynecol Oncol. 1997;67(2):162–5.
5. Wetta LA, Matthews KS, Kemper ML, Whitworth JM, Fain ET, Huh WK, Kendrick JE, Straughn Jr JM. The management of cervical intraepithelial neoplasia during pregnancy: is colposcopy necessary? J Low Genit Tract Dis. 2009;13(3):182–5.
6. Frega A, Scirpa P, Corosu R, Verrico M, Scarciglia ML, Primieri MR, Palazzo A, Iacovelli R, Moscarini M. Clinical management and follow-up of squamous intraepithelial cervical lesions during pregnancy and postpartum. Anticancer Res. 2007;27:2743–6.
7. Owens GL, Kitchener HC. Pre-malignant disease in the genital tract in pregnancy. Best Practice & Research Clinical Obstetrics & Gynecology 2106;33:33–43.
8. Bentley J. Society of Canadian Colposcopists. Colposcopic management of abnormal cervical cytology and histology. J Obstet Gynaecol Can. 2012;34(12):1188–206.
9. Wang R, Li X, Qian M, Niu J, You I. The natural history of cervical intraepithelial neoplasia and the clinical significance of p16(INK4a) protein as a marker of progression in cervical intraepithelial neoplasia. Zhonghua Fu ChanKe Za Zhi. 2015;50(3):210–5.
10. Douvier S, Filipuzzi L, Sagot P. Management of cervical intra-epithelial neoplasm during pregnancy. Gynecol Obstet Fertil. 2003;31(10):851–5.

11. Hopkins MP, Morley GW. The prognosis and management of cervical cancer associated with pregnancy. Obstet Gynecol. 1992;80(1):9–13.
12. Blomfield P. Cervical neoplasia in pregnancy. Cancer. 2012;14(1):34–5.
13. Demeter A, Sziller I, Csapó Z, Szánthó A, Papp Z. Outcome of pregnancies after cold-knife conization of the uterine cervix during pregnancy. Eur J Gynaecol Oncol. 2002;23(3): 207–10.
14. Weismiller DG. Triage of the abnormal Papanicolaou smear and colposcopy in pregnancy. In: Apgar, Bradman, Spitzer, editors. Colposcopy-principles & practice. Philadephia Saunders Elsevier. 2002. p. 391–98.
15. McIntyre-Seltman K, Lesnock JL. Cervical cancer screening in pregnancy. Obstet Gynecol Clin North Am. 2008;35(4):645–58.
16. Broderick D, Matityahu D, Dudhbhai M, Alter S. Histologic and colposcopic correlates of ASCUS pap smears in pregnancy. J Low Genit Tract Dis. 2002;6(2):116–9.
17. Paraskevaidis E, Koliopoulos G, Kalantaridou S, Pappa L, Navrozoglou I, Zikopoulos K, Lolis DE. Management and evolution of cervical intraepithelial neoplasia during pregnancy and postpartum. Eur J Obstet Gynecol Reprod Biol. 2002;104(1):67–9.
18. Zoundi-Quango O, Morcel K, Classe JM, Burtin F, et al. Uterine cervical lesions during pregnancy: diagnosis and management. J Gynecol Obstet Biol Reprod. 2016;35(3):227–36.
19. Yost NP, Santoso JT, McIntire DD, Iliya FA. Postpartum regression rates of antepartum cervical intraepithelial neoplasia II and III lesions. Obstet Gynecol. 1999;93(3):359–62.
20. Massad S, Einstein MH, Huh WK, KAtki A, et al. Updated Consensus guidelines for management of abnormal cervical cancer screening tests and cancer precursors. J Low Genit Tract Dis. 2013;17:S1–27.
21. Cruickshank M. Colposcopic appearances during pregnancy, the menopause and the effects of exogenous hormones. CME J Gynecol Oncol. 2005;10:26–30.
22. Yang KY. Abnormal pap smear and cervical cancer in pregnancy. Clin Obstet Gynecol. 2012;55(3):838–48.

CIN: Ablative Therapies

14

Veena Rahatgaonkar

The active management of Cervical Intraepithelial Neoplasia (CIN) is necessary to halt the progression of disease and prevent development of invasive carcinoma. CIN can be treated either by ablative or by excisional methods.

Different methods of ablative treatment are

- Cryotherapy
- Electrocoagulation
- Cold coagulation
- Laser ablation

14.1 Principle of Ablative Treatment

Ablative therapy eradicates the abnormal epithelium with minimal topographical changes in the cervix [1–4].

14.2 Prerequisites for Ablation

The primary concern in treating CIN by ablative methods is whether the treatment is adequate to eradicate the CIN lesion completely or not. Therefore the following prerequisites must be fulfilled before proceeding for ablative treatment.

1. Invasive carcinoma must be ruled out.
2. Lesion should be fully visible.

V. Rahatgaonkar, MD, DGO
Department of Obsterician and Gynecologist and Colposcopist,
Deenanath Mangeshkar Hospital and Research Center, Pune, India
e-mail: ven_rah@yahoo.com

S. Mehta, P. Sachdeva (eds.), *Colposcopy of Female Genital Tract*,
DOI 10.1007/978-981-10-1705-6_14

3. There should not be any evidence of glandular dysplasia.
4. Clinical expertise in these techniques is essential.
5. Patient should be compliant for a follow-up.

14.3 Methods of Ablative Treatment

14.3.1 Cryotherapy

Cryotherapy was first introduced in the United States by Crisp [5]. It is also known as cryocautery or cryosurgery. The technique uses a cryoprobe with a tip made of highly conductive metal usually silver and copper that makes direct contact with ectocervical lesion. Rapid freezing of tissue is caused due to substantial drop in temperature which is achieved when a compressed refrigerant gas is allowed to expand through a small aperture in the cryoprobe.

14.3.2 Principle

Rapid freezing causes cellular necrosis by intra and extracellular crystallization leading to cell dehydration, thermal shock, vascular stasis, and protein denaturation. Neoplastic cells are damaged due to rapid freezing and slow thawing.

14.3.3 Equipment

Cryotherapy requires less financial investment for equipment, maintenance, and repair. Equipment required is as follows:

1. Cryotherapy unit with cryoprobes
2. Gas cylinder.

14.3.4 Cryotherapy Unit with Cryoprobes (Figs. 14.1 and 14.2)

The cryotherapy unit consists of a cryotherapy gun attached to a flexible gas conveying tube, a pressure gauge showing the cylinder gas pressure, an outlet silencer, a gas trigger to allow the release of gas from reservoir to cryoprobe at high pressure and a cryoprobe.

Cryoprobes are of two types; flat tip and a probe with 2 mm endocervical extension. Silver and copper are the best materials to use in probe tips because high conductivity produces both a better freezing effect and a more effective local cryonecrosis [6]. The size and shape of the probe affect the depth of cryonecrosis [7].

The 19 and 25 mm mini-cone tips are recommended for the required depth of cryonecrosis.

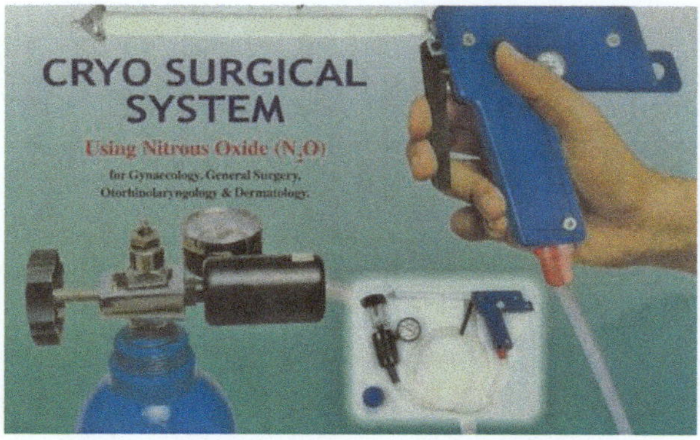

Fig. 14.1 Cryotherapy unit

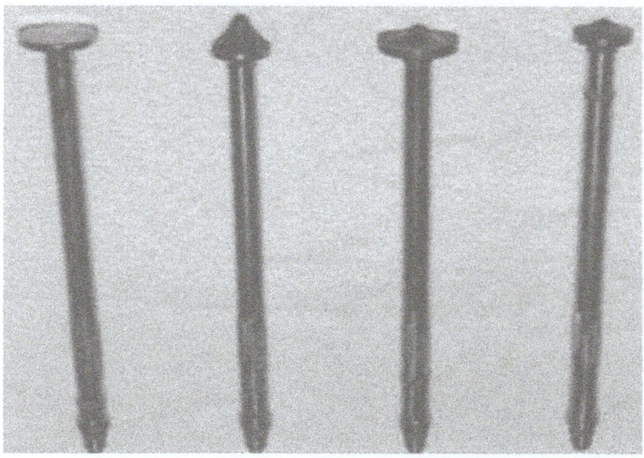

Fig. 14.2 Cryotherapy probes

14.3.4.1 Gas Cylinder

Gases selected for cryotherapy should have their freezing point below the cryogenic range from −20 to −30 °C needed for tissue destruction. Nitrous oxide (N_2O) and carbon dioxide are used for cryotherapy as these gases provide excellent thermal transfer when circulating in the probe tip (Fig. 14.3) [8, 9].

Nitrous oxide produces lower temperatures to a greater depth than carbon dioxide [10]. The comparison of depth of tissue destruction is shown in Table 14.1.

14.3.5 Eligibility Criteria for Cryotherapy

- Lesion should be on the ectocervix and visible in its entire extent. No extension of lesion is noted in the endocervical canal or vagina.
- The lesion can be adequately covered by the cryotherapy probe and it should not extend 2 mm beyond the tip of the cryotherapy probe.
- The CIN lesion should be confirmed by colposcopy or biopsy.

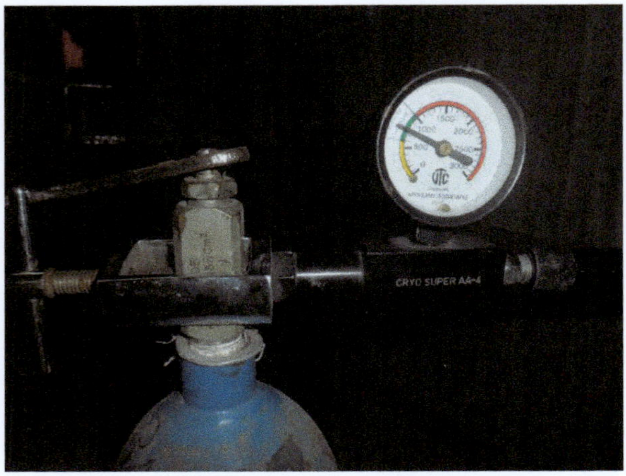

Fig. 14.3 Gas cylinder

Table 14.1 Depth of tissue destruction

Depth of destruction	Gas	Temperature
3 mm	Carbon dioxide	–68 °C
5 mm	Nitrous oxide	–89 °C

14.3.6 Exclusion Criteria

1. Pregnancy

   Cryotherapy is not to be carried out in pregnant women as the risk of pregnancy loss is greater when it is performed during pregnancy.

   During pregnancy, a follow-up of CIN lesions with colposcopy in each trimester is done but therapy is delayed up to 12 weeks postpartum [11].
2. Invasive carcinoma

   Cryotherapy should not be done before invasion is ruled out. There should not be suspicion of glandular dysplasia.
3. Pelvic inflammatory disease (PID)

   It is advisable to delay the cryotherapy until the infection has been treated and resolved completely. The risk of postoperative infection after cryotherapy is minimal but can be increased if the procedure is carried out in women with pelvic inflammatory disease, sexually transmitted cervicitis like chlamydia or gonorrhea, vaginal trichomoniasis, and bacterial vaginosis.
4. Marked atrophic changes of the cervix

   In old women, if there is a marked atrophy due to estrogen deficiency, the staining of the outer margin of the lesion is indistinct. In such conditions, cryotherapy may be carried out after a course of topical estrogen treatment and colposcopic reassessment.
5. Menstruation

   Cryotherapy is not to be done during menstruation.

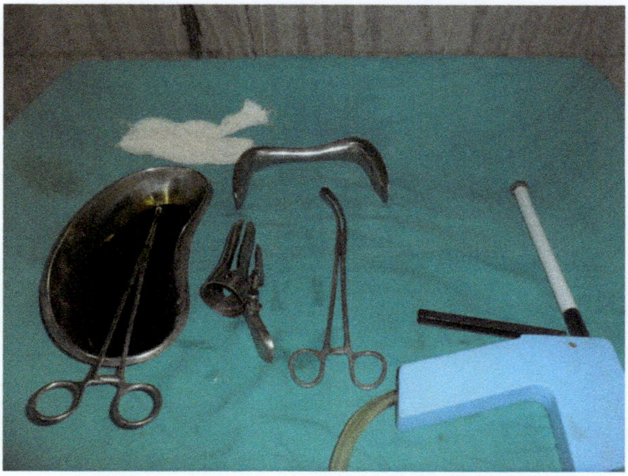

Fig. 14.4 Instrument trolley for cryotherapy

14.3.7 Technique of Cryotherapy

Before proceeding to cryotherapy, the health provider must confirm that the patient is eligible for the therapy as per the eligibility criteria. An informed consent is taken. The clinician should explain the procedure to the patient and reassure her. The procedure is carried out under colposcopic guidance without anesthesia (Fig. 14.4).

Woman should be placed in a dorsal lithotomy position and Cusco's speculum is inserted to expose the cervix. The cryoprobe surface is wiped with saline or coated with water-soluble lubricating jelly to provide good contact and firm application of the cryoprobe tip to the cervix and an optimal lowering of the tissue temperature. While applying cryoprobe, care is taken so that the vaginal walls are not in contact with the cryoprobe. No anesthesia is required except in very anxious patients who may be given NSAID 30 min prior to the procedure.

The probe should cover the lesion completely. The gas trigger in the cryogun is released and the gas escapes with a hissing noise. The gas circulating through the cryoprobe withdraws heat from the cervix till the freezing temperature is reached. As freezing progresses, ice forms on the cervix and on the cryoprobe. The rapidity of the ice-ball formation and efficacy of the procedure depend on:

- Adequate pressure of gas in the tank or reservoir
- Proper and firm application of the probe on the cervix
- Cryogenic gas used [9] (Fig. 14.5)

Nitrous oxide based cryotherapy achieves a temperature of about −89 °C and carbon dioxide based system achieves −68 °C at the core of the tissue that is at the center of the ice ball. The temperature at the edge of the frozen tissue may be around −20 °C.The minimum temperature of the probe tip for effective tissue freezing should be −60 °C. An adequate freezing is achieved when the margin of the ice ball

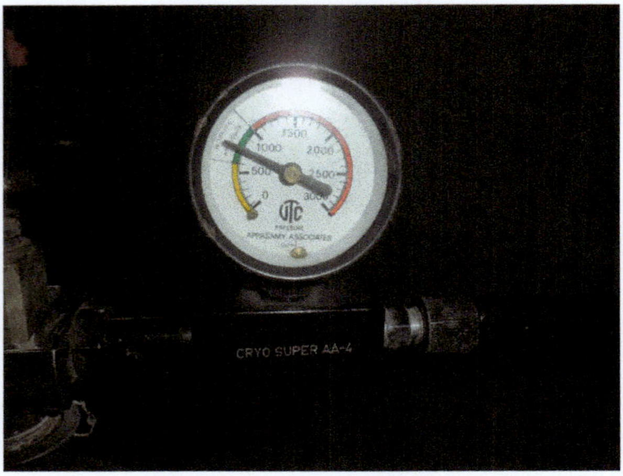

Fig. 14.5 Needle in pressure gauge should be in the *green* region

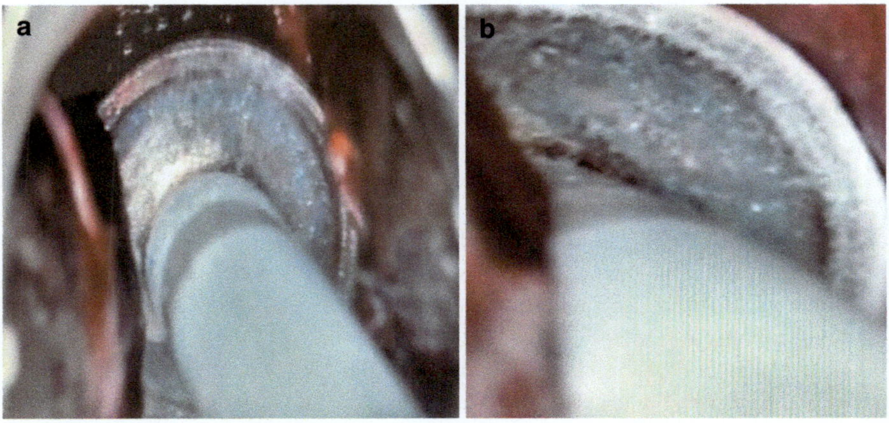

Fig. 14.6 Cryotherapy in progress (**a**, **b**)

extends 4–5 mm past the outer edge of the cryotip; this will ensure that cryonecrosis occurs down to at least 5 mm depth [9].

The two methods of cryotherapy are as follows:

1. Single freeze: In this method, cryogenic gas is applied continuously.
2. Double freeze: It consists of two sequential "freeze–thaw" cycles; each cycle consists of 3 min of freezing followed by 5 min of thawing (3 min freeze–5 min thaw–3 min freeze–5 min thaw).

The double freeze technique produces more tissue destruction than the single freeze cycle [6, 12].

When thawing is completed, the ice on the cryoprobe is totally cleared and then the probe is removed by gently rotating on the cervix. After the procedure, the cervix is examined for any bleeding (Fig. 14.6).

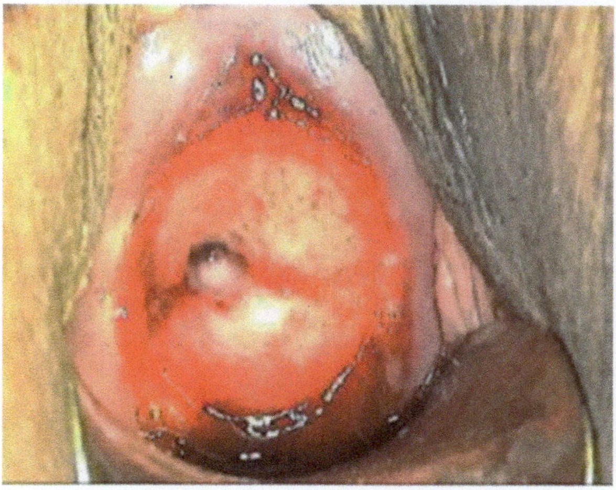

Fig. 14.7 Cervix immediately after cryotherapy

(a) Cryoprobe in firm contact with the cervix, process of freezing in progress
(b) Ice formation at the center and at the edge of the probe tip
(c) Appearance of the cervix immediately after cryotherapy (Fig. 14.7)

14.3.8 Cleaning of Cryoprobe and Cryogun

The cryotip is washed with clean water until visibly clean. The high-level disinfection (HLD) of cryotip is done by boiling in water for 20 min or soaking the cryotip in chemical disinfectant for 20 min and then rinsed with water. It is critical that the hollow part of the cryotip is completely dry before it is used for the next case; otherwise the water would freeze and the probe could crack.

14.3.9 Adverse Effects

- Uterine cramping may occur during or shortly after treatment.
- Rarely vasovagal syncope may occur during the procedure in anxious patients.
- Profuse watery vaginal discharge is seen for 2–4 weeks after the therapy. So after cryotherapy, the vagina should not be packed to allow secretions to escape.

14.3.10 Long-Term Complications (Table 14.2)

- Postoperative infection: It is rare and can be reduced by an adequate treatment of STD before cryotherapy.
- Cervical stenosis: It is seen in less than 1 % of cases.
- Failure of therapy and the recurrence of CIN.

Table 14.2 Complications of cryotherapy [13]

Complication	Frequency
Posttreatment severe bleeding	Rare
Pelvic inflammatory disease (PID) and cervical infections	<5 %
Long-term complications	
Cervical stenosis	<1 %
Fertility impairment Obstetrical outcomes	No effect

Table 14.3 Cure rate by cryotherapy [13]

Grade of CIN	% cure rate
CIN 1	94 %
CIN 2	91 %
CIN 3	84 %
Overall CIN1+	*88 %*
Overall CIN2+	*86 %*

14.3.11 Follow-Up After Cryotherapy

Women should be instructed not to use tampons or vaginal douche for 4 weeks and advised abstinence for 6 weeks. Patients should report to the health provider if they have any of the following symptoms:

- Severe lower abdominal cramps
- Foul-smelling discharge
- Heavy bleeding
- Fever more than 2 days

Healing takes place within 6 weeks after the treatment. Follow-up with VIA or cytology is done 6 and 12 months after cryotherapy. Thereafter, yearly follow-up is done for 3 years. If no abnormality is detected for 3 years, the patient is referred for routine screening program.

14.3.12 Cryotherapy and HIV

In HIV positive women, HIV1 virus is shed in vaginal secretions after cryotherapy, which may increase, the transmissibility of HIV. Therefore condoms should be distributed after cryotherapy free of cost in settings where HIV infection is endemic.

14.3.13 Efficacy of Cryotherapy

Cryotherapy in low-grade lesion is effective with a success rate as high as 94 %, but in high-grade lesions, the cure rate is 84–86 % (Table 14.3).

14.3.14 Causes of Failure of Cryotherapy

1. *Pretreatment assessment of lesion is not correct* (poor diagnostic workup).
   Cryotherapy fails to treat an extensive high-grade lesion with the involvement of the deeper cervical glands and clefts. If the linear extent of the lesion is more, e.g., when lesion occupies more than three quadrants of the cervix, it will not be effectively treated by cryotherapy.
2. *Faulty technique*
   It is essential to maintain good contact between the probe tip and the tissue throughout the procedure. Poor contact means relatively a large variation in the temperature achieved within the ice ball and therefore variable effectiveness in the target tissue leading to failure of the therapy.
   The pressure of the gas in the reservoir tank should be sufficient to provide an effective flow of the refrigerant through the probe tip for the required duration of treatment. The minimum gas pressure shown on the gauge should be 40 kg/cm^2. If the gas tank pressure is not checked before starting the procedure and if it is low, there will be insufficient freezing and no required extent of cryonecrosis and hence failure of therapy will occur.

14.3.15 Management of Women in Cryotherapy Failures

Treatment failure is seen in 5–10 % of treated women. In therapy failures, a biopsy of all persistent lesions should be done to rule out unsuspected invasive carcinoma, and then re-treatment with cryotherapy, LEEP, or cold-knife conization is done as appropriate [14].

14.3.16 CO_2 Laser Vaporization

In CO_2 laser vaporization, boiling of intracellular water causes vaporization of tissue. The incineration of the protein and minerals leads to charring of the treated area [15].

14.3.17 Technique

CO_2 laser is mounted on the colposcope. The vaporization is started from the posterior lip and at a margin of 5 mm from the edge of the lesion till the depth of cervical glands, which is identified by the appearance of yellow collagen matrix.

The depth of tissue destruction is 6–7 mm. The vapor produced during the procedure is removed by a suction pump. The depth of tissue destruction depends on

- Power of laser beam
- Duration of exposure by laser beam
- Spot size of beam [16]

The procedure is completed within 15–20 min.

14.3.18 Advantages

1. The depth and extent of tissue destruction is controlled accurately.
2. Laser vaporization removes the lesion at the same time of treatment while in other ablative techniques, the removal of the lesion with tissue necrosis occurs 1–2 weeks later.
3. Healing occurs rapidly with minimal fibrosis.
4. Watery discharge lasts for 1 week as against the cryotherapy where it lasts for 4 weeks.
5. Postoperative infection is rare due to blood and lymphatic vessels getting sealed at the time of surgery.
6. Excellent cure rates. Excellent healing with cure rates by CO_2 laser vaporization quoted by Wright et al. are 97.6 %, 95 %, and 94.7 % for CIN I, CIN II, and CIN III, respectively [17].
7. There are no effects on reproductive function.

14.3.19 Disadvantages

High cost of equipment and its maintenance and high degree of expertise are required for the therapy.

14.3.20 Electrocautery

It is the oldest method of management of CIN. It is an outpatient procedure and does not require anesthesia. It involves radial strokes from the cervical canal to the periphery of the cervix with a resistance-type heating instrument. The treatment is not very effective as depth of tissue destruction is only 2–3 mm [4, 5].

14.3.21 Electrodiathermy

The procedure is carried out in an operation theater under general anesthesia. In this procedure, the whole transformation zone and the adjacent columnar epithelium are destroyed to a depth of 1–1.5 cm using a needle and a ball electrode. Healing is complete within 4 weeks, and sanguineous discharge may occur 3–4 weeks following the procedure. The results are comparable to other forms of local destructive therapy and the cure rate ranges from 88 to 98 % [18].

14.3.22 Cold Coagulation

Cold coagulation is a more feasible, sustainable, and affordable method for the treatment of cervical precancerous lesions [19].

It was introduced by Kurt Semm in 1996. This terminology is a misnomer as in this technique, CIN lesion is treated using a heated metallic probe. It is an OPD procedure and does not require anesthesia [4, 5].

14.3.23 Principle

Abnormal tissue destruction is done by thermal damage.

14.3.24 Prerequisites for Cold Coagulation

They are as follows:

1. Type 1 transformation zone (TZ1)
2. Lesion involving less than 75 % of the transformation zone
3. No evidence of invasive cancer

14.3.25 Equipment Required

- Colposcope
- Cervical speculum
- Light source
- Semm's cold coagulator

14.3.26 Semm's Cold Coagulator [20, 21]

It is a compact electronic device working on 220 V. The temperature range is 60–120 °C. It has a Teflon-coated small metallic probe (Fig. 14.8).

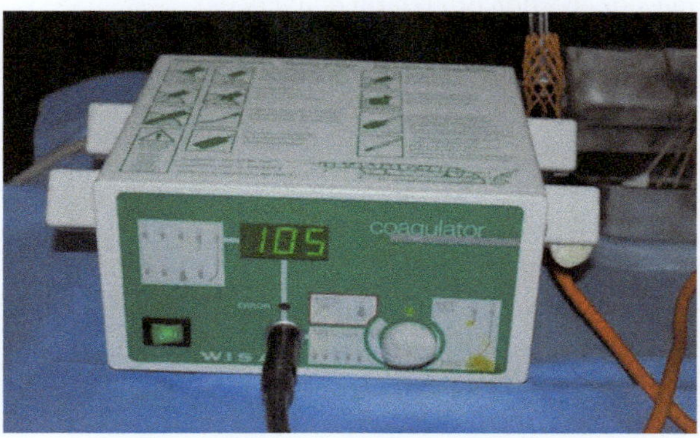

Fig. 14.8 Semm's cold coagulator

14.3.27 Procedure

The procedure is carried under colposcopic guidance. No anesthesia is required. The patient is taken in a modified lithotomy position. The extent of the lesion is marked with colposcopy. A probe is applied to the cervix at a temperature of 105 °C for 40 s without touching the vagina. Three to four overlapping applications are done to treat the entire transformation zone. The used probe is cleaned and sterilized by heating up to 120 °C for 45 s.

The depth of the tissue destruction depends on

1. *Temperature of heat application*
   The higher the temperature, higher is the depth of tissue destruction.
2. *Length of exposure*
   Longer length of exposure leads to more tissue destruction. The depth of tissue destruction exceeds 4 mm after an application for 40 s. With multiple applications, the depth of tissue destruction increases to 7 mm.

14.3.28 Post Procedure Advice

1. The woman should be informed that she may have a mild blood-stained discharge after the procedure.
2. She should be given a course of antibiotics after the therapy.
3. Abstinence for 1 month is advised.
4. The patient should report to the health provider if she develops symptoms like fever, foul-smelling discharge, bleeding or severe abdominal pain.

14.3.29 Complications

Complications are rare. Sometimes immediate problems may occur like pain, abdominal cramps, bleeding or vaginal burns. Late complications are PID and cervical stenosis (1 %). There are no adverse effects on obstetric outcome like increased rates of abortion or preterm delivery.

14.3.30 Follow-Up

Colposcopy and Pap smear are done 6 months after the procedure.

Conclusion

CIN is treated by local ablative or excisional techniques both of which have similar cure rates. The ablative methods are preferred in younger women which are more conservative. Ablative methods are relatively noninvasive and can be carried out on an outpatient basis without anesthesia. Cryotherapy is a simple and effective method for treating selected cases of CIN that can be used in a single-visit approach as "see and treat policy".

Key Points

CIN is treated by various ablative methods. Ablative methods are relatively noninvasive and can be carried out on an outpatient basis without anesthesia.

The prerequisites for ablative techniques are that invasive carcinoma must be ruled out, lesion should be fully visible, there should not be any evidence of glandular dysplasia, clinical expertise in these techniques is essential, and the patient should be compliant for a follow-up.

Cryotherapy is a simple and effective method for treating selected cases of CIN. It can be used in resource poor settings, in a single-visit approach as "see and treat policy."

Laser vaporization removes the lesion at the same time of treatment while in other ablative techniques, the removal of the lesion with tissue necrosis occurs 1–2 weeks later. The depth of tissue destruction can be controlled accurately, and healing occurs rapidly with minimum fibrosis.

Semm's cold coagulator causes destruction of abnormal tissue by thermal damage with temperatures as high as 105 °C.

References

1. Richart R. Cervical cancer precursors and their management. In: Rock JA, Thompson JD, editors. TeLinde's operative gynecology. 8th ed. Philadelphia: Lippincott-Raven; 1997. p. 1385–412.
2. Hatch KD, Hacker FN. Intraepithelial disease of the cervix, vagina and vulva. In: Berek JS, Adashi EY, Hillard PA, editors. Novak's gynecology. 12th ed. Hong Kong: Williams and Wilkins; 1996. p. 447–86.
3. Herbst AL. Intraepithelial neoplasia of the cervix : etiology, screening, diagnostic techniques and management. In: Mishell DR, Stenchever MA, Droegemueller W, Herbst AL, editors. Comprehensive gynecology. 3rd ed. Maryland Heights: Mosby; 1997. p. 801–34.
4. Coppleson M, Atkinson KH, Dalrymple JC. Cervical squamous and glandular intraepithelial neoplasia: clinical features and review of management, colposcopy : a scientific and practical approach to cervix, vagina and vulva in health and diseases, 3rd ed. Thomas Spring field; 1986. p. 111–64.
5. Krebs HB. Premalignant lesions of the cervix. In: Copeland LJ, editor. Textbook of gynecology. 2nd ed. Philadelphia: WB Saunders; 2000. p. 1225–60.
6. Charles EH, Savage EW, Hacker N, Jones NC. Cryosurgical treatment of cervical intraepithelial neoplasia. Gynecol Oncol. 1981;12(1):83–8.
7. Boonstra H, Aalders JG, Koudstaal J, Oosterhuis JW, Janssens J. Minimum extension and appropriate topographic position of tissue destruction for treatment of cervical intraepithelial neoplasia. Obstet Gynecol. 1990;75(2):227–31.
8. Campion Michael J. Preinvasive disease. 1984:173–80.

9. Sellors JW, Sankaranarayanan R. Colposcopy and treatment of cervical intraepithelial neoplasia: a beginner's manual. Published by International Agency for Research On Cancer, 2003. Treatment of cervical intraepithelial neoplasia by cryotherapy. p. 95–102.
10. Mariategui J, Santos C, Taxa L, Jeronimo J, Castle PE. Comparison of depth of necrosis achieved by CO2- and N2O-cryotherapy. Int J Gynaecol Obstet. 2008;100(1):24–6.
11. American College of Obstetricians and Gynecologists. ACOG Practice Bulletin number 66, September 2005. Management of abnormal cervical cytology and histology. Obstet Gynecol. 2005;106(3):645–64.
12. Campion Michael J. Preinvasive disease. In: Berek JS, Hacker NF, editors. Practical gynecologic oncology. 4th ed. Philadelphia: Lippincott Williams & Wilkins; 2005. p. 265–309.
13. Sauvaget C, Muwonge R, Sankaranarayanan R. Meta-analysis of the effectiveness of cryotherapy in the treatment of cervical intraepithelial neoplasia. Int J Gynaecol Obstet. 2013;120(3):218–23.
14. Sellors JW, Sankaranarayanan R; IARC. Treatment of cervical intraepithelial neoplasia by cryotherapy. 2003:102.
15. Bellina JH, Bandieramonte G. Applications in gynecology, principles and practice of gynecologic laser surgery. New York: Plenum Publishing Corporation; 1984. p. 111–64.
16. Baliga S. Principles and practice of colposcopy. In: Cervical Intraepithelial neoplasia: management options. p.185–7.
17. Cecil Wright V. Laser vaporization of the cervix for the management of cervical intraepithelial neoplasia, chapter 12. In: Baggish MS, editor. Basic and advanced laser surgery in gynecology. 1985. p. 229.
18. Byrne P, Nawa G, Woodman CBJ. Premalignant lesions of the lower genital tract, chapter 20. In: John Studd, editor. Progress of obstetrics and gynecology, vol. 6. 1987. p. 365.
19. Loobuyck HA, Duncan ID. Destruction of CIN I and CIN II with Semm cold coagulator: 13 years' experience with a see and treat policy. BJOG. 1993;100(5):465–8.
20. Semm K. A new instrument for cold coagulation of benign cervix erosions. Geburtshilfe Frauenheilkd. 1966;26(5):657–63.
21. Haddad N, Hussein I, Blessing K, Kerr-Wilson R, Smart G. Tissue destruction following cold coagulation of the cervix. J Gynecol Surg. 2009;4(1):23–7.

Excisional Procedures for Treatment of Intraepithelial Lesions

15

Mala Srivastava and Ankita Srivastava

Cervical intraepithelial neoplasia (CIN) is a spectrum of disease that precedes invasive squamous cell carcinoma of the cervix [1, 2]. Histopathologically it means there is a disordered pattern of squamous cell maturation and nuclear atypia. Whenever the density of cells increases and the cytoplasmic glycogen reduces, then the diagnosis of CIN is made as a preinvasive lesion which is graded as CIN 1, 2 or 3 depending on the severity of the lesion.

The predictions of the progression and regression of cervical preinvasive lesions are influenced by many factors; however, it is known that low-grade lesions have high regression rates and low progression rates, while high-grade lesions have a greater risk of progression if left untreated. So, the patients with preinvasive lesions of the cervix can be divided into two subgroups: those with low-grade cervical intraepithelial neoplasia (HPV changes and CIN 1 changes) and those with high-grade cervical intraepithelial neoplasia (CIN 2–3/CIS). In 2006, a panel of experts developed consensus guidelines for the treatment of CIN for each of these two subgroups which were again upgraded in 2012 [3].

Cervical intraepithelial neoplasia (CIN) arises in the transformation zone at the squamocolumnar junction (SCJ). The process of metaplasia progresses from the squamocolumnar junction, towards the external os and over the columnar epithelium, to establish the transformation zone. The pathology of CIN begins during the reproductive age group, when metaplasia is very active. After menopause, when the metaplasia is less active, a woman has a lesser risk of developing CIN.

If left without treatment, most CIN 1 and some CIN 2 lesions will regress spontaneously. For all practical purposes, more than 90 % of all CIN lesions are caused by human papillomavirus (HPV) infection.

M. Srivastava (✉)
Institute of Obstetrics and Gynaecology, Sir Ganga Ram Hospital, New Delhi, India
e-mail: malasrivastava2001@yahoo.co.in

A. Srivastava
Sri Aurobindo Institute of Medical Sciences, Indore, India

S. Mehta, P. Sachdeva (eds.), *Colposcopy of Female Genital Tract*,
DOI 10.1007/978-981-10-1705-6_15

Table 15.1 Treatment modalities for CIN

Observation
Local excision
Electrocauterisation
Cryosurgery
Laser cauterisation
Cold coagulation
Loop electrosurgical excision procedure (LEEP)
Conisation (using knife or laser)
Hysterectomy

In a review of more than twelve series in which 4000 patients suffering from CIN were followed up by biopsy, Mitchell showed that 45 % of these lesions regressed, 31 % persisted and 23 % progressed to a higher lesion. Of all those patients in whom the lesion progressed, 14 % progressed to CIS and only 1.4 % progressed to invasive carcinoma of the cervix [4]. The spontaneous regression possibility of biopsy-proven CIN 1 is 60–85 %. The regressions usually occur within a 2-year follow-up with cytology and colposcopy [5].

In contrast, a review by Holowaty et al. of 353 patients suffering from CIN 3/CIS from several series found that 127 (36 %) progressed to invasive carcinoma of the cervix. It is usually accepted that low-grade lesions have a high spontaneous regression rate and that most lesions will regress within a 2-year follow-up period [6].

15.1 Treatment Options

Nowadays, many treatment options for CIN are available (Table 15.1). The decision about the choice of therapy for CIN depends on the age of the patient and desire for fertility. No therapy is 100 % effective, but the benefit/risk ratio should be explained so that the patient can take a reasonable decision regarding her therapy and well-being [7].

The management of low-grade CIN lesions includes conservative treatment by ablation or excision of the transformation zone, or they can undergo follow-up without treatment.

It is known that both conservative treatment and observation with no treatment are reasonable options for women with CIN 1, and with no evidence to support that one is better than the other, a woman's preference to be treated should be considered important in the decision-making on an individual basis [8–10].

When choosing a technique for treating a low-grade cervical lesion, the ablative techniques have more than 90 % cure rates, but with the ease of loop electrosurgical excision procedure (LEEP), it remains a very common treatment for low-grade lesions [11–13]. Besides after LEEP, the tissue is also available for histopathology.

The patients with high-grade lesions (CIN 2–3/CIS) require treatment according to the 2012 consensus guidelines.

15.2 Limitations of Ablative Therapy for CIN

- Not suitable for microinvasive or invasive cancer of the cervix
- Not suitable for lesions that are reaching into the endocervical canal
- Endocervical curettage positive for disease
- Noncompatibility of cytology with biopsy results
- Lesions with size more than 2.5 cm or covering two quadrants [14].

The ablative techniques for treating CIN lesions are appropriate only when the extent of the disease is known; colposcopy with biopsy is consistent with preinvasive cervical disease; and invasive carcinoma is not detected. If these criteria are not met, an excisional procedure should be performed.

The excisional techniques are LEEP either as a cone, cold knife conisation (CKC) or carbon dioxide (CO_2) laser conisation.

15.3 Indications for Excisional Therapy

- Endocervical curettings are positive for intraepithelial lesion or microinvasive carcinoma.
- Cytological and histopathological diagnosis are not consistent with each other.
- The entire transformation zone is not accessible.
- Microinvasive carcinoma diagnosed by biopsy.
- Cytology- or biopsy-proven premalignant or malignant glandular epithelium [15].

Excisional methods of treatment of CIN include

1. LEEP/LLETZ
2. Conisation by cold knife
3. Conisation by laser.

15.4 Large Loop Excision of the Transformation Zone (LLETZ)

The *large loop excision of the transformation zone* (LLETZ) and the *loop electrosurgical excision procedure* (LEEP) are both used to describe an excision of the transformation zone with electrocautery. The thin wire loops that excises the tissue and provides a histopathologic specimen has become the therapy of choice. It treats the transformation zone similar to ablative techniques, and it also provides a tissue specimen for histopathological diagnosis as in surgical conisation. The LEEP can be performed as an outpatient procedure (Table 15.2).

Local infiltration at 12, 3, 6 and 9 o'clock positions of the cervix is done. Alternatively paracervical block can begin. The procedure should be performed under colposcopic guidance so that the visualisation of the area to be removed is

Table 15.2 Procedure of LEEP technique

1. Colposcopy is performed and the disease is delineated. Figure. 15.1 shows the instruments required for performing colposcopy
2. Local anaesthesia is given
3. The cautery machine is turned on with cut/blend adjusted to 25–50 W. The various sizes of loops can be used (Fig. 15.2 and 15.3)
4. The coagulation is set to 60 W when the ball electrode is used
5. Excision of the lesion is done using the LEEP procedure (Fig. 15.4)
6. The base of the cone is coagulated (Fig. 15.5)
7. Monsel's paste is placed on the cut edge

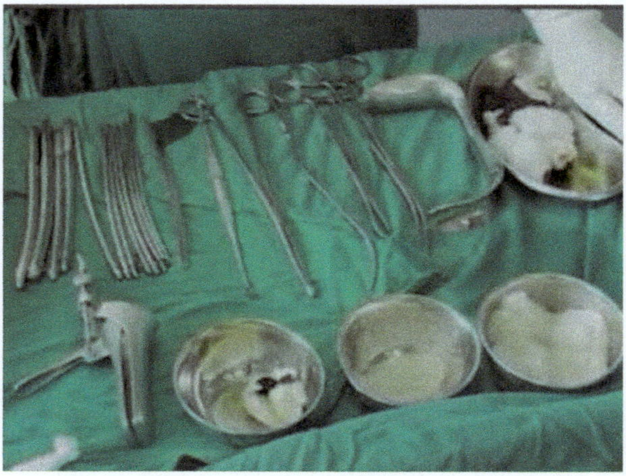

Fig. 15.1 Trolley for colposcopy

facilitated. The transformation zone is excised to a depth of 6–7 mm, extending 4–5 mm beyond the diseased area. A 60–80 W setting in the cut mode on the electrocautery machine allows a smooth excision of the lesion (Figs. 15.3 and 15.4).

If the lesion is large, the anterior and posterior portions of the lesion can be excised in separate passes to avoid using excessively large loops. After the removal of the specimen, the bleeding areas can be cauterised using the ball electrode or hemostatic paste; Monsel's solution (ferrous subsulfate) can be applied to the cervix (Figs 15.4 and 15.5).

15.5 Indications of LEEP

Indications of LEEP include

- When good visualisation or access to the entire transformation zone is difficult
- An atrophic or stenotic cervix flushed with the vaginal wall
- Large lesions extending widely on the cervix
- Lesions going into the endocervical canal
- Lesions extending on to the vaginal epithelium

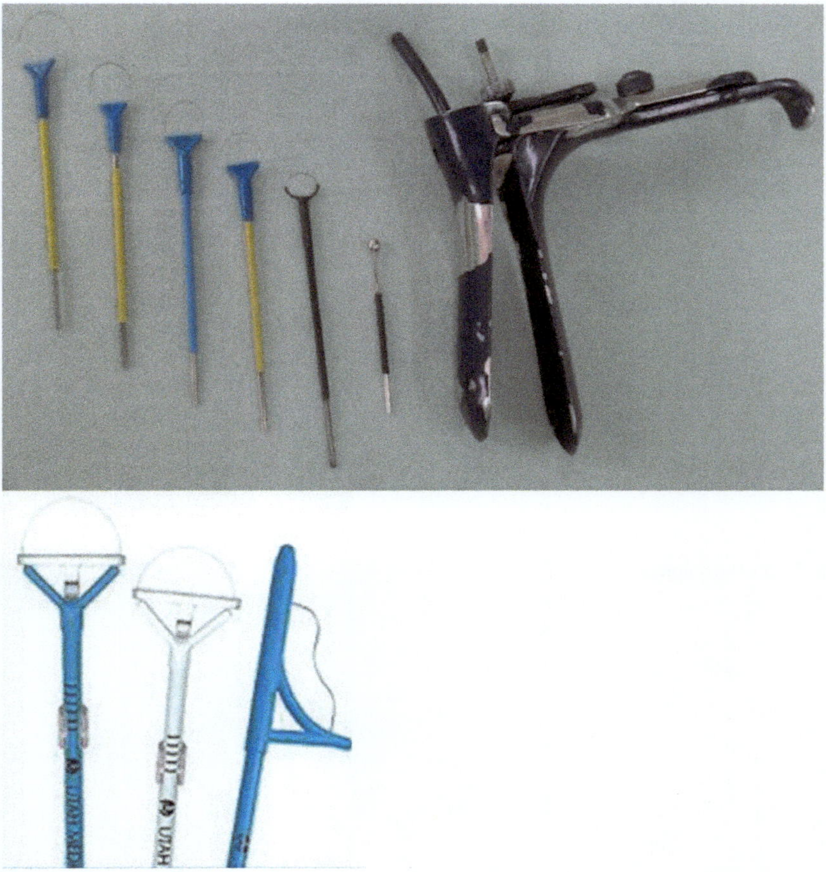

Fig. 15.2 Loops of various sizes

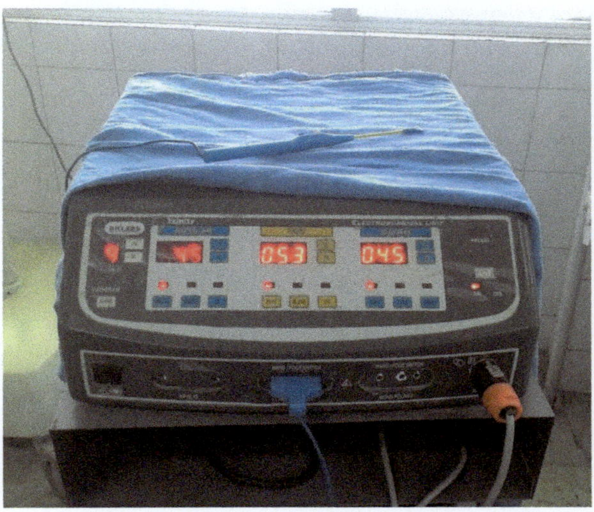

Fig 15.3 Electrocautery unit

Fig. 15.4 Loop excision

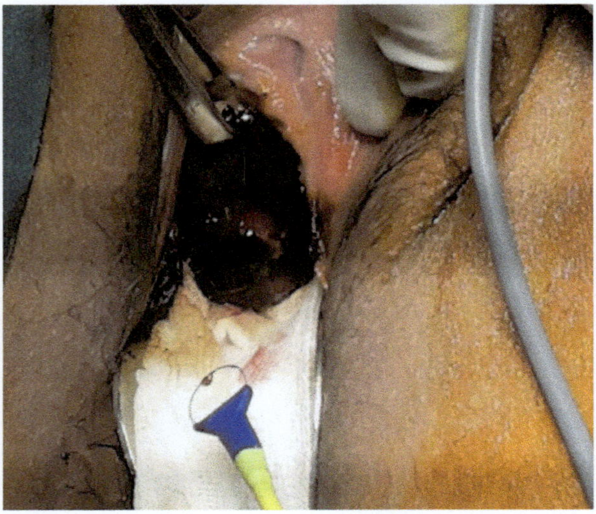

Fig. 15.5 Ball cautery

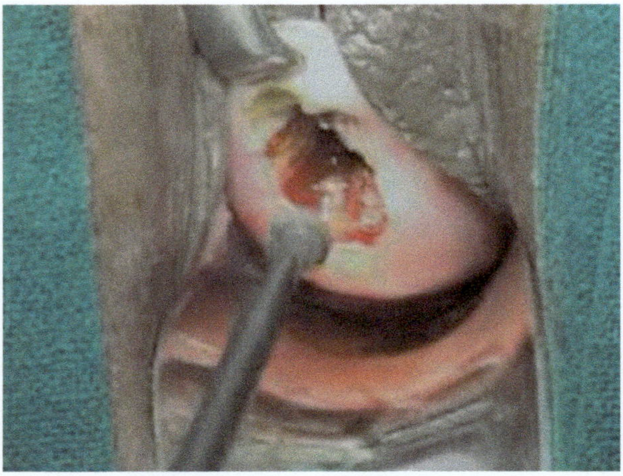

The LEEP procedure has become popular for the treatment of high-grade CIN lesions as it is easily available. The advantage of the LEEP over ablative procedures is that there is a specimen available for histopathology.

Two problems have evolved with the use of LEEP procedures; first, the removal of excessive tissue, and second, the danger of overtreatment. The advantages of performing colposcopy and treatment at one visit avoid patients lost to follow-up in noncompliant populations and decreased expense from repeated visits. The incidence of negative specimens in see-and-treat series varies from 14 to 32.5 % [16, 17]. The negative specimens were related to smaller lesions and younger women. Factors which are contributing to a higher rate of negative see-and-treat specimens include the liberal use of colposcopy to evaluate low-grade lesions on Pap smear. This is relevant for young women who desire fertility preservation. The see-and-treat approach is appropriate for noncompliant patients with a high-grade lesion on LBC/Pap smear that is unequivocal on colposcopy.

15.6 Advantages of LEEP

1. It can be done as an OPD procedure.
2. Tissue is available for histopathological evaluation.
3. See-and-treat can be done at the same sitting.
4. No repeated visits are required.

Cold knife cone biopsy has the advantage of obtaining an intact specimen. This is important in cases of microinvasive cancer or glandular dysplasia as the specimen obtained by cold knife gives a better idea regarding the depth of the invasion and margin status. The difficulty of using LEEP for excising a cone is that, at times, broken specimens are obtained which are difficult for pathological evaluation.

15.7 Conisation

Conisation of the cervix has a prominent role in the treatment of CIN. Before the advent of colposcopy, conisation was the only method of evaluating an abnormal Pap test. Conisation, being both a diagnostic and a therapeutic method, has the distinct advantage over ablative procedures of providing tissue for biopsy to rule out invasive cancer [18–21].

Conisation is indicated for the evaluation of women with HSIL or AGC-adenocarcinoma in situ and may be considered under the following circumstances: [5]

1. Margins of the lesion cannot be seen with colposcopy.
2. The entire squamocolumnar junction (SCJ) is not visible at colposcopy.
3. Endocervical curettage (ECC) is positive for CIN 2 or CIN 3 histologically.
4. There is a lack of correlation between the results of cytology, biopsy and colposcopy.
5. Microinvasion is suspected depending on biopsy, colposcopy or cytology findings.
6. The colposcopy cannot rule out invasive cancer.

Lesions which have positive margins are likely to recur after conisation [18–20]. About 23.6 % of patients with endocervical gland involvement recurred compared to the 11.3 % without gland involvement [22]. When compared with conisation, LEEP is the simpler technique, and short-term results are similar to those obtained with conisation or laser excision [23, 24].

In a prospective study examining the long-term effects of LEEP, conisation and laser excision, no difference in the recurrence of dysplasia or in pregnancy outcomes was found [25].

15.8 Procedure of Conisation

Conisation means the removal of ectocervical lesions and a portion of the endocervix in a cone-shaped manner (Fig. 15.6).

Fig 15.6 Cone biopsy

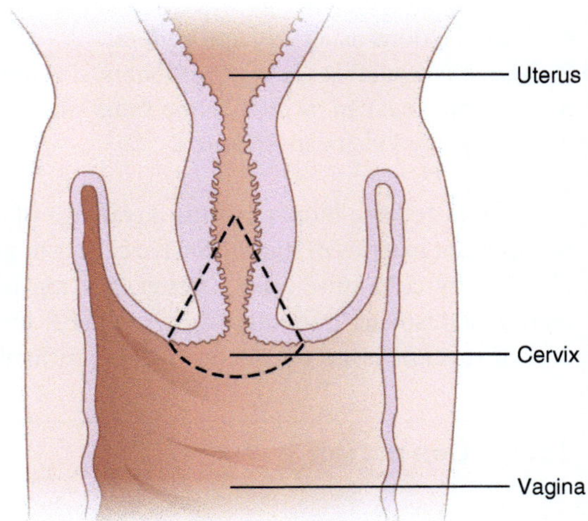

Fig 15.7 Sutures at 3 and 9 o'clock positions to minimise bleeding during conisation

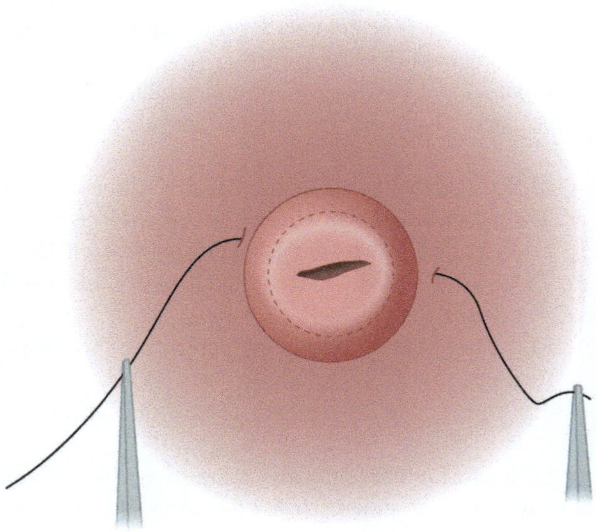

It is performed under general anaesthesia in a lithotomy position after the bladder is emptied. The cervix is exposed, and the vaginal side walls are retracted with preferably insulated Cusco's speculum with a smoke extractor. After demarcating the limits of the lesion on the ectocervix by colposcopy, the limits of the base of the cone on the cervix can be determined.

The descending cervical branches of the uterus are ligated with a figure-of-eight suture at the 3 and 9 o'clock positions (Fig 15.7). A uterine dilator or sound is placed in the endocervical canal to orient the surgeon to assess the depth and direction of the canal.

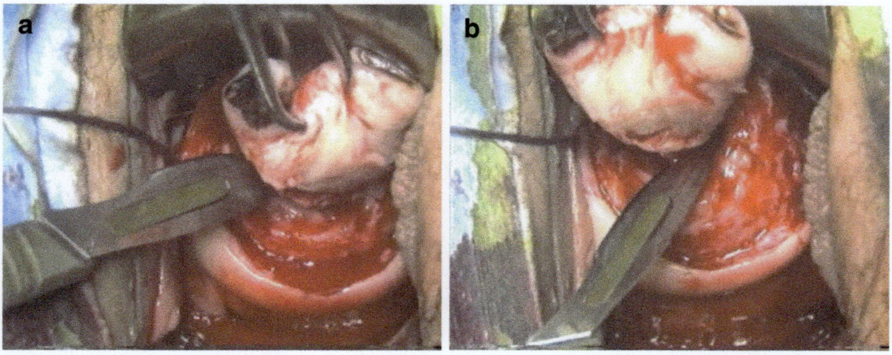

Fig 15.8 (**a**, **b**) Technique of cone biopsy

Fig 15.9 Crater after cone biopsy

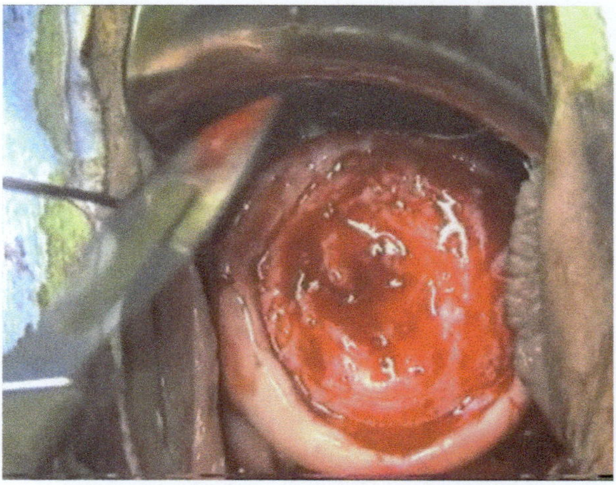

An incision is put on the lower or the posterior lip of the cervix. A circumscribing incision is made 2–3 mm around the entire cervix. The blade is directed cephalad at 45° angle (Fig 15.8a, b). After removal of the cone, an orientation suture is put at 12 o'clock position. Haemostasis is achieved by the suturing of the isolated vessel or coagulation (Fig 15.9).

15.9 Disadvantages of Conisation

1. Dysmenorrhea.
2. Inadequate postoperative surveillance, e.g. Pap smear.
3. Flap might conceal a residual disease.

Many surgeons use laser as an instrument instead of a knife in performing cone biopsy of the cervix.

In some centres, conisation of the cervix is used as a diagnostic as well as a therapeutic procedure for patients who are young and desire fertility [7].

15.10 Procedure of Laser Conisation (Table 15.3)

If margins after conisation rule out invasive cancer, then these patients have almost a 100 % disease-free follow-up.

Laser conisation needs a local or general anaesthesia and can be performed in the outpatient setting. Besides, the laser cone specimens have cautery artefact which may make histopathological diagnosis difficult. Since LEEP is more efficient, has widespread availability and is more easily performed, it has replaced laser cone in all the centres. If appropriate power settings are used, LEEP excision produces minimal cautery artefact [26].

15.11 Treatment Complications

Both laser and LEEP are associated with bleeding, but the rates of complications are low. Post-treatment cervical/vaginal bleeding occurs in 2–7 % of LEEP cases [16, 26–28] and requires hospitalisation in only 1–2 %. Long-term side effects of these procedures are minimal. Only 1.3–9 % patients undergoing LEEP have unsatisfactory colposcopy, and 1.3–3.8 % has cervical stenosis after the LEEP [27].

The risk of cervical stenosis and hydro-hematometra is higher in women who have a LEEP that extends 1.5 cm or more into the endocervical canal and in women who have had past history of ablative therapy.

Two case–control studies revealed that after comparing with controls, patients with a history of a LEEP had no higher rate of prematurity or caesarean delivery [29, 30].

The effect on fertility is difficult to obtain, but there is no clear association between decreased fertility and LEEP (Tables 15.4 and 15.5).

Table 15.3 Laser conisation

Instruments	CO_2 laser, colposcope
Power output	25–30 W
Power density	1400 W/cm^2
Spot size	0.5 mm
Operating mode	Continuous
Lateral margins	5 mm around the lesion
Endocervical margin	Excised surgically
Haemostasis	By sutures
Anaesthesia	Either general or local

Table 15.4 Major complications of conisation

Immediate	Delayed
Haemorrhage	Bleeding (10–14 days after operation)
Uterine perforation	Stenosis of the cervix
Anaesthetic risk	Infertility
	Cervical incompetence
	Increased risk of preterm delivery
	Premature rupture of membranes

Table 15.5 Comparison of haemorrhage between laser and knife conisation

Author	Laser (%)	Author	Knife (%)
Wright et al. [31]	12.2	Larsson et al.	14.8
Baggish et al.	2.5	Bostofte et al.	17.0
Larsson et al.	2.3	Jones et al. [33]	10.0
Bostofte et al. [32]	5.0	Luesley et al.	13.0

15.11.1 WHO Guidelines for the Treatment of CIN 2/3 and Adenocarcinoma In Situ (2014)

15.11.1.1 Strong Recommendation

Use LEEP over no treatment.

Use cryotherapy over no treatment.

Use cold knife conisation over no treatment.

Use cryotherapy over cold knife conisation in patients for whom either cryotherapy or cold knife conisation can be used.

Use LEEP over cold knife conisation in patients for whom either LEEP or CKC is appropriate to use.

15.11.1.2 Conditional Recommendation

For women with histologically proven diagnosis of adenocarcinoma in situ, regardless of HIV status, use CKC over LEEP.

15.11.2 CIN in Pregnancy

The same screening and diagnostic procedure, e.g. Pap smear/LBC, HPV testing and colposcopy, can be used to evaluate patients during pregnancy. The cold knife conisation should only be done during pregnancy when an invasive cancer is suspected and could not be excluded by colposcopy-directed biopsy. The patients follow-up with preinvasive lesion during pregnancy should be reevaluated by colposcopy after 6–8 weeks postpartum when there is involution of the uterus and cervix [34].

15.12 Treatment of Recurrent Dysplasia

A follow-up of women treated for CIN is mandatory to identify treatment failures or patients with recurrent CIN. Predictors of recurrent CIN include:

- Women who are more than 40 years old
- Positive margins of the specimen
- Glandular lesions of the cervix
- Large lesions

ASCCP guidelines of 2012 recommend co-testing at 12 and 24 months for women treated for high-grade lesions (CIN 2/3). If both of these tests are negative, then retesting is recommended after 3 years, and if it is negative, then she returns to routine screening. If any of the tests is abnormal, colposcopy with endocervical sampling is to be done.

A repeat diagnostic excisional procedure can be done for women with recurrent or persistent CIN 2/3. In women in whom such a procedure is not feasible and in whom fertility is not desired, hysterectomy is acceptable.

Data have shown an increased prevalence of CIN in women with decreased levels of micronutrients like vitamin C, folic acid, vitamin B6/12 and lycopene. According to the available evidence, a diet rich in these micronutrients may prevent the development of CIN though their roles in the treatment of CIN is controversial [35].

15.13 Hysterectomy

Hysterectomy is considered a treatment of last resort for recurrent high-grade CIN. In a study of 38 cases of invasive CA in the cervix occurring after hysterectomy amongst 8,998 women, there have been incidences of bleeding, infection and other complications, which is higher with hysterectomy than with other means of treating CIN [36]. There are various conditions in which hysterectomy is an appropriate method of treating CIN:

1. Microinvasion
2. CIN 3 at the endocervical margins of cone specimen in selected patients
3. Patients with poor compliance for follow-up
4. Some other gynaecologic conditions requiring hysterectomy, e.g. fibroids, prolapsed uterus and endometriosis
5. Histologically confirmed recurrent high-grade CIN

Conclusion

The ultimate goal of the management is to eliminate all cases of cancer in the cervix which cannot be realised completely. But there have been significant advances in the diagnosis and management of preinvasive lesions of the cervix. By carefully choosing treatment procedures for all individual patients, gynaecologists can avoid unnecessary discomfort and cost from overtreatment and undertreating or misdiagnosing a malignant condition.

References

1. Richart RM. Natural history of cervical intraepithelial neoplasia. Clin Obstet Gynecol. 1967;10:748.
2. McIndoe WA, McLean MR, Jones RW, et al. The invasive potential of carcinoma in situ of the cervix. Obstet Gynecol. 1984;64:451.
3. Wright Jr TC, Massad LS, Dunton CJ, et al. 2006 consensus guidelines for the management of women with cervical intraepithelial neoplasia or adenocarcinoma in situ. J Low Genit Tract Dis. 2007;11:223–39.
4. Mitchell MF, Schottenfeld D. The natural history of cervical intraepithelial neoplasia and management of the abnormal papanicolaou smear. In: Rubin SC, Hoskins WJ, editors. Cancer of the cervix. 1st ed. Philadelphia: Lippincott-Raven; 1996. p. 103–13.
5. Garcia F, Hatch KD, Berek JS. Intraepithelial disease of the cervix, vagina and vulva, 15th ed. Berek and Novak's. Berek & Novak's Gynecology. Lippincott Williams & Wilkins, Philadelphia; 2015. p. 574–618.
6. Holowaty P, Miller AB, Rohan T, To T. Natural history of dysplasia of the uterine cervix. J Natl Cancer Inst. 1999;91:252.
7. Creasman WT. Preinvasive disease of the cervix. In: DiSaia PJ, Creasman WT, editors. Clinical gynaecologic oncology, 7th ed. Mosby Elsevier publishers, Philadelphia; 2007. p. 1–36.
8. Bjork S, Hagstrom HG. Of what significance is abnormal results of smear test? Anxiety because of insufficient information in connection with abnormal results of cervical smear test. Lakartidningen. 2001;98:2796.
9. Jones MH, Singer A, Jenkins D. The mildly abnormal cervical smear: patient anxiety and choice of management. J R Soc Med. 1996;89:257.
10. Wilkinson C, Jones JM, McBride J. Anxiety caused by abnormal results of cervical smear test: a controlled trial. BMJ. 1990;300:440.
11. Benedet JL, Miller DM, Nickerson KG. Results of conservative management of cervical intraepithelial neoplasia. Obstet Gynecol. 1992;79:105.
12. Kaufman RH, Irwin JF. The cryosurgical therapy of cervical intraepithelial neoplasia. Am J Obstet Gynecol. 1978;131:381.
13. Hatch KD, Shingleton HM, Austin JM, et al. Cryosurgery of cervical intraepithelial neoplasia. Obstet Gynecol. 1981;57:692.
14. Treatment of cervical intraepithelial neoplasia. Connor J, Hartenbach E. Glob. libr.women's med; 2008. doi: 10.3843/GLOWM.10228
15. From American College of Obstetricians and Gynecologists: Technical Bulletin, No. 183, 1993.
16. Ferenczy A, Choukroun D, Arseneau J. Large loop excision procedure for squamous intraepithelial lesions of the cervix: advantages and potential pitfalls. Obstet Gynecol. 1996;87:332.
17. Alvarez RD, Helm CW, Edwards RP, et al. The prospective randomized trial of LLETZ versus laser ablation in patients with cervical intraepithelial neoplasia. Gynecol Oncol. 1994;52:175.
18. Chappatte OA, Byrne DL, Raju KS, Nayagam M, Kenney A. Histological differences between colposcopic-directed biopsy and loop excision of the transformation zone (LETZ): a cause for concern. Gynecol Oncol. 1991;43(1):46–50.
19. Baggish MS. A comparison between laser excisional conization and laser vaporization for the treatment of cervical intraepithelial neoplasia. Am J Obstet Gynecol. 1986;155(1):39–44.
20. Larsson G, Gullberg B, Grundsell H. A comparison of complications of laser and cold knife conization. Obstet Gynecol. 1983;62(2):213–7.
21. Luesley DM, McCrum A, Terry PB, Wade-Evans T, Nicholson HO, Mylotte MJ, Emens JM, Jordan JA. Complications of cone biopsy related to the dimensions of the cone and the influence of prior colposcopic assessment. Br J Obstet Gynaecol. 1985;92(2):158–64.
22. Demopoulos RI, Horowitz LF, Vamvakas EC. Endocervical gland involvement by cervical intraepithelial neoplasia grade III. Predictive value for residual and/or recurrent disease. Cancer. 1991;68(9):1932–6.
23. Mitchell MF, Tortolero-Luna G, Cook E, Whittaker L, Rhodes-Morris H, Silva E. A randomized clinical trial of cryotherapy, laser vaporization, and loop electrosurgical excision for treatment of squamous intraepithelial lesions of the cervix. Obstet Gynecol. 1998;92(5):737–44.

24. Duggan BD, Felix JC, Muderspach LI, Gebhardt JA, Groshen S, Morrow CP, Roman LD. Cold-knife conization versus conization by the loop electrosurgical excision procedure: a randomized, prospective study. Am J Obstet Gynecol. 1999;180(2 Pt 1):276–82.
25. Mathevet P, Chemali E, Roy M, Dargent D. Long-term outcome of a randomized study comparing three techniques of conization: cold knife, laser, and LEEP. Eur J Obstet Gynecol Reprod Biol. 2003;106(2):214–8.
26. Herzog TJ, Williams S, Adler LM, et al. Potential of cervical electrosurgical excision procedure for diagnosis and treatment of cervical intraepithelial neoplasia. Gynecol Oncol. 1995;57:286.
27. Wright TC, Richart RM. Loop excision of the uterine cervix. Curr Opin Obstet Gynecol. 1995; 7:30.
28. Prendiville W. Large loop excision of the transformation zone. Clin Obstet Gynecol. 1995; 38:622.
29. Haffenden DK, Bigrigg A, Codling BW, et al. Pregnancy following large loop excision of the transformation zone. Br J Obstet Gynaecol. 1993;100:1059.
30. Blomfield PI, Buxton J, Dunn J, et al. Pregnancy outcome after large loop excision of the cervical transformation zone. Am J Obstet Gynecol. 1993;169:620.
31. Wright VC, Riopelle MA, Rubinstein E, Rylander E, Joelsson I. CO2 laser and cervical intraepithelial neoplasia. Acta Obstet Gynecol Scand Suppl. 1984;125:1–36.
32. Bostofte E, Berget A, Falck Larsen J, Hjortkjaer Pedersen P, Rank F. Conization by carbon dioxide laser or cold knife in the treatment of cervical intraepithelial neoplasia. Acta Obstet Gynecol Scand. 1986;65(3):199–202.
33. Jones 3rd HW. Treatment of cervical intraepithelial neoplasia. Clin Obstet Gynecol. 1990;33(4):826–36.
34. Connor JP. Noninvasive cervical cancer complicating pregnancy. Obstet Gynecol Clin North Am. 1998;25:331.
35. Palan PR, Chang CJ, Mikhail MS, et al. Plasma concentrations of micronutrients during a nine-month clinical trial of beta-carotene in women with precursor cervical cancer lesions. Nutr Cancer. 1998;30:46–52.
36. Shafi MI. The management of cervical intraepithelial neoplasia. In: Jordan J, Singer A. The cervix. Blackwell; New York; 2006.

Colposcopy of Vulva and Vagina

16

Divya Pandey and Sumita Mehta

16.1 Colposcopy of Vulva

The colposcopic examination of vulva, also known as vulvoscopy, forms an integral part of gynecological examination and is an important component of the screening process for lower genital tract disease [1]. It is a helpful tool in the identification of subclinical and premalignant lesions. For the purpose of diagnosis of vulvar lesions, the vulvar biopsy remains the gold standard. But the anatomic structure of vulva is entirely different from the cervix because it has a mucosa as well as skin [2]. Vulvoscopy is not as good a predictor of preinvasive lesions as colposcopy of the cervix because

- The vulvar skin has keratinized stratified squamous epithelium which renders the underlying dermis vascularity not clearly visible even colposcopically.
- Vulvar intraepithelial neoplasia (VIN) disorders have a multifocal character, thus limiting the usefulness of colposcopy.

16.1.1 Anatomical Definition

Vulva consists of female genital organs: mons pubis, labia majora, labia minora, clitoris with prepuce and frenulum, and vestibule along with the glandular structure openings in it (Fig. 16.1) [3].

D. Pandey, MS (✉)
Department of Obstetrics and Gynecology,
Vardhman Mahavir Medical College and Safdarjung Hospital, Delhi, India
e-mail: dr_devya1@yahoo.co.in

S. Mehta, DGO, DNB, MAMS, MICOG
Department of Obstetrics and Gynecology, Babu Jagjivan Ram Memorial Hospital, Delhi, India

S. Mehta, P. Sachdeva (eds.), *Colposcopy of Female Genital Tract*,
DOI 10.1007/978-981-10-1705-6_16

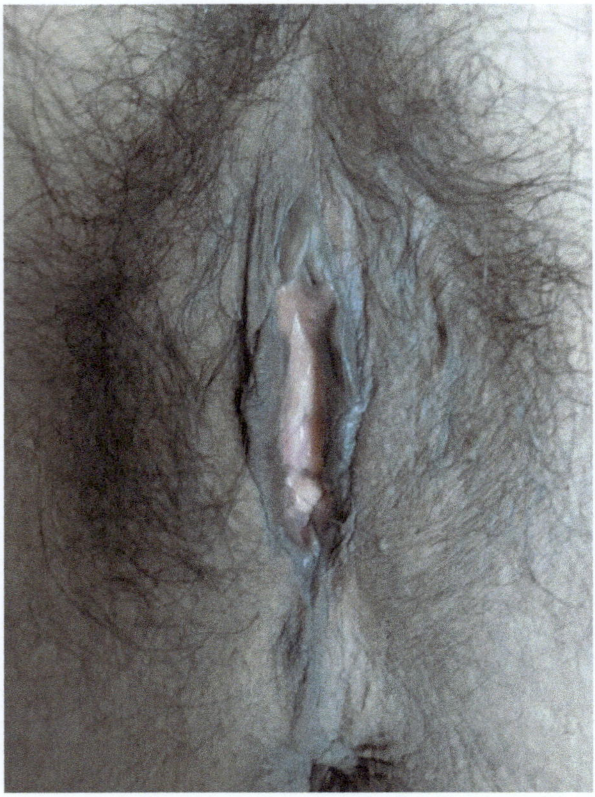

Fig. 16.1 Anatomical extent of vulva, showing hair-bearing skin on mons pubis, lateral parts of labia majora, and perianal area

16.1.2 Colposcopic Definition

The colposcopic definition of vulva refers to the external urethral orifice, the perineum, the perianal region, and the anus (Figs. 16.1 and 16.2) [3].

16.1.3 Histological Variation and Its Basis

Due to the different embryological origins of various vulvar parts, the histology also varies. Vulva has an ectodermal origin with keratinized stratified squamous epithelium which lacks glycogen in the epidermis and mesodermal dermis (with its reticular and papillary layer). In contrast, vestibule has an endodermal origin and is covered by nonkeratinized squamous epithelium, which is relatively thinner with abundant mucus-secreting glands [4]. Mons pubis, outer parts of labia majora, and perianal area are covered with hair follicle-bearing skin. The skin in this part has rich sebaceous glands along with sweat glands.

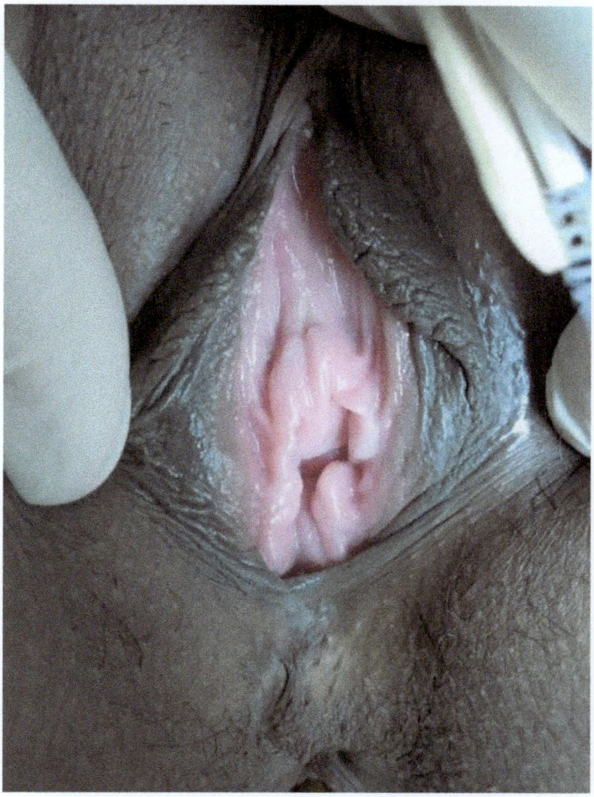

Fig. 16.2 Non-hair-bearing skin after retracting labia showing medial part of labia majora, labia minora, and clitoris

16.1.4 Basis of Colposcopy of Vulva

Colposcopic features depend on the specific parts of the vulva. It is widely variable for different vulvar parts and varies even from person to person. This is the reason behind the different appearances of histologically similar lesions in different parts of the vulva. The features are based on the fact that epithelial thickness directly affects the skin thickness, and hence its opacity thus obscuring the clear view of the underlying vascularity [4]. Moreover any pigmentation on the vulvar skin can also mask the clear view. This is in contrast to the colposcopy of the cervix where specific vascular patterns are pronounced and form a reliable colposcopic finding.

While acetowhitening is the most frequent colposcopic appearance along with leukoplakia, the atypical vessel pattern can be seen in invasive carcinoma [5].

Punctation and mosaic patterns are less common on most of the vulvar region except the inner parts of labia minora where the layer of keratin is thinner and in the vestibular part where the keratin is absent [4].

16.1.5 Indications for Colposcopy of Vulva

- Pruritus vulvae to rule out subclinical papilloma infection, intraepithelial lesion (VIN), or early malignant lesion
- Vulvodynia
- Condyloma of cervix and/or vagina
- Cervical or vaginal intraepithelial lesions (CIN/VAIN)
- To delineate a visible lesion (VIN, cancerous growth, or Paget's disease).

16.1.6 Contraindications

- The use of local medication just before the procedure
- Acute vulvar infection or presence of vulvitis

Any visible growth of a nonhealing ulcer on vulva must be biopsied to rule out tuberculosis and malignancy even in young patients.

16.1.7 Colposcopic Appearance of Vulva

The following points are to be looked for during vulvoscopy: [6]

- Color changes
- Topography
- Surface contour
- Angioarchitecture

16.1.7.1 Color Changes

Lugol's iodine application shows a clearly demarcated vulvovaginal line (Fig. 16.3) owing to glycogenated vaginal epithelium. Due to the nonglycogenated nature of the vulvar epithelium, there is no role of iodine application in vulvoscopy. 5% acetic acid application results in acetowhite response extending a few millimeters lateral from vulvovaginal line, but it never involves the fourchette. There has been no correlation between the degree of acetowhitening and primary histopathology. A special note should be made of generalized depigmentation (due to loss of melanin as in vitiligo) or localized whiteness (due to transient loss of pigment as in a scar of a healed ulcer) [6].

White lesions may be seen in non-neoplastic epithelial disorder, HPV lesion, and in VIN. To differentiate, biopsy is a must.

Red lesion on vulva is due to increased vascularity and vasodilatation as in infections (candidiasis) and inflammation (dermatitis and eczema), thinning of epidermis (in postmenopausal age-group), and neovascularization seen in malignancy. Diffused redness is suggestive of benign pathology, while an isolated red lesion is invariably a feature of neoplasia.

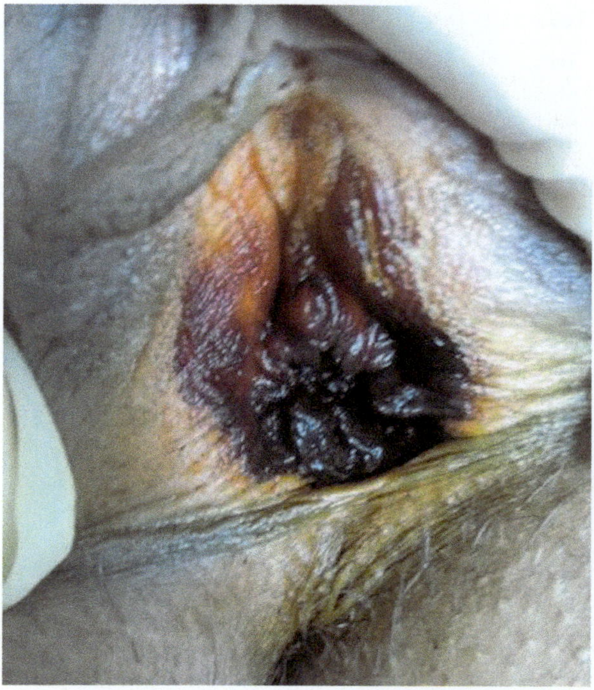

Fig. 16.3 Vulva after Lugol's iodine application showing demarcated iodine-positive vaginal epithelium from nonglycogenated keratinized vulvar epithelium

Dark lesion is due to melanin, which is a result of increased melanin production in epidermal melanocytes which is then extruded toward the papillary dermis as a result of a mechanism known as "melanin incontinence" leading to an occasional pigmented appearance of the VIN lesion. Thus dark lesions are seen in VIN, hyperpigmentation, nevi, lentigo, and malignant melanoma.

16.1.7.2 Topography

Acetowhitening beyond normal limits or isolated acetowhite areas are abnormal findings. It can be unifocal, multifocal, or with a multisite involvement [6].

16.1.7.3 Surface Contour

The surface contour is mentioned in the context of the level of surrounding skin and can be differentiated into:

- Raised above the skin surface – papule, pustule, proliferative, vesicular
- At the level of the skin – acetowhitening, pigmentation, macula
- Below the level of the skin – ulcer or erosion.

In reproductive age-group females, papillary and villiform features (also called micropapillomatosis) are present in contrast to those in postmenopausal and prepubertal age-groups. These micropapillomatosis may be mildly acetowhite. They may sporadically merge and can be misinterpreted as HPV infection.

Table 16.1 Definition of primary vulvar lesions

Term	Definition
Macule	Small (<1.5 cm) area of color change; no elevation and no substance on palpation
Patch	Large (>1.5 cm) area of color change; no elevation and no substance on palpation
Papule	Small (<1.5 cm) elevated and palpable lesion
Plaque	Large (>1.5 cm) elevated, palpable, and flat-topped lesion
Nodule	A large papule (>1.5 cm) often hemispherical or poorly marginated; may be located on the surface of, within, or below the skin; may be cystic or solid
Vesicle	Small (<0.5 cm) fluid-filled blister; fluid is clear
Bulla	Large (>0.5 cm) fluid-filled blister; fluid is clear
Pustule	Pus-filled blister; fluid is white or yellow

Source: Lynch et al. [7]

Table 16.2 IFCPC (2011) terminology of the vulva; definitions of *secondary morphology presentation* [8]

Term	Definition
Eczema	A group of inflammatory diseases that are characterized by the presence of itchy, poorly marginated red plaques with minor evidence of microvesiculation and/or subsequent surface disruption
Lichenification	Thickening of the tissue and increased prominence of skin markings. Scale may or may not be detectable in vulvar lichenification. Lichenification may be bright red, dusky red, white, or skin-colored in appearance
Excoriation	Surface disruption (notably excoriations) occurring as a result of the "itch-scratch" cycle
Erosion	A shallow defect in the skin surface; absence of some, or all, of the epidermis down to the basement membrane; the dermis is intact
Fissure	A thin linear erosion of the skin surface
Ulcer	Deeper defect; absence of the epidermis and some, or all, of the dermis

Source: Bornstein et al. [8]

According to the International Federation for Cervical Pathology and Colposcopy (IFCPC) colposcopic terminology of the vulva, the definitions of primary lesion types are mentioned in Tables 16.1 and 16.2 [7].

16.1.7.4 Angioarchitecture

Due to the presence of surface keratinization, the terminal vessels are rarely visible. However atypical vessels and prominence of vessels may be features in invasive cancers. Punctation and mosaic patterns are evaluated in the same manner as in the colposcopic evaluation of cervix.

Various types of lesions cannot be differentiated on the basis of gross appearance and distribution of lesions on vulva. Vulvoscopy only helps in localizing the lesion for biopsy or mapping the extent of the lesion during excision.

Table 16.3 IFCPC 2011 terminology of vulva (including anus)

Normal findings	Micropapillomatosis		
	Sebaceous glands (Fordyce spots)		
	Vestibular redness		
Abnormal findings	Lesion type	Lesion color	Secondary morphology
	Macule	Skin-colored	Eczema
	Patch	Red	Excoriation
	Papule	White	Purpura
	Plaque	Dark	Scarring
	Nodule		Ulcer
	Cyst		Erosion
	Vesicle		Fissure
	Bulla		Wart
	Pustule		
Miscellaneous findings	Trauma		
	Malformation		
Suspicion of malignancy	Gross neoplasm		
	Ulceration		
	Necrosis		
	Bleeding		
	Hyperkeratosis		
Abnormal colposcopic findings	Acetowhite epithelium		
	Punctation		
	Atypical vessels		
	Surface irregularities		
	Abnormal anal squamocolumnar junction		

Source: Bornstein et al. [8]

16.1.8 Colposcopic Terminology of Vulvar Lesions

The IFCPC in 2011 has suggested the clinical/colposcopic terminology of the vulva (including the anus) (Table 16.3) [8].

16.1.9 Technique of Colposcopy of Vulva

The first vulvar examination is done with naked eye followed by low-power magnification. The technique is almost similar to that of colposcopy of the cervix. The patient is put in a lithotomy position. The examiner must be gentle but thorough. The vulva should be examined in a systematic fashion to include the mons pubis, labia majora, labia minora, clitoral prepuce, clitoris, perineal, and anal region.

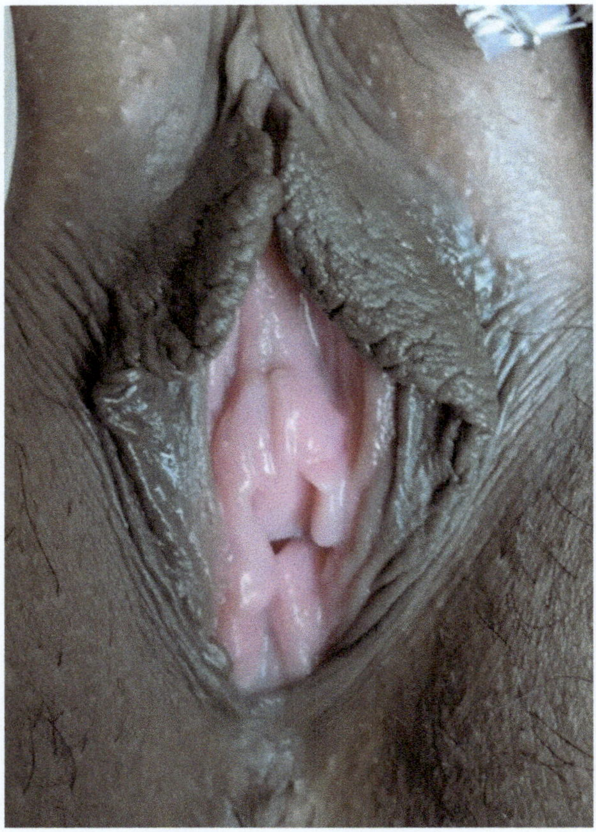

Fig. 16.4 Labial separation for the adequate exposure of entire vestibule

The gland openings (Bartholin and Skene) and urinary meatus should also be noted. If the patient is co-operative, the examination must include the colposcopic examination of the anal canal with the use of a proctoscope. The application of normal saline or a water-based jelly negates the keratinizing effect, thereby assisting in the easy visualization of abnormal vessels over the vulva.

16.1.9.1 Steps of Vulvoscopy [9]

- Visual inspection
- Acetic acid application
- Collins test
- Biopsy
- Documentation

16.1.9.2 Visual Inspection

A thorough visual examination of the entire vulva should be done. All structures should be properly examined including the non-hair-bearing parts which require labial separation for the adequate exposure of the entire vestibule (Fig. 16.4). The adequate inspection will help in the identification of fields of redness, leukoplakia,

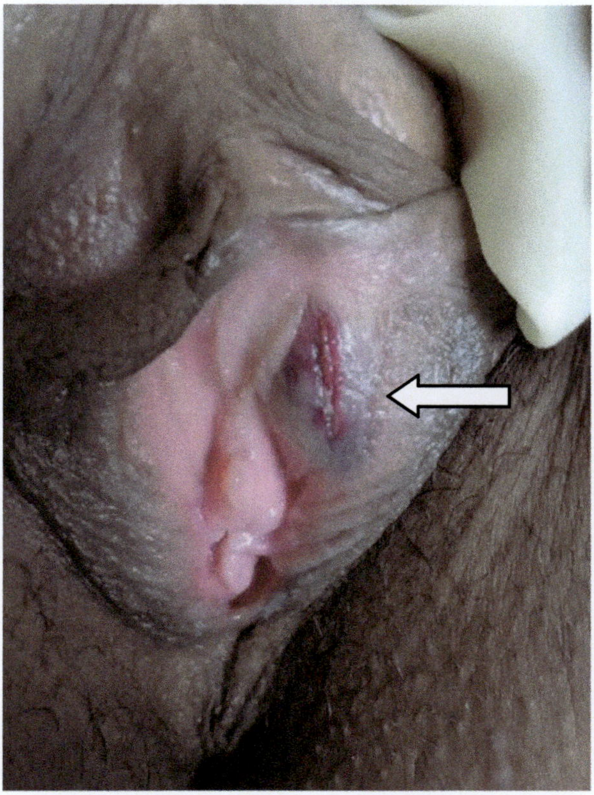

Fig. 16.5 Small vulvar hematoma on medial side of the left labia minora

ulceration, atrophy, and pigmentation apart from genital warts and invasive cancers. Other findings of benign conditions like folliculitis, genital molluscum, etc., should also be noted (Figs. 16.5, 16.6, 16.7, and 16.8).

A water-soluble lubricant or a simple application of normal saline can help complete the examination by negating the drying of the keratinizing feature of the vulvar skin thereby increasing the visibility of the abnormal vascular pattern. This is similar to normal saline application in colposcopy of cervix.

16.1.9.3 Acetic Acid Application

Due to presence of keratinization, more concentrated (i.e., 5 %) freshly prepared acetic acid is required (in contrast to 3 % for cervix). Also prolonged application for 5 min is required to highlight abnormal areas. This can be done by compressing a swab/gauze soaked in 5 % acetic acid against the vulvar skin.

Acetic acid can cause acetowhitening of normal skin at the vestibule, but it never extends to the fourchette. There is a normal papillary pattern seen on vestibule of reproductive age-group females, but this pattern is absent in postmenopausal and prepubertal girls (Fig. 16.9). HPV lesions can appear acetowhite with micropapillary surface pattern. Vulvar ulcer and any inflammatory condition of vulva including trauma from intercourse can cause acetowhitening (Figs. 16.10, 16.11, and

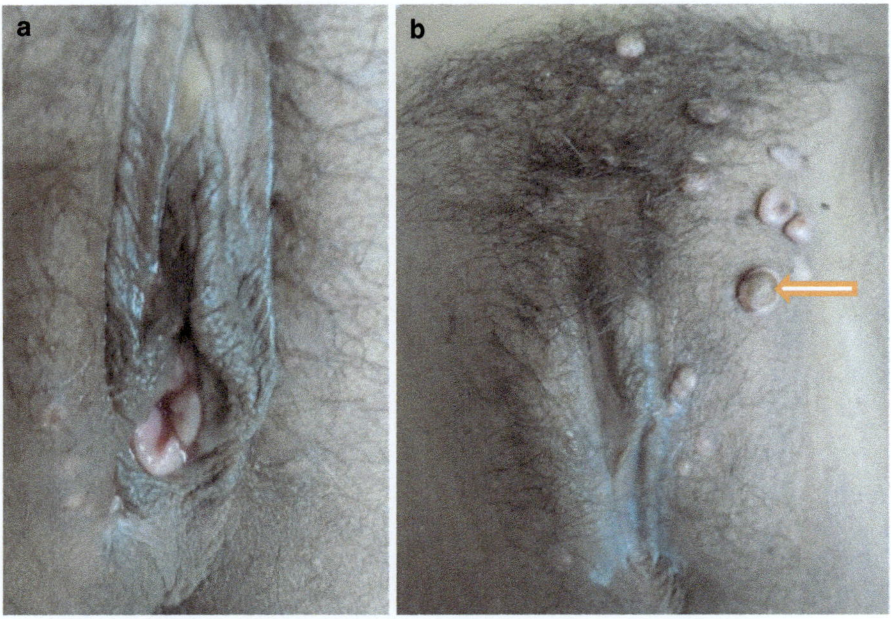

Fig. 16.6 (**a**, **b**) Genital molluscum lesions

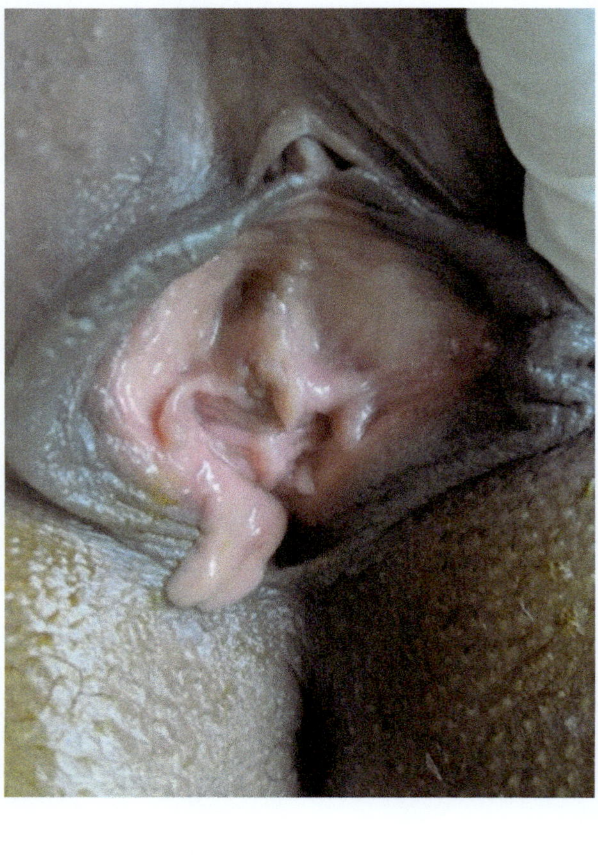

Fig. 16.7 Mucosal tag on the medial side of labia minora; a normal finding

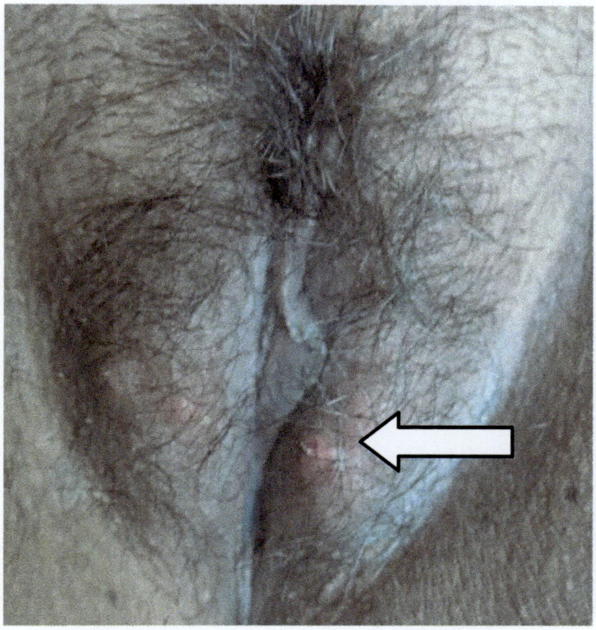

Fig. 16.8 Vulvar folliculitis

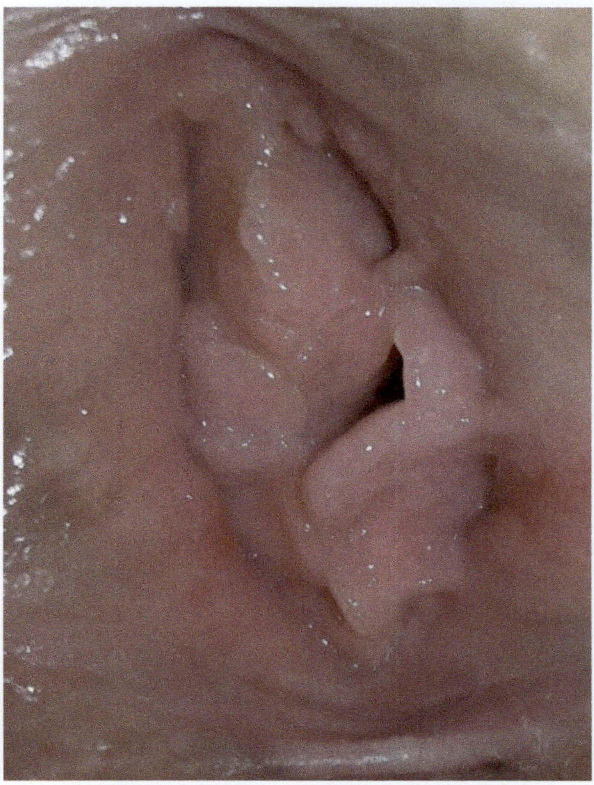

Fig. 16.9 Normal villiform pattern of labia minora; this pattern is often confused with HPV infection

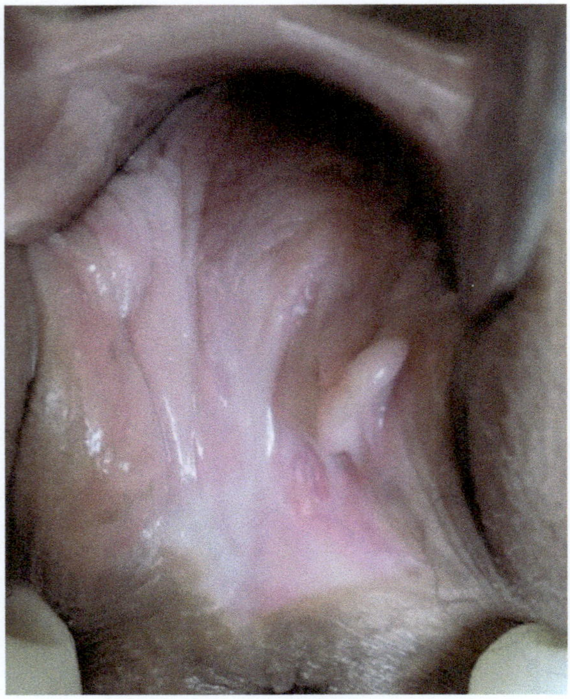

Fig. 16.10 Acetowhitening at the posterior fourchette extending to the posterior vaginal wall

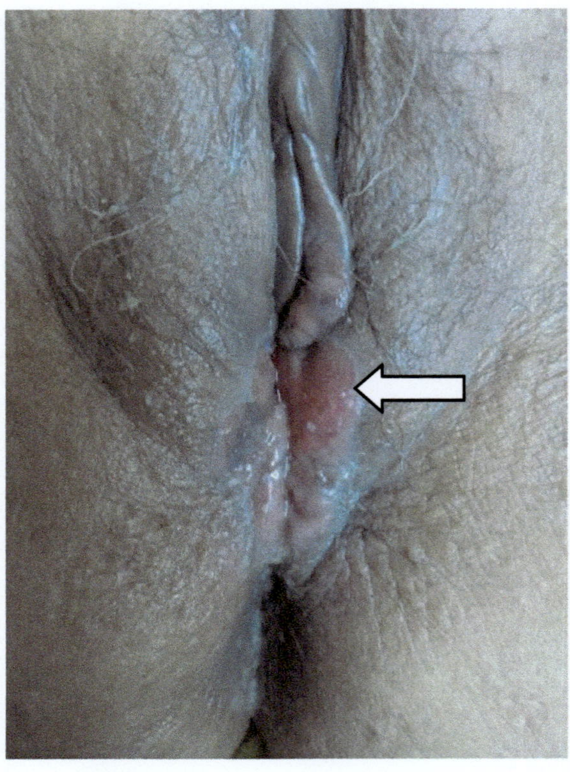

Fig. 16.11 Vulvar ulcer

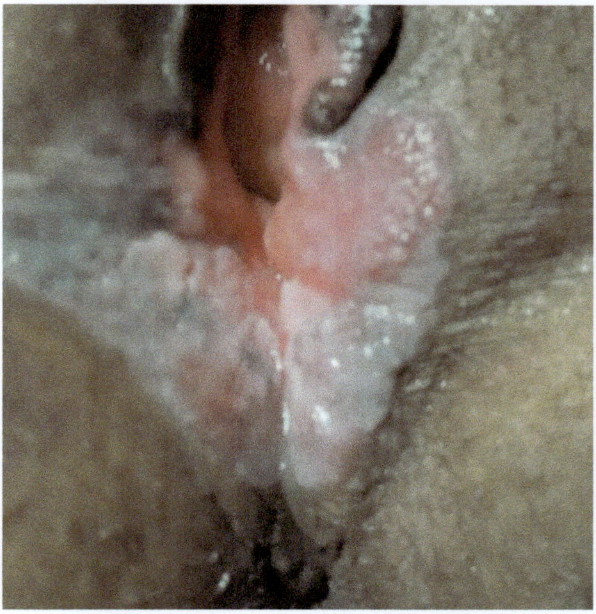

Fig. 16.12 Acetowhitening in vulvar ulcer after acetic acid application

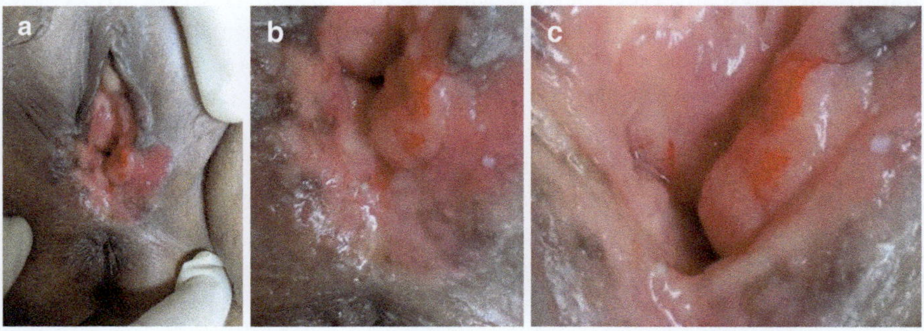

Fig. 16.13 (**a**) Atypical vessels and growth over vulva. (**b**) Colposcopic view of growth. (**c**) Atypical vessels on vulvar lesion

16.12). One should also look for punctation and mosaic which can appear on the medial side of labia minora. It is better to start from the lowermost magnification (6x) for the quick survey of the vulva, thereafter proceeding to higher magnifications. Note the satellite lesions also.

Owing to keratinization, the terminal vessels of the dermis are not visible, but atypical vessels are a feature of invasive carcinoma (Fig. 16.13a–c). Beyond normal limits, acetowhitening (Fig. 16.9) is an abnormal finding. Besides this, surface contour and angioarchitecture are also noted.

16.1.9.4 Collins Test

This test is performed by using 1 % aqueous solution of toluidine blue, a blue nuclear stain that stains the surface cell nuclei in vivo. Thus increased nuclear activity can be picked up by this test. A positive test is seen not only in neoplastic condition but also in ulcers, vulvar bruising, reparative changes, and parakeratosis [3, 10]. Collins test has an important role to differentiate VIN from hyperplastic nonneoplastic disorders. Moreover, it also delineates the vulvar biopsy site.

Procedure: 1% of aqueous solution of toluidine blue is applied to the skin after cleansing the skin off of any ointment or medication. It should be applied for 2 min. Then the epithelium is rinsed with 1 % acetic acid. The stain is then completely washed off from the normal skin of vulva. As the surface vulvar skin is devoid of nuclei, it does not take the stain. But in conditions where the nuclear activity is raised as in dysplasia, the stain is retained which appears as blue dots easily seen by colposcope. This test thus helps in delineating the optimal site for biopsy.

16.1.9.5 Biopsy

After the localization of the lesion through vulvoscopy, biopsy is a must for a complete diagnosis as most of the vulvar disorders lack characteristic features.

Indications for biopsy include rapidly growing lesions, areas of bleeding and ulceration, lesions not responding to treatment, asymmetrical lesions, suspicious area of any color, and large multicentric lesions. Biopsy is done under a local anesthesia by injecting 1 % lignocaine in subepithelial and subdermal areas using a fine gauge needle. At least a 5-mm-thick tissue should be obtained. Keyes punch biopsy forceps are especially good and are available in 3–5 mm sizes (Fig. 16.14) [6]. Biopsy is taken involving the dermis tissue in the specimen. Ulcerated lesions should be biopsied at the raised edge, and multiple biopsies should be taken if the lesion has a complex appearance. Monsel's solution (ferric bisulphate) can be applied to control bleeding, and the defect can be left open for healing [10]. Large biopsy defects need to be closed with interrupted absorbable sutures. The location of biopsies should be indicated on a vulvar diagram, and multiple biopsies should be sent separately for a pathologic evaluation [10].

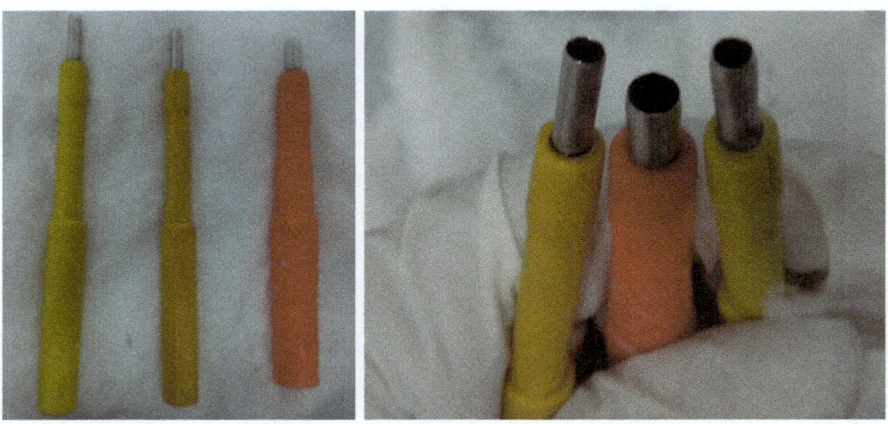

Fig. 16.14 Keyes vulvar punch biopsy forceps

16.1.9.6 Documentation

It should be done in a simple schematic vulvar diagram showing the labia majora, minora, vestibule, perineum, and anus. The lesion location should be marked in the diagram (Fig. 16.15a–c).

The photographic camera/video camera/video printer attached to the colposcope can provide a more objective documentation. The digital color imaging colposcopy system can be used to provide the best digital documentation.

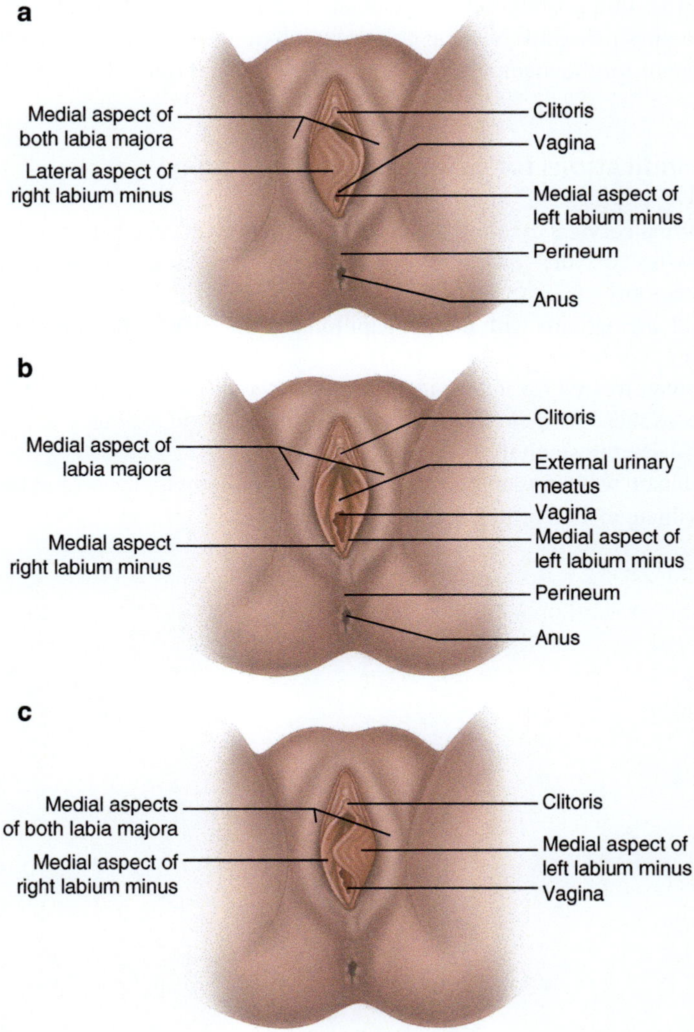

Fig. 16.15 (**a**) Showing the lateral aspect of the right labium minus and medial aspect of the left labium minus. (**b**) Showing the medial aspect of both labia minora. (**c**) Showing the lateral aspect of the left labium minus and medial aspect of the right labium minus

16.2 Colposcopy of Vagina

16.2.1 Anatomical Basis of Vaginal Colposcopy

The vaginal epithelium extends from the vulvovaginal junction (Hart's line) to the original squamocolumnar junction cranially. The normal vaginal epithelium is non-keratinized stratified squamous epithelium. It looks pink with a specific surface contour owing to the presence of extensive rugae in a reproductive age-group patient (Fig. 16.16). In a postmenopausal woman, these rugae and folds are lost, and the color becomes pale pink. Vaginal colposcopy requires the use of an iris hook and a dental mirror for the manipulation of vaginal rugae and folds (Fig. 16.17a, b).

16.2.2 Indications for Colposcopy of the Vagina

- Abnormal cervical cytologic report incongruent with cervical colposcopy
- Follow-up of the patients with abnormal cervical cytology after total hysterectomy
- To evaluate patients with human papillomavirus (HPV) infection of the vulva or cervix
- In women treated for vulvar intraepithelial neoplasia or high-grade CIN/cancer cervix as these women are at risk of multifocal genital lesions
- Unexplained postcoital bleeding
- To evaluate women with history of exposure to diethylstilbestrol in utero
- To evaluate visible or palpable vaginal lesions.

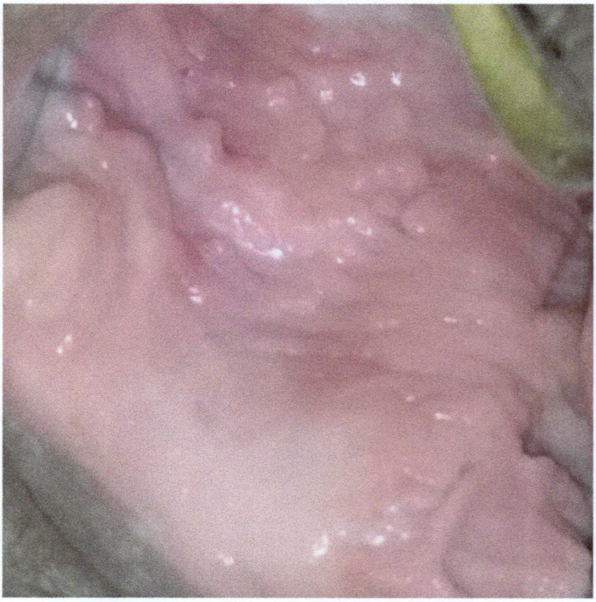

Fig. 16.16 Normal vaginal rugosities

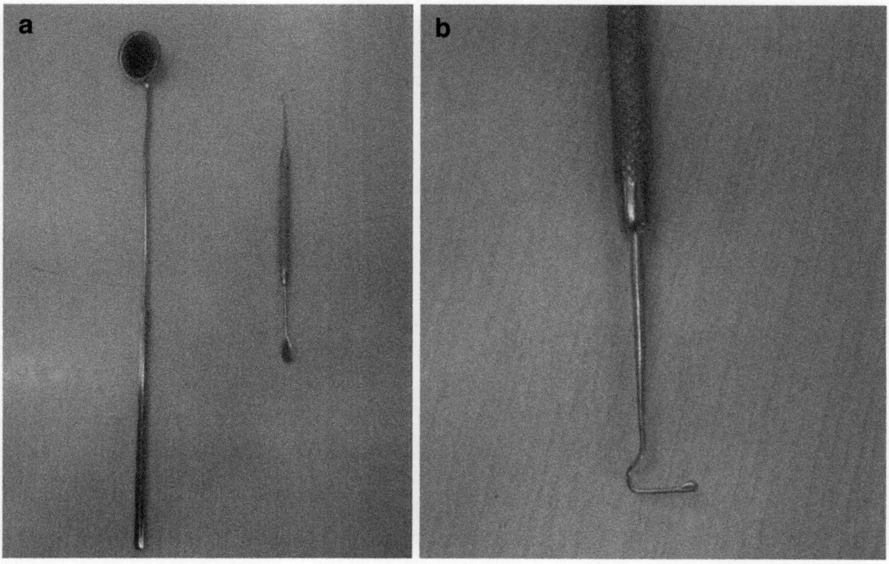

Fig. 16.17 (**a**, **b**) Iris hook and dental mirror

16.2.3 Contraindications

Vaginal colposcopy should not be done in the presence of an acute infection of the lower genital tract, menstrual bleeding, and the use of any vaginal medications within the last one week. In case of severe atrophic changes (as in postmenopausal age-group), the patient is subjected to colposcopy after pretreatment with estrogens. The colposcopic examination of the vagina should be deferred in case of surgery on the lower genital tract in the last one month as it may interfere with the procedure or findings.

16.2.4 Colposcopic Terminology of Vaginal Lesions

IFCPC in 2011 has suggested the clinical/colposcopic terminology of the vagina (Table 16.4) [8].

16.2.5 Technique of Colposcopy of Vagina

16.2.5.1 Steps of Colposcopy of Vagina

- Visual inspection
- Acetic acid application
- Biopsy
- Documentation

Table 16.4 Clinical/colposcopic terminology of vagina (IFCPC 2011)

General assessment	Adequate/inadequate for the reason (inflammation, scar)	
Normal colposcopic findings	Mature Atrophic	
Abnormal colposcopic findings	*General principles*	Upper third/lower two-thirds
		Anterior/posterior/lateral
	Grade 1(minor)	Thin acetowhite
		Fine mosaic and punctation
	Grade 2 (major)	Dense acetowhite
		Coarse mosaic and punctation
	Suspicious for invasion	Atypical vessels
		Additional signs: fragile vessels, irregular surface, necrosis, ulceration, tumor
	Nonspecific	Lesion staining by Lugol's iodine
		Leukoplakia
		Columnar epithelium
Miscellaneous findings	Erosion, condyloma, polyp, cyst, endometriosis, inflammation	

16.2.5.2 Visual inspection

The patient is placed in a lithotomy position in a colposcopy chair. Start with the vulvoscopy (colposcopy of the vulva) followed by vaginal colposcopy. The speculum is then gently used to retract the cervix laterally, forward, and backward to visualize the fornices properly. An iris hook or a tissue-dissecting forceps or a long swab stick can be used to manipulate the cervix and to examine the vaginal mucosa in detail. The saline application will help in clearing off the discharge and make lesions clearer.

16.2.5.3 Acetic Acid Application

After the application of 3 % acetic acid, the lateral walls are visualized first followed by the anterior and posterior vaginal walls, which are seen best by withdrawing the Cusco's speculum. Alternatively, Sim's speculum along with the anterior vaginal wall retractor can be used as per the convenience of the operator. The lateral vaginal wall retractor can ease the process, if available.

16.2.5.4 Documentation

The documentation is done in an especially designed line diagram [10] (Figs. 16.18 and 16.19) or through a photo documentation through the video colposcope.

16.2.5.5 Vaginal Biopsy

Vaginal dysplastic changes are less specific in appearance compared with cervical intraepithelial lesions. Biopsy can be done from any suspicious lesion using a sharp biopsy forceps or scalpel with blade no.11. The knife is required especially for the lesion in the fornix. Vaginal mucosa needs to be stabilized using an iris hook or a cotton swab stick, and the punch must be at right angle to the mucosal fold for

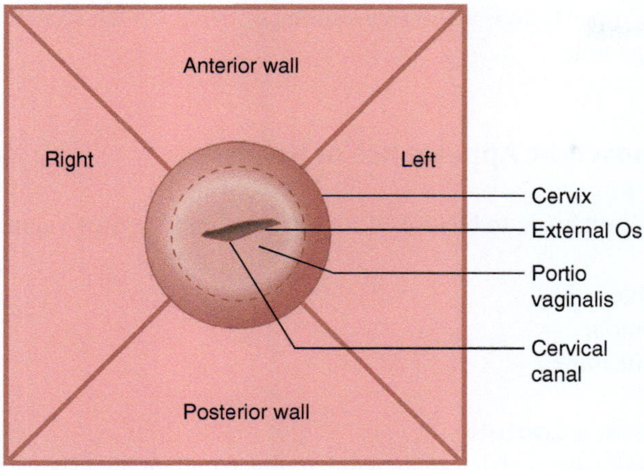

Fig. 16.18 Line diagram for the documentation of vaginal colposcopy findings

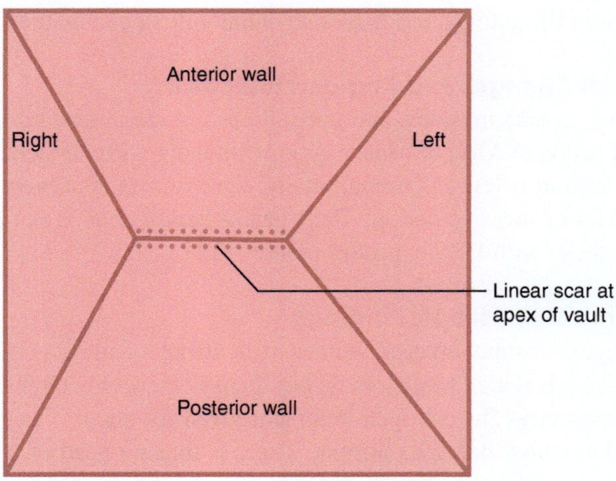

Fig. 16.19 Line diagram for the documentation of vaginal colposcopy findings in a hysterectomized female

preventing slippage. The upper two-thirds of the vagina has less sensation and so can be biopsied without anesthesia, while biopsy of lower third of vagina requires local anesthesia. To control bleeding, Monsel's paste or silver nitrate can be used. Sutures using 2-0 or 1-0 chromic catgut/Vicryl can also be applied. For a small amount of bleeding, even a tight vaginal packing may suffice [11].

If multiple biopsies are taken, they should be sent in different containers for histopathology. Biopsies should be properly labeled so as to identify the distance from the vaginal introitus. Rest of the colposcopic findings are noted and recorded/

documented. Proper follow-up and scheduling of the next visit should be mentioned in the discharge note.

16.2.6 Colposcopic Appearance of Vagina

The following points are to be looked for during colposcopy of vagina:

- Color changes
- Surface contour
- Angioarchitecture

16.2.6.1 Surface Contour

Vagina is a highly distensible organ owing to the abundant underlying loose connective tissue and vascularity. This provides a specific surface contour in the form of multiple rugae and folds. Owing to the presence of rugosities and folds, there is an irregular surface contour of vagina. Because of this, the grade of lesion appears to be higher than the original histopathology. For the in-depth examination of vagina in the presence of these folds, iris hook and dental mirror can be used.

16.2.6.2 Color Changes and Angioarchitecture

Acetowhitening, coarse mosaics, and punctations are common findings in vaginal intraepithelial lesion (VAIN) or cancer. Acetowhitening without a coarse mosaic or punctation is seen in severe inflammation and condylomas, and biopsy is essential to rule out VAIN or invasive cancer. The transformation zone is not present in the vagina except those with DES exposure in utero [11].

16.2.6.3 Other Colposcopic Findings

Atrophic changes: Postmenopausal women with atrophic vaginitis have prominent subepithelial vessels which bleed easily, but there is no acetowhitening or atypical vessels on colposcopy. The estrogen treatment given for about 2 weeks reverts the condition, and cytology becomes normal. There is thus no need of biopsy in these cases. In contrast to this, in *radiation-induced atrophy* in patients who have received radiotherapy for cervical or endometrial cancer, the epithelium is although thin but shows atypical blood vessels and negative iodine uptake. Biopsy is a must in these cases to rule out malignancy.

Keratosis: It is a common finding in females with uterovaginal prolapse and on prolonged estrogen therapy. However the atypical vessels are absent. It can be seen with human papillomavirus infection [12]. The HPV infection can present as an exophytic papillary form, flat-raised lesions, or as spiked lesions.

Atypical vessels, irregular surface contour, or ulcer: These are the common findings of malignancy. In general, angiotexture is more pronounced, dilated, and coarser in adenocarcinomas as compared to squamous cancer. But this needs to be established by biopsy.

Key Points

- Indications for vulvoscopy include pruritus vulvae, vulvodynia, and intraepithelial lesions of the cervix and vagina.
- During vulvoscopy, color changes, topography, surface contour, and angio-architecture of all the parts of the vulva should be noted.
- Vulvar biopsy remains the gold standard for the diagnosis of vulvar lesions as VIN is multifocal and the keratinized stratified squamous epithelium makes it difficult to visualize the underlying dermis vascularity.
- Collins test can help in identifying the site of vulvar biopsy as the areas with increased mitotic activity.
- Indications for vaginal colposcopy include unexplained postcoital bleeding, HPV infection of vulva or cervix, and after treatment of women with VaIN or CIN.
- The findings during colposcopy of vulva or vagina should be described using the latest terminology described by IFCPC.
- Documentation of the lesions found during colposcopy is essential and can be done using schematic diagrams.

References

1. Van Beurden M, Van de Vange N, deCraen AJ, Tjong-A-Hung SP, ter Schegget J, et al. Normal findings in vulval examination and vulvoscopy. Br J Obstet Gynaecol. 1997;104:320–4.
2. Micheletti L, Bogliatto F, Lynch PJ. Vulvoscopy: review of a diagnostic approach during clarification. J Reprod Med. 2008;53:179–82.
3. Batra A, Nigam S, Das SK. Colposcopy practice and atlas, 1st ed. CBS Publishers & Distributors Pvt Ltd; Delhi. 2014. p. 17–36.
4. Michael S. Baggish. Colposcopy of the cervix, vagina, and vulva: a comprehensive textbook, 1st ed. Mosby; Elsevier. 2003.
5. Burke L, Antonioli DA, Ducatman BS. Colposcopy-text and atlas. Norwalk: Appleton & Lange; 1991. p. 133–52.
6. Coppleson M, Pixley EC. Colposcopy of vulva and vagina. In: Coppleson M, editor. Gynecologic oncology. Fundamental principles and clinical practice, vol. 1. 2nd ed. New York: Churchill Livingstone; 1992. p. 325–39.
7. Lynch PJ, Moyal-Barraco M, Scurry J, Stockdale C. 2011 ISSVD Terminology and classification of vulvar dermatological disorder: an approach to clinical diagnosis. J Low Genit Tract Dis. 2012;16(4):339–44. doi:10.1097/LGT.0b13e3182494e8c.
8. Bornstein J, Sideri M, Tatti S, et al. 2011 Terminology of the vulva of the International Federation for Cervical Pathology and Colposcopy. J Low Genit Tract Dis. 2012;16(3):292.
9. Kesic V. Colposcopy of the vulva, perineum and anal canal. EAGC course book of colposcopy. Available online http://www.gyncph.dk/procedur/ref/gyn/vulvoscopi_chapter14_eagc.pdf.
10. Shakuntala Baliga B. Principles and practice of colposcopy. 2nd ed. New Dehi: Jaypee Publications; 2011. p. 177–96.
11. Mayeaux EJ, Thomas Cox J. Modern colposcopy textbook and atlas, 3rd ed. American Society for Colposcopy and Cervical Pathology, Lippincott Williams & Wilkins; Wolter Kluwers. 2011.
12. Gagne HM. Colposcopy of the vagina and vulva. Obstet Gynecol Clin North Am. 2008;35(4):659–69. doi:10.1016/j.ogc.2008.10.002:x.

Part IV

Case Discussion

Cases

17

Sweta Balani

Case 1

A 40-year-old parous woman in a stable relation came to the clinic with a Pap smear report of inflammatory and high-risk HPV report, positive. She is very anxious, as she has been told that this virus causes cancer of the uterus.

On examination

Per speculum – The cervix shows ectropion.

Per vaginam – Uterus normal size, mobile, non-tender, fornix free.

Q.1 What will be your next step?

Answer – The patient should be counseled that usually HPV infection is transient and clears on its own within 1–2 years. Women with HPV positive and cytology negative should be followed with either

1. Repeat co-testing in 12 months
2. Immediate HPV genotype-specific testing for HPV 16/18

Q.2 This patient opted for co-testing after 1 year. The report showed normal Pap smear and HPV 18 positive. How will you proceed?

Answer – Colposcopy is indicated in this patient.

S. Balani, MS
Department of Obstetrics and Gynecology, Sant Parmanand Hospital, Delhi, India
e-mail: swetagarima@gmail.com

S. Mehta, P. Sachdeva (eds.), *Colposcopy of Female Genital Tract*,
DOI 10.1007/978-981-10-1705-6_17

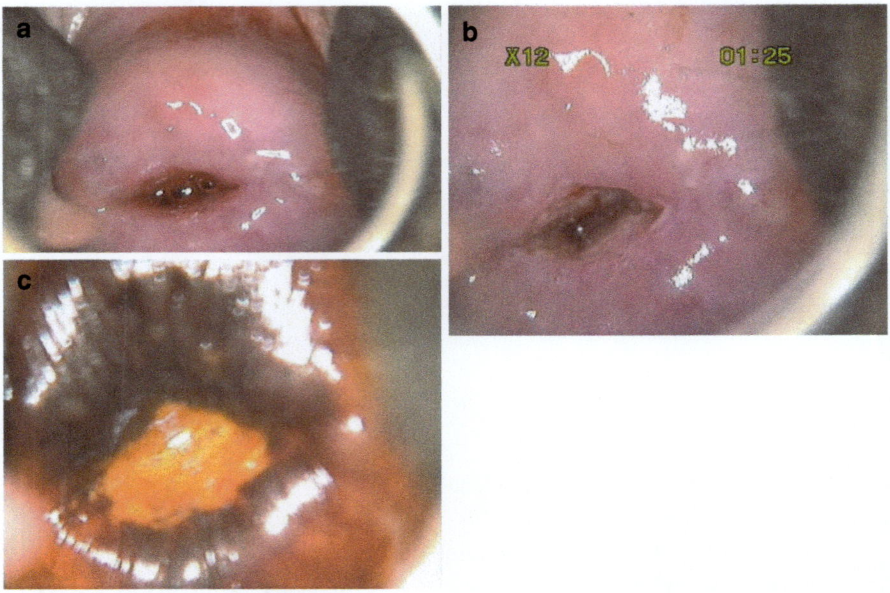

Fig. 17.1 (**a**) After saline application. (**b**) After acetic acid application. (**c**) After Lugol's iodine application

Q.3 Colposcopy images are shown. Describe the findings (Fig. 17.1)**.**

Answer 3 – This is an adequate colposcopy with a completely visible squamocolumnar junction (SCJ), Type 1 transformation zone (TZ) with no colposcopic abnormal finding.

Q.4 After 1 year, repeat HPV 18 was positive and LBC was negative – persistent HPV infection. How will you counsel this lady? What will be the follow-up?

Answer – The patient needs to be counseled regarding persistent infection with high-risk HPV, but she has a normal Pap test with a normal colposcopy so she will require a regular follow-up with a yearly co-testing.

Further this patient can undergo triage with E6/7mRNA depending on the facilities available. The partners of this patient should also be examined for HPV infection.

Case 2

A 32-year-old lady, P1L1, last childbirth – 5 years.

The routine cytology screening shows Atypical squamous cell of undetermined significance (ASCUS).

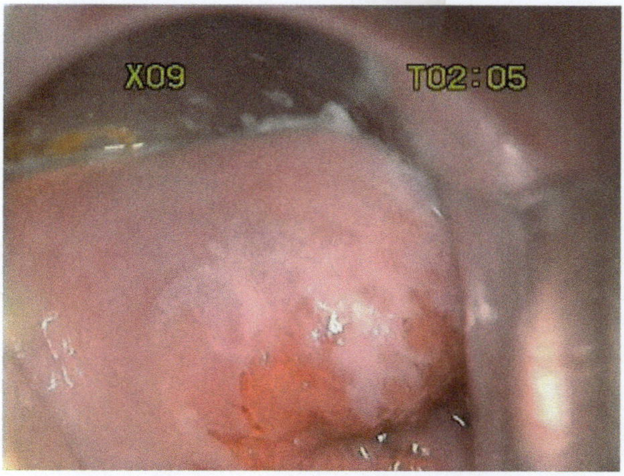

Fig. 17.2 Colposcopy after the application of acetic acid

Q.1 What will be your next step?
Answer 1 – Women with ASCUS on cervical cytology should be triaged with the high-risk HPV DNA testing. If negative for high-risk HPV DNA, then repeat cytology at 12 months. If positive for high-risk HPV DNA, then refer for colposcopy.

Q.2 The patient underwent high-risk HPV DNA testing, which came as positive. Colposcopy was done. Describe the colposcopy findings (Fig. 17.2).

Answer 2 – It is an adequate colposcopy with a completely visible SCJ. Many tongues of the acetowhite epithelium with ill-defined margins and flat surface are seen on the transformation zone, occupying two quadrants of the cervix, with no vascular abnormality. These findings are consistent with low-grade lesions.

Q.3 How will you manage this patient?
Answer 3 – Women with positive HPV with ASCUS are at an increased risk of Cervical intraepithelial neoplasia (CIN) 3 (11 %) within 2 years of referral for colposcopy. This patient needs excision/ Loop electrosurgical excision procedure (LEEP) rather than surveillance.

Q.4 The Histopathological examination (HPE) report shows mild dysplasia with clear margins. How will you follow up this patient?
Answer 4 – The patient should be checked in 1 month for healing. Followed by co-testing in 9–12 months. If two consecutive screens are negative, then the patient should undergo routine screening.

Case 3

A 28-year-old woman was referred to the clinic with an abnormal smear. Her two previous smears were negative. Her periods were regular with a combined oral contraceptive pill she used for contraception. She had no history of post-coital bleeding or vaginal discharge. She is in a stable relationship and has one child delivered by cesarean section (Fig. 17.3).

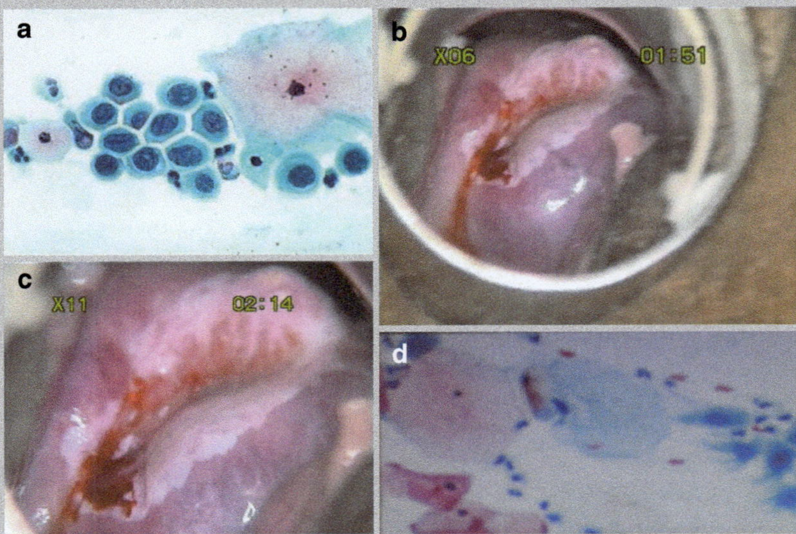

Fig. 17.3 (**a**) HSIL. (**b**) After the application of acetic acid. (**c**) Magnified view. (**d**) Normal smear

Q.1 Describe the smear.

Answer – The nuclei show a markedly increased nuclear/cytoplasmic ratio, anisocytosis (variation in size), hyperchromatism (increased intensity of staining), irregularity of nuclear chromatin, and irregular nuclear membranes. These are features of a high-grade intraepithelial lesion (HSIL).

Q.2 Colposcopy was done for this patient. Describe the findings.

Answer – Colposcopy is adequate, with SCJ not visible (Type 3 TZ). There is a dense acetowhite area with sharp borders involving all four quadrants in the TZ; the upper margin of the lesion is not visible. These findings are suggestive of a high-grade lesion.

Q.3 What is the risk of invasion in this high-grade lesion?
Answer – The risk of invasion is approximately 30 % over 5 years for CIN III.

Q.4 What will be your modality of treatment – excisional treatment (LEEP/ cone biopsy) or ablative treatment?
Answer – This patient should undergo a cone biopsy going well beyond the lesion, considering that it is a high-grade lesion involving a large area whose upper margin is not visible.

Q.5 Unfortunately, a loop excision of TZ (LEEP/ Large loop excision of transformation zone (LLETZ)) confirmed CIN III, which was incompletely excised at the endocervical margin. Does she require repeat excision?
Answer – Such patients are known to have a slightly increased risk of recurrent CIN [1] but re-treatment is not required unless the cytology indicates a persistent or recurrent high-grade disease.

Q.6. Six months later, a further smear was taken at colposcopy. Describe the findings.
Answer – This is a normal smear with predominantly superficial and intermediate cells, with normal nucleic cytoplasmic ratio.

Q.7 How will you follow up this patient?
Answer – She should be kept under six monthly follow-ups by both cytology and colposcopy. After a 1-year follow-up, and with two consecutive negative reports of cytology as well as colposcopy, she can return to the routine screening program.

Case 4

A 56-year-old postmenopausal lady P3L3 came with complaints of pyuria and lower abdominal pain for 1 year. She had an increasing frequency of micturition for 2 months and is a known diabetic and hypertensive on medication. menopausal since 8 years, no h/o PMB.

On examination: She is obese, P/S – cervix hypertrophied, nabothian follicles on the anterior lip of the cervix, Pap smear taken

P/V – Uterus AV, NS, FF (Fig. 17.4)

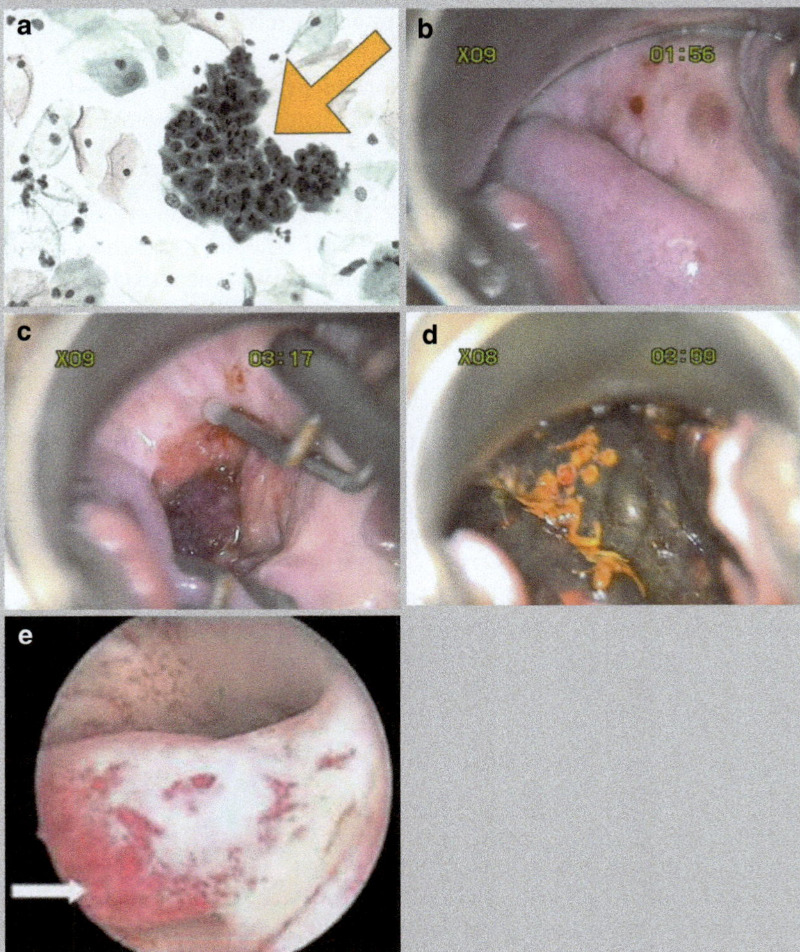

Fig. 17.4 (**a**) Atypical glandular cells. (**b**) After saline application. (**c**): Visualization of SCJ with endocervical retractor. (**d**) After Lugol's iodine application. (**e**) Hysteroscopic view

Q.1 The Pap smear report showed atypical glandular cells (AGC). How often do you see a Pap smear report like this? What is its importance?

Answer – Cervical glandular dysplasia is 100 times less common than its squamous counterpart. It is becoming increasingly important due to an increase in detection;

earlier age (median age 35) at presentation where fertility is an issue. Most CGIN arise within 1 cm of the squamocolumnar junction and are associated with other small lesions (skip lesions). There is an underlying adenocarcinoma in 40 % of cases.

Q.2 What are the causes of AGC on a Pap smear?
Answer – This report of AGC can be seen in high-grade and low-grade squamous lesions, adenocarcinoma in situ, adenocarcinoma, endometriosis, Arias-Stella reaction, endometrial polyp, fallopian tube malignancy, and also ovarian cancer.

Q.3 How will you manage this patient?
Answer – This patient needs investigations such as urine routine and culture, blood sugar test, HbA1c test, and a transvaginal ultrasonography. In view of AGUS on Pap smear, colposcopy and endocervical curettage are needed.

Q.4 Transvaginal sonography (TVS) showed the uterus is normal sized with an endometrial thickness of 10 mm with bilateral ovaries normal. Colposcopy was done. Describe the colposcopic findings.
Answer 4 – Adequate colposcopy with SCJ not visible (Type 2 TZ). No lesion on ectocervix seen. No abnormal vessels. No iodine-negative areas seen. On using the endocervical retractor, complete SCJ was visible, with no abnormal findings.

Comment
Colposcopy is recommended in all women with AGUS. However, glandular lesions are often difficult to detect by colposcopy particularly if they exist along with squamous lesions. The mosaic pattern, punctation, and leukoplakia are not seen with glandular lesions. Before the application of acetic acid, the adenocarcinoma often has a dull, pale orange or yellow appearance. The appearance of AIS is often even more subtle. After the acetic acid is applied, the only abnormality may be the acetowhitening of the columnar villi.

Q.5 How will you further manage this case?
Answer – This patient should undergo the evaluation of the cervical canal and uterine cavity (thick endometrium on TVS) by hysteroscopy and endocervical curettage.

Q.6 Hysteroscopy showed normal endocervical canal with hyperplasic endometrium with increased vascularity together with an endometrial polyp arising from the fundus. The biopsy showed disorderly arranged endometrial glands. A few of the glands are dilated. On histopathology at places crowding of glands with atypia seen. How will you treat this patient?
Answer – This patient needs hysterectomy with bilateral salpingo-oophorectomy.

Case 5

A 32-year-old lady P1L1 came from a remote village with the complaint of postcoital bleeding.

Visual inspection with acetic acid (VIA) was done in the Out patient department (OPD) which was positive

Q.1 Colposcopy was done for this patient. Describe the finding (Fig. 17.5)**.**

Answer 1 – Colposcopy is adequate with partially visible SCJ (Type 2 TZ). There is a small (grade 1) lesion on the posterior lip at 6 o'clock position inside the TZ. The entire lesion is seen.

Q.2 How will you manage this lady?

Answer 2 – This lady should be managed by a colposcopy-directed biopsy followed by a cryotherapy as the follow-up of this patient cannot be ensured.

Q.3 Cervical punch biopsy showed CIN I. What is the next step?

Answer 3 – The patient should be followed up at 9–12 months with VIA/Pap smear/colposcopy for 2 years. If the two consecutive follow-ups are negative, the patient can be sent to routine screening.

Comment

Most of the CIN I lesions are transient. Only 10–15 % will progress to higher lesion. CIN I should be treated if follow-up cannot be ensured (as in low-resource setting) or the lesion persists for 2 years or worsens in size or grade.

Case 6

A 50-year-old female presented with a history of postmenopausal spotting.

On examination: PS – Cx and vagina normal, PV – uterus normal size, fornix free. Transvaginal USG showed normal size uterus, ET – 3 mm, B/L ovaries normal

Q.1 The Pap smear report is HSIL. What will be the next step?

Answer – This patient should undergo a colposcopy.

Q.2 The colposcopy picture is shown. Describe the finding (Fig. 17.6)**.**

Answer – Colposcopy shows menopausal cervix, SCJ not visualized (Type 3 TZ); unsatisfactory colposcopy.

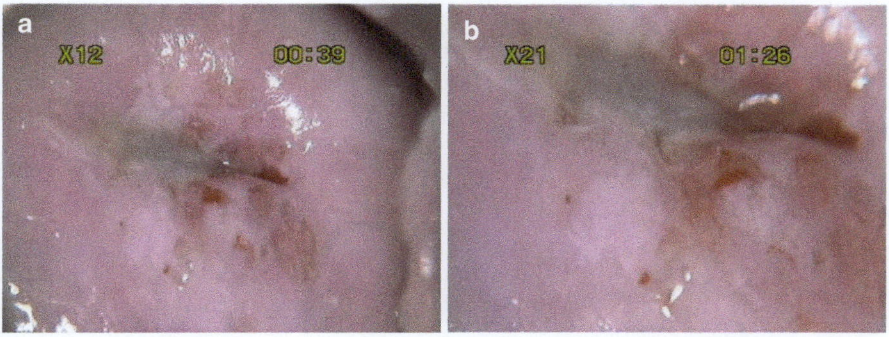

Fig. 17.5 (**a**) After application of acetic acid. (**b**) Magnified view

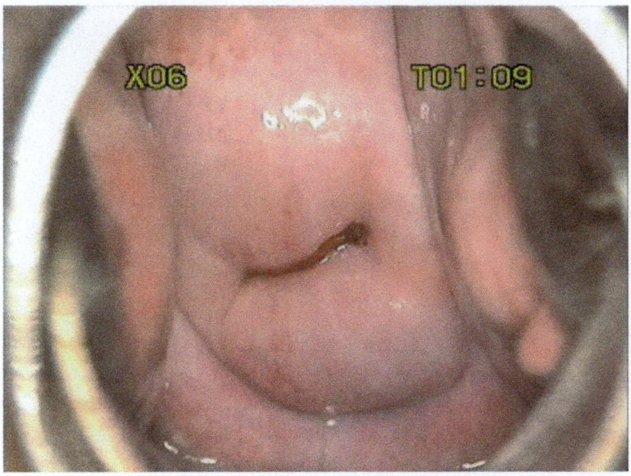

Fig. 17.6 After saline application

Q.3 Is there any means to convert this unsatisfactory colposcopy to satisfactory colposcopy?

Answer – The short course of oral estrogen for 1 week or vaginal application for 2–3 weeks can help in 30 % of cases. In this case where cytology shows a high-grade lesion, waiting may not be possible, and one can use misoprostol 400 μg, 4–6 h before colposcopy; this might open the os.

Q.4 In spite of all these efforts, the colposcopy remains unsatisfactory. What will be your next step?

Answer – This lady should undergo cone biopsy with Type 3 excision of the transformation zone.

Q.5 The histopathology shows CIN II with negative margins. How will you follow up this patient? Till what age you will screen this lady?
Answer – This patient should have a yearly follow-up for at least 10 years. A combined cytological evaluation together with an HPV test will significantly increase the safety of the follow-up surveillance. If these screenings are negative, then the routine screening for another 10 years even after the age of 65 years is recommended.

Case 7
A 28-year-old primigravida with 28 weeks of pregnancy presented with excessive vaginal discharge.

The examination showed the hypertrophied cervix with ectropion and copious discharge. A high vaginal swab was taken for bacterial culture and a course of metronidazole was given with vaginal pessary.

A week later on examination, the discharge was less but the cervix still showed an ectropion. A Pap smear was taken which was reported as low-grade squamous intraepithelial lesion (LSIL).

Q.1 How will you manage this case?
Answer 1 – It is recommended that pregnant patients with an abnormal smear should undergo colposcopy. The colposcopy should be done by an experienced colposcopist as the cervical changes together with pregnancy may make the examination and interpretation difficult.

Q.2 Colposcopy pictures are shown. Describe the finding (Fig. 17.7).
Answer 2 – The colposcopy is adequate with visible SCJ and Type 1 TZ. There is a metaplastic epithelium, with no abnormal finding.

Q 3 What is your plan of management?
Answer – Subsequent follow-up with cytology is recommended 6 weeks after the delivery.

Case 8
A 38-year-old P1L1 presented with a routine cytology smear showing LSIL.

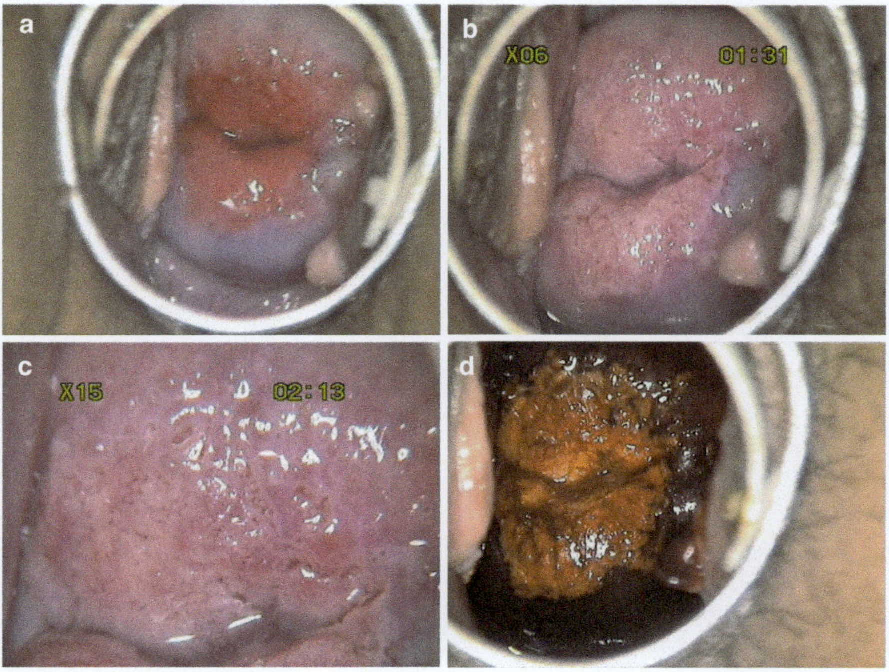

Fig. 17.7 (**a**) After saline application. (**b**) After acetic acid application. (**c**) Magnified view. (**d**) After Lugol's iodine application

Q.1 What will be your next step? Why?
Answer – The patient should undergo colposcopy as the risk of high-grade CIN is 40–68 %; hence immediate colposcopy is more cost-effective than repeat cytology (TOMBOLA study).

Q.2 Colposcopy pictures are shown. Describe findings (Fig. 17.8)**.**
Answer 2 – This is an adequate colposcopy, with completely visible SCJ (Type 1 TZ) with dense acetowhite area on the anterior lip, from 10 o' clock to 1 o'clock position. The lesion has sharp margins with coarse mosaic at the SCJ, with poor iodine uptake suggestive of a high-grade lesion.

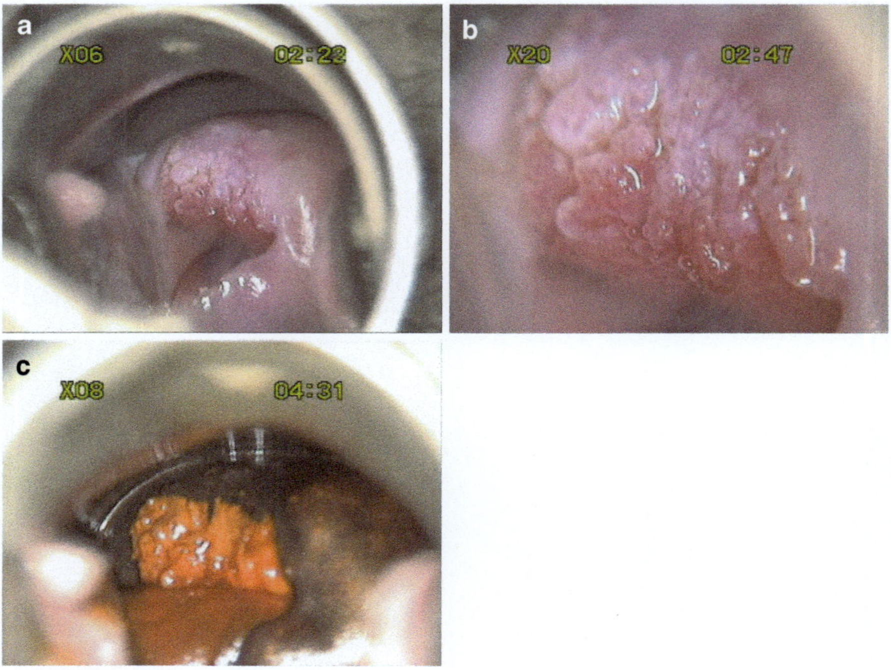

Fig. 17.8 (**a**) After acetic acid application. (**b**) Magnified view. (**c**) After Lugol's iodine application

Q.3 Single-pass LLETZ from the anterior lip was carried out. The histopathology revealed CIN II; the endocervical margins were free but ectocervical margins were involved. What will be your next step?
Answer – This patient should be followed up by cytology and colposcopy in 6 months for the first 2 years; if normal, then annually for 10 years.

Reference

1. Flannelly G, Bolger B, Fawzi H, De Lopes AB, Monaghan JM. Follow up after LLETZ: could schedules be modified according to the risk of recurrence? BJOG 2001;108(10):1025–30.

Appendices

Preparation: 5 % Acetic Acid

Ingredients

Glacial acetic acid	5 ml
Distilled water	95 ml

Preparation

Carefully add 5 ml of glacial acetic acid to 95 ml of distilled water and mix thoroughly.

It is important to dilute the acid as undiluted acid can cause chemical burns if applied to the epithelium.

Storage

Unused acetic acid should be discarded at the end of the dy. Always freshly prepared acetic acid should be used.

Label

5 % dilute acetic acid

Preparation: Lugol's Iodine

Ingredients

Potassium iodide	10 g
Distilled water	100 ml
Iodine crystals	5 g

S. Mehta, P. Sachdeva (eds.), *Colposcopy of Female Genital Tract*,
DOI 10.1007/978-981-10-1705-6

Preparation

Dissolve 10 g potassium iodide in 100 ml of distilled water.
Slowly add 5 g iodine crystals while shaking.
Filter and store in a tightly stoppered brown bottle.

Storage

One month

Label

Lugol's iodine solution

Preparation: Monsel's Paste

Monsel's paste is a thick, sticky, fast-acting compound that is used to cover bleeding areas on the cervix to stem the flow of blood. It can be useful after cryotherapy, punch biopsy, and loop electrosurgical excision procedure (LEEP).

Ingredients	Quantity
1. Ferric sulfate base	15 g
2. Ferrous sulfate powder	A few grains
3. Sterile water for mixing	10 ml
4. Glycerol starch	12 g

Preparation

Add a few grains of ferrous sulfate powder to 10 ml of sterile water in a glass beaker and shake.
Dissolve the ferric sulfate base in the solution by stirring with a glass stick. The solution should become crystal clear.
Weigh the glycerol starch in a glass mortar. Mix well.
Slowly add the ferric sulfate solution to the glycerol starch, constantly mixing to get a homogeneous mixture.
Place in a 25 ml brown glass bottle.

Note: Most clinics prefer to leave the stopper of the bottle loose, to allow the mixture to evaporate until it has a sticky paste-like consistency and looks like mustard. This may take 2–3 weeks, depending on the environment. The top of the bottle can then be secured for storage. If necessary, sterile water can be added to the paste to thin it.

Label	Monsel's paste	
	Store in a cool place	
	For external use only	
	Use by: [day/month/year] (1 year from date of preparation)	

As it is a caustic product that can damage tissues if left too long, no vaginal packing should be used after application.

Format for Reporting VIA and VILI

1.	Clinic/serial/unique number	[·][·] [·][·]	
2.	Date of testing (day (two digits)-month (two digits)-year (two digits)):	[·][·]-[·] [·]-[·][·]	
3.	Name: ______________________________		
4.	Address: ______________________________		
	______________________________		
5.	Age (in years)	[·][·]	
6.	Education (1, nil; 2, primary; 3, middle; 4, high school; 5, college; 9, not known)	[·]	
7.	When did you have your last menstruation? (1, less than 12 months ago; 2, more than 12 months ago)	[·]	
8.	Marital status: (1, married; 2, widowed; 3, separated; 8, other; 9, not known)	[·]	
9.	Age at marriage or first sexual intercourse: (99, if not known)	[·][·]	
10.	Total number of pregnancies/miscarriages:	[·][·]	
11.	Do you suffer from the following? (use Y to indicate if the response is yes; otherwise, leave blank):		
	Excessive vaginal discharge	[·]	
	Itching in the external anogenitalia	[·]	
	Ulcers in the external anogenitalia	[·]	
	Lower abdominal pain	[·]	
	Pain during sexual intercourse	[·]	
	Bleeding after intercourse	[·]	
	Intermenstrual bleeding	[·]	
	Low backache	[·]	
12.	Visual examination findings? (use Y to indicate if the response is yes; otherwise, leave blank):		
	Squamocolumnar junction fully seen	[·]	
	Cervical polyp	[·]	
	Nabothian follicles	[·]	
	Cervicitis	[·]	
	Leukoplakia	[·]	
	Condyloma	[·]	
	Growth	[·]	
13.	Findings 1 min after application of 5 % acetic acid (VIA) (1, negative; 2, positive; 3, positive – invasive cancer)	[·]	
14.	If VIA positive, does the acetowhite lesion extend in to the endocervical canal? (1, yes; 2, no)	[·]	
15.	If VIA positive, how many quadrants are involved in the acetowhite lesion(s)? (1, two or less; 2, three; 3, four quadrants)	[·]	
16.	Diagram (Draw the location of the squamocolumnar junction with a dotted line and the acetowhite/iodine non-uptake area(s) as a continuous line)		

	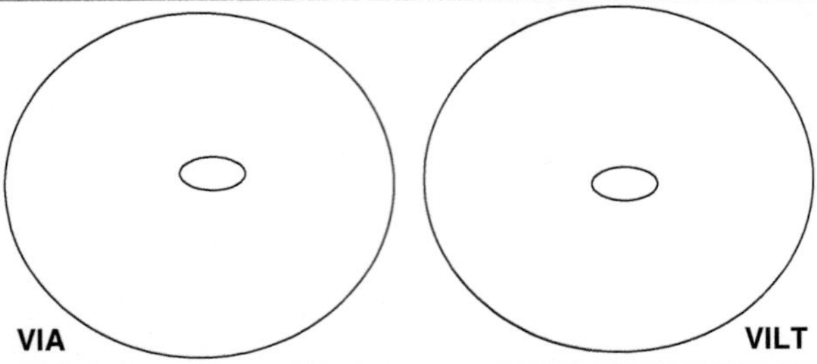		
17.	Findings after application of Lugol's iodine (VILI) (1, negative; 2, positive; 3, positive – invasive cancer)	[·]	
18.	If invasive cancer, stage (1, IA; 2, IB; 3, IIA; 4, IIB; 5, IIIA; 6, IIIB; 7, IVA; 8, IVB; 9, not known)	[·]	
19.	Biopsy taken? (1, yes; 2, no)	[·]	
	(If yes, indicate the biopsy site(s) in the diagram with "x" mark)		
20.	Action taken: (1, advised follow-up after 5 years; 2, advised medication for cervicitis and follow-up after 6 months; 3, referred for colposcopy; 4, referred for immediate treatment; 5, referred for staging and treatment of invasive cancer; 7, other, specify ____________________)	[·]	

Courtesy: International Agency for Research on Cancer

Colposcopic Terminology of the Cervix (IFCPC 2011)

Section	Pattern
General assessment	Adequate or inadequate for the reason (e.g., cervix obscured by inflammation, bleeding, scar)
	Squamocolumnar junction visibility: complete, partial, not visible
	Transformation zone (TZ) types 1, 2, 3
Normal colposcopic findings	Original squamous epithelium: mature, atrophic
	Columnar epithelium: ectopy/ectropion
	Metaplastic squamous epithelium: nabothian cysts, crypt (gland) openings
	Deciduosis in pregnancy
Abnormal colposcopic findings	*Location of the lesion*: inside or outside TZ; location by clock position
	Size of the lesion: number of cervical quadrants, size as percentage of the cervix
	Grade 1 (*minor*): thin acetowhite epithelium, irregular, geographic border, fine mosaic, fine punctation
	Grade 2 (*major*): dense acetowhite epithelium, rapid acetowhitening, sharp border, inner border sign, ridge sign, coarse mosaic, coarse punctation, cuffed crypt openings
	Nonspecific: leukoplakia (keratosis, hyperkeratosis), erosion
	Lugol's staining (Schiller's test): stained or unstained

Section	Pattern
Suspicious for invasion	Atypical vessels
	Additional signs: fragile vessels, irregular surface, exophytic lesion, necrosis, ulceration, tumor or gross neoplasm
Miscellaneous findings	Congenital TZ, condyloma, polyp (endo- or exocervical), inflammation, stenosis, congenital anomaly, posttreatment consequence, endometriosis

2011 IFCPC Colposcopic Terminology of the Cervix: Addendum

Excision treatment types	*Excision types 1, 2, 3*
Excision specimen dimensions	*Length*: the distance from the distal or external margin to the proximal or internal margin *Thickness*: the distance from the stromal margin to the surface of the excised specimen *Circumference* (optional): the perimeter of the excised specimen

Source: Bornstein J, Bentley J, Bosze P, Girardi F, Haefner H, Menton M, Perrotta M, Prendiville W, Russell P, Sideri M. Colposcopic terminology of the International Federation for Cervical Pathology and Colposcopy. Obstet Gynecol 2012;120:166–72.

Colposcopic Terminology of Vaginal Lesions (IFCPC2011)

General assessment	Adequate/inadequate for the reason (inflammation, scar, bleeding)	
	Transformation zone	
Normal colposcopic findings	Squamous epithelium:	
	Mature	
	Atrophic	
Abnormal colposcopic findings	*General principles*	Upper third/lower two thirds
		Anterior/posterior/lateral
	Grade 1 (minor)	Thin acetowhite
		Fine mosaic and punctation
	Grade 2 (major)	Dense acetowhite
		Coarse mosaic and punctation
	Suspicious for invasion	Atypical vessels
		Additional signs: fragile vessels, irregular surface, necrosis, ulceration, tumor
	Nonspecific	Lesion staining by Lugol's iodine
		Leukoplakia
		Columnar epithelium (adenosis)
Miscellaneous findings	Erosion, condyloma, polyp, cyst, endometriosis, inflammation, vaginal stenosis, congenital transformation zone	

Clinical/Colposcopic Terminology of the Vulva (Including the Anus) (IFCPC 2011)

Basic definitions	*Various structures*:		
	Urethra, Skene duct openings, clitoris, prepuce, frenulum, pubis, labia majora, labia minora, interlabial sulcus, vestibule, vestibular duct openings, Bartholin's duct openings, hymen, fourchette, perineum, anus, anal squamocolumnar junction (dentate line)		
	Composition:		
	Squamous epithelium: hairy/nonhairy, mucosa		
Normal findings	Micropapillomatosis		
	Sebaceous glands (Fordyce spots)		
	Vestibular redness		
Abnormal findings	Lesion type	Lesion color	Sec morphology
	Macule	Skin colored	Eczema
	Patch	Red	Excoriation
	Papule	White	Purpura
	Plaque	Dark	Scarring
	Nodule		Ulcer
	Cyst		Erosion
	Vesicle		Fissure
	Bulla		Wart
	Pustule		
Miscellaneous findings	Trauma		
	Malformation		
Suspicion of malignancy	Gross neoplasm		
	Ulceration		
	Necrosis		
	Bleeding		
	Exophytic lesion		
	Hyperkeratosis		
Abnormal colposcopic findings	Acetowhite epithelium		
	Punctation		
	Atypical vessels		
	Surface irregularities		
	Abnormal anal squamocolumnar junction		

Definitions of Primary Lesion Types (IFCPC Vulva Terminology)

Term	Definition
Macule	Small area (<1.5 cm) of color change; no elevation and no substance on palpation
Patch	Large (>1.5 cm) area of color change; no elevation and no substance on palpation
Papule	Small (<1.5 cm) elevated and palpable lesion
Plaque	Large (>1.5 cm) elevated, palpable, and flat-topped lesion
Nodule	A large papule (>1.5 cm) often hemispherical or poorly marginated; may be located on the surface, within or below the skin; may be cystic or solid

Term	Definition
Vesicle	Small (<0.5 cm) fluid filled blister; fluid is clear
Bulla	Large (>0.5 cm) fluid filled blister; fluid is clear
Pustule	Pus-filled blister; fluid is white or yellow

Definitions of Secondary Morphology Presentation (IFCPC Vulva Terminology)

Term	Definition
Eczema	A group of inflammatory diseases that are characterized by the presence of itchy, poorly marginated red plaques with minor evidence of microvesiculation and/or subsequent surface disruption
Lichenification	Thickening of the tissue and increased prominence of skin markings. Scale may or may not be detectable in vulvar lichenification. Lichenification may be bright red, dusky red, white, or skin-colored in appearance
Excoriation	Surface disruption (notably excoriations) occurring as a result of the "itch-scratch cycle"
Erosion	A shallow defect in the skin surface; absence of some, or all, of the epidermis down to the basement membrane; the dermis is intact
Fissure	A thin linear erosion of the skin surface
Ulcer	Deeper defect; absence of the epidermis and some, or all, of the dermis

Source: Bornstein J, Sideri M, Tatti S, Walker P, Prendiville W, Haefner HK. 2011 Terminology of the vulva of the International Federation for Cervical Pathology and Colposcopy. J Lower Genital Tract Dis.2012;16(3):290–95.

Reid Score and Its Interpretation

Colposcopic signs	Zero point	One point	Two points
Color	Low-intensity acetowhitening; (indistinct transparent or translucent), beyond the margin of transformation zone, pure snow-white color with intense surface shine	Intermediate shade – gray/white color and shiny surface (most lesions should be scored in this category)	Dull, opaque, oyster white; gray
Lesion margin and surface configuration	Microcondylomatous or micropapillary contour, flat lesions with indistinct margins (feathered or finely scalloped), angular, jagged lesions, satellite lesions beyond the margin of the transformation zone	Regular-shaped, symmetrical lesions with smooth, straight outlines	Rolled, peeling edges, internal demarcations between areas of differing colposcopic appearance – a central area of high-grade change and peripheral area of low-grade change

Colposcopic signs	Zero point	One point	Two points
Vessels	Fine/uniform-caliber vessels, closely and uniformly placed, vessels beyond the margin of transformation zone, vessels within microcondylomatous or micropapillary lesions, poorly formed patterns of fine punctation/mosaic	Absent vessels	Well-defined coarse punctation or mosaic, sharply demarcated, and randomly and widely placed
Iodine staining	Positive iodine uptake (mahogany brown). Negative uptake of insignificant lesion, i.e., yellow staining by a lesion scoring three points or less. Negative areas beyond the margin of transformation zone (parakeratosis)	Partial iodine uptake – variegated, speckled appearance	Negative iodine uptake of significant lesion, i.e., yellow staining by a lesion already scoring four points or more on the first three criteria

Score:
0–2: *likely to be CIN 1*
3–4: *overlapping lesion, likely to be CIN 1 or 2*
5–8: *likely to be CIN 2–3*.

Swede Score

	0	1	2
Aceto uptake	Zero or transparent	Shady, milky (not transparent or opaque)	Distinct, opaque white
Margins/surface	Diffuse	Sharp but irregular, jagged, geographical satellites	Sharp and even, difference in surface level incl. "cuffing"
Vessels	Fine, regular	Absent	Coarse or atypical
Lesion size	<5 mm	5–15 mm Two quadrants	>15 mm Three to four quadrants Endocervically undefined
Iodine staining	Brown	Faintly or patchy yellow	Distinct yellow

The total Swede score ranges between 0 and 10

Interpretation of Swede Score

Swede score	Remarks
<5	Likely benign, no need for biopsy
5–7	High grade, biopsy confirmation
>8	See and treat – diagnostic excision

CPI Antony Rowe
Chippenham, UK
2018-10-25 23:38